Carol Schaufel recounts her life with remarkable detail, as she demonstrates how her life, and her being, was not, and is not, defined by a wheelchair. As a lifelong friend of Carol, I laughed, I cried and I remembered many of the incidents she relates in her story. This book is an uplifting message to anyone facing adversity in their lives that what you think may define you as a person is only a portion of what makes you the person you really are.

Les Ryshkus
Retired Copy Editor

~~~

I loved the book. Your autobiography is truly an inspiration for anyone to read. I am so grateful you decided to put your story into words. Your hard work and determination is a fine example for us all.

Louie Ferraro
Pharmacist

~~~

Carol is a survivor! The only way Carol has survived, considering her debilitating health condition, is because of her strong capable character and personality, which had to make up for the incapacity of her body. She also had the strong support and love of her family and friends. Considering all of Carol's heath issues, and virtually no muscle strength, with ability of moving less than a pound, nothing in this world has stopped Carol! She did everything a fully capable normal human being could have done... going to college, holding down a job, hardships, traveling the world, getting married, and more! I still believe, to this day, at her age, and confined even more so to her wheelchair, there is virtually nothing in this world that can stop this woman from doing what she wants to do! Carol's life story has a great deal to teach all of us about what is important in life! Live it; Love it; BE it!

Author Anita Meyer
Author of three books:
The Primordial Language,
In Search Of The Holy Language,
and Beyond The Bible Code.
Criminologist.
Religious procurement specialist.

Reviews

BY THE GRACE OF GOD AND YOU - A Chair Does Not a Person Make

This is a true story about someone that rose above a multitude of life obstacles, to have a successful and rewarding life.

While reading this book, I felt that I was transported to her home and was sitting, over coffee, listening to her tell her story.

Carol's story is an inspiration for all that experience setbacks in their life. The "Eveready Bunny" has nothing on Carol.

Sylvia Bahling RN
Kenosha WI

~~~

Carol is a true inspiration to able-bodied people as well as disabled. She has touched on so many things in her book that a person would never even think of. She has done so much in her life, proving that no disability was going to hold her back! A 'must-read' for all!

Susan Nielsen, published author.

BY THE GRACE OF GOD AND YOU
A Chair Does Not a Person Make

Carol Schaufel

Edited by
LK Kelley

DragonEye Publishing

BY THE GRACE OF GOD AND YOU
A Chair Does Not a Person Make
Copyright © 2014 Carol Schaufel

Cover portrait by artist, George Pollard

Editor: LK Kelley

First Edition
First Printing September 20, 2014

ISBN 13: 978-1-61500-057-9 Paperback

(Author Previously Published through CreataSpace 2013-
ISBN 13: 978-1492754091 - Paperback)

Library of Congress Control Number: 2014950090

~~~~~~~~

Other formats
ISBN 13: 978-1-61500-058-6 E-book

Visit our Website
www.DragonEyePublishers.com

Published by DragonEye Publishing

Dedicated with love to my parents, Steve, kids, grandkids, sister & family, friends, relatives coworkers, caregivers and strangers, all those who have touched my life in so many ways
Thank you

∼ Foreword ∼

I can't quite remember when I first met Carol Schaufel. I'm sure, if I asked her, she would remember. She demonstrates here with uncanny ability the details of a life spent in, but not defined by, a wheelchair.

Carol and I were classmates at Orthopedic School, a school that served students with all kinds of disabilities. We didn't look at things we couldn't do, but rather at how we could do things that *others* thought we might not be able to do. Whether it was sports, playing at recess, or just communicating with those students who had less ability to convey what was on their minds.

Carol demonstrates here how she used her ability, rather than her disability, to become a teacher, a counselor and, more importantly, a success in life.

I found myself not only laughing, but also crying, as I read her story and remembered many of the events she so wonderfully recalls. Even if you don't know Carol, you will get to know her as you read her remarkable story - her victories far outnumber her defeats in life.

This book should be read by anyone who thinks they have insurmountable obstacles in their lives. It is a story of hope, of overcoming those obstacles and succeeding in life not matter the roadblocks set in front of you.

Les Ryshkus
Retired Copy Editor

~ About the Author ~

I originally self-published my book, since there were different packages which included assistance. I sold about 200 books, but learned that self-publishing has its hazards. I had book signings at such places as Barnes and Nobles. The book signings were fun, and I learned a lot from other authors. Some were self-published, and some were not. At my fourth signing, I met an Author, Anita Meyer, who told me that her publisher might be interested in my book. I met her, again, at a fifth book signing in a Racine church. Anita told me she would e-mail him that same night, and I followed it with my own e-mail the next day. I agreed, and Publisher Michael Kiser, provided me with a book Editor, LK Kelley, who is knowledgeable, and is also a published author.

Since the writing of this book, I am now on the Kenosha County Commission on Aging, assisting with the needs of the elderly in our community along with legislative advocacy. I am also pleased to be on the Board of Society's Assets which is an independent living center serving five counties in Southeast Wisconsin.

TABLE OF CONTENTS

~ Introduction ~

I loved watching *"Ghost Whisperer"* on television. I especially enjoyed the way it started saying that the main character, Melinda, was just an average person who grew up in a small town, married, and was just like everyone else except that she saw ghosts!

My situation was very similar. I had a very normal life going to school, completing a Master's degree, and getting married. I worked for 39 years as a teacher and vocational rehabilitation counselor. Life was average, except that I never remember a time when I could dress myself, or use the bathroom without assistance. I stopped walking at the age of four, and gradually became weaker at regular intervals, until I stopped growing. Twelve years before I retired, I also lost the ability to feed myself.

I had multiple limitations. My family, friends, caregivers, coworkers and strangers were my natural supports. I adapted to multiple technologies, which became my tools to living my life instead of just existing. I did not want people to see me differently. I only wanted people to see that I just did things differently. It made me happy when people would stop seeing my wheelchair, and asked me to do things that they knew I could not do, but they forgot that I could not do them. For much of my life, I have used a motorized wheelchair, a mouthstick, or Dragon Dictate to type with my voice, and another device, a Sicare, that helped me to turn lights on and off, dial my phone, and unlock, and open my front door.

I was fortunate to have the support of my parents for 38 years before I organized myself to try independent living. In the process, I discovered that there was no such thing as independent living. One morning, in order to go to work, eight different people touched my life:

- a caregiver who helped me to get up and ready;
- a 15 year-old boy, who lived upstairs, and kindly pushed me through the snow to the bus stop;
- the bus driver,
- a secretary,
- a couple of probation officers,
- as well as a stranger who opened a door.

Whenever I needed someone to help, or assist me in my life, it seemed like someone was always there, and often it even might have been you!

This is the story of my life, what happened, the obstacles that I needed to overcome, the support that I received, and the deaths of so many old and young individuals from whom I learned many things. I recalled the laughter and tears we shared, and how, as a child, I saw, and adjusted to my changing, physical limitations. There were also the struggles of being seen as an adult when having to be taken care of as a child. When I left home at 38, my parents were lost as I changed from being dependent on them, to their being dependent on me. Forgive me if this is not chronologically correct, or if I have filled in details due to my failing memory. I am 67 now, you know! (Note: If I feel a person might be a bit uncomfortable from my story, I will change their name).

Enjoy reading my story, because I have faith that *anyone* can do *anything* by just making up their minds to do it.

If one is creative, not afraid to try, or fail and can adapt to things differently than the general population, then one can do it. If one does not mind being stared at occasionally, because they look different doing everything, then one can do it.

This is a thank you to everyone in my life—past, present and future. I am so grateful that you were/are/will be there!

~ 1 ~
Background

It was one of those rainy days. The room was a little dark and dreary. Nothing was on TV, so, I decided to clean some of my drawers. My attendant placed my three high school yearbooks in front of me on my bed, but I only attended two years of high school—my junior and senior years. I started with the 1963 yearbook, which would have been my sophomore year. Why did I have this book? I started turning the pages with my mouthstick, but didn't remember anyone specific. I turned another few pages and then I saw it—a half-page, fuzzy, black and white picture of Tim. He was one of the 15 friends and classmates that died before I was 20 years old.

I leaned my mouthstick next to my arm so that I could grab it later. My mind began clearing up that fuzzy picture. Why did Tim die in his senior year of school? I knew he had a limp from polio when he was in fourth grade, and I was in the first grade at the Orthopedic School. I had such a crush on him. I vaguely remember something about a tumor moving up his spine between his lungs, but I can't remember for sure. But, I do remember that he was handsome, funny, and used a wheelchair before he died.

Several of my other classmates had already died. Kathy who had died at the age of 12 of kidney failure was sweating urine the day she died, as there was no dialysis at the time. Ronnie, who died at the age of 16, had Muscular Dystrophy. Ronnie's body was distorted, so the mortician wanted to break Ronnie's bones to fit him flat into the coffin comfortably. I often thought, because my knees are contracted, and my back is curved, that the same would happen to me.

The one thing very special about Ronnie was that he was the only person I knew who could touch his nose with the tip of his tongue. He had very little other movement in his body. And, then, there was Dennis who died of a heart problem, along with many others.

From about the age of six years-old, I watched Muscular Dystrophy telethons. I knew that I was supposed to die by the age of 15, and I knew that I built up barriers between myself, and all around me. I did ~ 11 ~not want anyone to hurt as much as I did when my friends died.

When I was older, my Mother admitted to me that she was afraid to love me. The diagnosis came after four years, and she did not know how she could handle my death after she had been through so much. She never saw herself as a strong person, but she was.

I'd like to tell you a bit about my family, if I may. My Mother, Shirley, and my Father, Ken, were nine and thirteen, respectively, when they met. My Mother was only five when her parents were divorced (almost unheard of in 1930). Her Mother, Tina, was not a person that liked to go out much, and eventually, married Harvey, ten years her junior, and taking over for his Father's 40-acre farm. That was a good spot for Tina, and she was a hard worker. Together, they ended up selling tomatoes to the Campbell Soup Company as well as growing 10 acres of gladiolas for local florists. Their gladiolas had 32 flowers as big as a man's fist per spike—beautiful along with having original colors. Their geraniums were huge, and the tomato plants, peppers, and geese kept them busy. My Mom's Mother and Stepfather had cats on their farm, and they became known as 'Grandma and Grandpa with the kitties!'

Bill, my Mother's Dad, only attended school until the fourth grade. He married Vivian, a woman 10 years his senior, and she had a daughter named Doris. Vivian set a beautiful table, and she was a great cook. My Grandfather was originally a coal miner, and at one point, was trapped for hours in a mine in southern Illinois. He lost part of his foot during the mining accident. Later, he said that he would never, again, do mining work. He taught himself to read and write as well as how to raise mink. He became one of the most sought after mink ranchers in the country. My other maternal Grandparents became known as 'Grandma and Grandpa with the mink!' They also loved to play cards, and often did this with my Father's parents, and, this is how my parents met. My Dad had totally no interest in my Mom at that time. I think she was probably more of a nuisance to him as all she did was sit, and wait while the parents finished their card games.

I actually have three sets of Grandparents. My Dad's Mom, Ida, was 6 foot tall—just like her boys. Ida married my Grandpa after her fiancé was shot to death the day after the World War I armistice was signed. (Soldiers in the field took a long time getting the word that the war was over—many died such a death). My Grandfather, John, (about 5'10") was in the Cavalry fighting Pancho Villa in Mexico. (Obviously, he never met Pancho Villa as he still had both his ears! Thank you, God). My Grandfather supported his wife, and two six-foot boys selling Watkins products—still excellent products today. Since my Dad's parents lived in town, they became known to the kids as 'Grandma and Grandpa in town'.

Mom lived with her Mother. My Mom attended Dublin School from the first through eighth grade. She was a fast learner, and had a chance to teach some of the classes helping students catch up in other grades. She walked two miles from the farm to Dublin School every day. When she was older, she lived in town with some friends so she could attend high school.

Eventually, however, my parents started going out on dates. My Dad was in high school, and received good grades without even picking up a book. My Mother had no siblings, but my Dad had one brother, Al, who was angry with my Dad, because Al would gas up the family car for his own dates. By the time he would be ready to leave, my Dad had already driven off with the car to pick up my Mom!

My Mom always teased my Dad, because even then he liked to drive fast, among other things. Mom was the "lookout" for the police so he wouldn't get a speeding ticket.

At the age of 16, my Mom became engaged to my Father, 20. He had graduated from High School, and was working at Johnson Motors, which later became known as Outboard Marine. Mom was young, yes, but both Dad and Al joined the Army Air Corp in 1941. World War II had begun.

Two years after Dad was in the service, Mom quit high school with only six weeks left to work in a curtain rod factory. All of her girlfriends had fiancés in the service, too. They all worked together. Women took over the jobs that men were doing.

It was really a surprise that I was born at all. Dad was in the Army Air Corp as a radar mechanic, and stationed in Honolulu, Hawaii (Pearl Harbor after the Japanese attack), and in the Air Corp for four years. His squadron was scheduled to go on an air attack on an island where 85% of his squadron was wiped out. Fortunately for my Dad (and me), he had his first kidney stone attack, and was put into the hospital, so he could not go on the mission. Again, *thank you God*!

When the war ended, both Al and Ken were ready to come home. Al had been stationed on an island in the Pacific where he was on office duty. Since the war had been over for a few days, it was devastating when he saw his buddies blown up by a bomb. He saw people running, and ran outside. An explosion occurred in front of him and, in a second, debris was forced over him killing buddies behind as well as in front of him. This attack on the Chinese front was a surprise. When Al's shock wore off, he still had the pencil that he was writing with in his hand—holding it tight near his head. Uncle Al would never talk about his service experience, but it seriously affected him both mentally and physically.

As soon as Grandma and Grandpa's in town boys came back from the Army Air Corp, they were ready to marry. Al chose March 1 as his wedding day, and Dad went with him. When Dad saw Mom, he told her, "Al will be married March 1. The only other date open for us to get married was March 30. I took it." That sounded like my Dad. Straight to the point—if you have something to do, just get it done! Mom was taken by surprise, but agreed to the adventure.

There was not much information on birth control in 1946. It wasn't something that was talked about. Mom disclosed that she had the opposite understanding of the rhythm method so I was born exactly 9 months and 15 days after their wedding!

~ Something is Wrong ~

"Wednesday's Child is full of woe"—and I was. It was 1947 on a mid-January Tuesday with a blizzard howling outside. Mom's labor began, and she slowly made her way to the hospital. Her pregnancy wasn't easy, and she lost all of her teeth (guess I robbed her calcium), and had false teeth by the age of 21.

My Dad was glad when I was finally born many hours later on Wednesday, January 15, 1947 at 9:15 a.m., and was 5 lbs. 6 oz. My parents wanted a boy, and I really surprised them! They quickly decided to name me Carol, since I was born just after Christmas.

Some people told them, "Her name should have been Susan, because her eyes are as dark as the center of 'a black-eyed Susan'."

My Dad brought my Mom some roses, gave her a kiss and went straight to work without sleep. He was a dedicated man. While Mom was sleeping, the nurses said that I was bald, and that baldness continued for 18 months!

Things began to look "wrong" when Mom was looking at my footprints, and wondered why they seemed to be curved. For a short period of time, my parents and I stayed with my Grandma and Grandpa's at their in-town home. I was thought to have colic, because I cried constantly, all night, every night! No one slept. And, doctor discovered that I was crying because I was hungry, because my lagging strength only allowed me to eat an ounce of my formula at a time. My doctor, Dr. Peckous, Sr., saved my life more than once! My tonsils are still part of me, because he said, "God put your tonsils there for some reason, and I think you are going to need them." As a side note, Dr. Peckous was also the doctor for the Chicago Bears

- the football team, not the bears in the Chicago zoo!

By the time we moved out of my Grandparents' house into a temporary housing project for returning service members, my parents were on a schedule of going to bed at 7:00 p.m. It allowed my parents a few hours asleep. With my problems, they were always minus five dollars, but my Grandparents in town helped.

We had a limited time to stay in the housing project, and Dad wanted to build his own house. He had building experience helping others. Except for plumbing and electrical, he could build just about anything at all. He borrowed $5000 from my Grandpa with the mink, and it took two years to finish the house while working fulltime at Johnson Motors. Of course, he had to work around the winter cold, and with different people's schedules that were helping him build it. Even Mom was on the roof helping him put on the shingles. Mom was "stuck" in the bathroom between the wall and tub, and almost became a "permanent fixture" when Dad installed the tub!

It took me six months before I could sit up by myself, but I did walk early at nine months even though my legs were never strong. My Mom described to me an incident that had happened.

"One day, when you were two, we were in a park by the lake having a picnic. You were standing next to a park bench, and your legs gave out. You had your tongue sticking out (more than likely talking). We rushed you to the hospital as you were bleeding badly from your mouth."

Dr. Peckous explained, 'If this little girl would have chopped her tongue just another quarter of an inch, she would never be able to speak!"

He had to stitch my tongue, or used gauze to hold my tongue together. Then he put me in a straitjacket, because sucking my thumb, at the time, could cause infection. To this day, I still have an inch scar on my tongue. But, I'm positive that this incident stopped me from sucking my thumb! God works in mysterious ways. To make matters worse, I also had a horrible case of chickenpox, which covered my entire body. When the doctor tried to give me some penicillin, I developed a case of hives. I had an allergic reaction causing terrible itching not only on my body, but also in my nose and throat. A straitjacket would've been good at that time, but they did not give it to me!

When I turned two, we moved into our house on the south side of Kenosha, Wisconsin. Dad had built a wonderful house! Of course, none of us knew that the steps were going to cause a problem in the future with three steps in the front, and two steps in the back. My Dad, finally, added a front porch with three steps. We worked that out later, but I now had my own room!

And, then, I was sick once again! My parents had taken me to too many doctors. The wife of one of my Dad's friends from the service put a little article in the newspaper in their town of Port Washington, Wisconsin. She wrote something about a little girl who was constantly sick. I received a couple hundred cards. I remember some of those cards, because my Mom saved them, and may still have a couple today. My favorite one was a sick little boy with his feet in a tub of water. You could tip the boy back and forth to help him soak his feet. Another one was a set of cards that I received one per day to make me guess from whom they came. On the seventh day, the person was revealed. I don't remember the name of the person, but it sure was fun! Mom wrote thank you notes, and I learned to print my first name on them.

One of the things my Mom wished the doctors could fix was to stop me from sleeping with my eyes open! So, that is why I was taken to the chiropractor. Spooky, huh? He did something to my back and neck, finally, I started sleeping with my eyes closed!

I was also taken to a healer, and that didn't work.

At four years old, I was still falling a lot and hitting my head. My Mom thought for sure I was going to have a learning disability.

Another time, I was playing with our dog in an add-on utility room while Mom was in the kitchen. There was a closed door between us while she washed the dishes. She heard an unusual noise, and stopped to check on me. The dog's chain had wrapped around my neck, and I turned blue. Mom quickly swirled the chain off my neck which spun the dog around backwards at the same rate of speed, and the poor dog was dizzy. . It was a close call for me, and I must have had an *extremely,* busy guardian angel. Perhaps even three—one for each shift!

Some of the doctors thought that I might have something called Muscular Dystrophy. My Grandfather "with the mink" drove us to the Mayo Clinic in Rochester, Minnesota. I don't remember the doctor, but I do remember that car. Grandpa always had a Cadillac, and it was usually pink. In the back seat, it had an arm rest that came down in the middle of the seat, and I could sit on it to see out of the window. On the way, my Grandma "with the mink" told me the story of *The Three Little Pigs* for the first time. As a matter of fact, she had to tell me a lot of times to make it all the way to Minnesota! I loved that story, especially the way she told it. That old huffing and puffing wolf!

Muscular Dystrophy was the specialist's diagnosis. Every doctor after that gave the same diagnosis without challenge. There was no sign of the disease in generations past. Why now? Why me? Why not me.

~ Recognizing Change ~

What was Muscular Dystrophy? Who knew? Who cared? I was only four years old! What was all the fuss? Why was Mom treating me differently?

The people next door were very nice who had four children, and later a fifth. I knew Patty and Buddy best. Patty was a few years older than me. She would come, and play with me almost every day until her Mother thought she was bothering my Mom too much. My Mom would see Patty at our back door, chin barely to the window, and asking, "Whatcha got to eat for me today?" Patty's brother, Buddy, played with me a lot, too. I would run around the house, and he would chase me. I would fall. Then, Buddy would stand me up again, and our chase began again. I noticed some differences in my body since I had begun to walk on my knees, now. My knees looked like the bottom of people's feet—with huge calluses. I found a little chair with no back on it that I put in front of me to use as a walker inside and outside which helped me meet more and more of our neighbors. In the summer, I would have a lot of company as well as investigated gardens, picking green beans and strawberries.

My Grandparents' in town babysat me more than anyone. My Grandma would play *Tiddlywinks* with me, and my Grandpa would play *Old Maid,* and try to cheat which would make me laugh. He would hold the old maid card loosely, and the rest of his cards tight so that I could not pull anything but the old maid. I wised up pretty fast! When we finished playing the games, my Grandfather would hold out his two fingers for me to grab onto so that I could walk on my knees to the kitchen table in a little nook which looked like a booth. My Grandma and I loved to put together about eight puzzles she kept in the same box, and I could separate six of them, and put them together easily. There were two puzzles that had no locking connections which were very hard for me. On these hard puzzles, Grandma would always sit with me, and finish them as we looked out the back window to see the lightning bugs in the garden.

When I was back home, I had a little rocking chair, and as I walked on my knees, I would back my feet underneath the chair, and sit down in it. As I got bigger, I couldn't figure out why I couldn't get my feet under that chair anymore. I recalled using some Encyclopedia books (my Mom got into great trouble with my Dad for buying those from a traveling salesman) stacking three of them, then two, and then one to make a staircase. I would go up the makeshift stairs on my knees, get to the top of my stairs, and try to go down all three books on the end. Well, it worked on the way down, but I could never get back up the three books! You'd think I could just go down the three steps I created instead of trying to jump up on the three, but, no. I didn't think of that!

Real staircases I handled differently. Going up was always hard, coming down was fun. I would wiggle my rear to the edge of the top step, and bounced my way down one step at a time. I would do this over and over again till I touched the bottom. I thought it was fine, but Mom and Dad always hollered at me when I did, because they thought it was dangerous. I began to take risks early.

I also liked to play in the closet with my clothing above my head. I had my dollhouse with a little wind up lady that would sweep like crazy. As I grew, I always wondered why my dresses kept hitting my head!

When winter came, my Mom took me for my first sled ride by putting me in a box. I fell off of course, and my face was cold in the snow. I couldn't breathe, and it seemed like a long time before she noticed that I was missing. I was really glad she finally rescued me, and please…no more sled rides with Mom?

I am not sure what happened to my first dog, but the summer that I was five, we got another dog, a very strong collie. There was a vacant lot next door on the south side of our house. Dad put his doghouse in the back of the lot. The dog was so strong, he could drag his doghouse with him to the front of the yard every night, and Dad would carry it back every morning! One day was the final straw as the dog chased a car with his doghouse attached. The dog caused the car to smash into the store across the street … there were no more dogs for a while. We would also fly kites in that same, vacant lot next door. My Dad would put my kite on a fishing pole, and it worked great!

In contrast, pretending that the electrical plug by our couch was a gumball machine didn't work well. I tried to push a penny between the prongs of the plug - the lamp was plugged into the socket. Sparks flew! I was scared! But, I was lucky enough not to get hurt - *or killed*! I was in serious trouble, yelling happened, but I *never did it again*! I was just lucky to be alive in order to 'never to do that again'!

We would visit my Grandma and Grandpa with the kitties. My parents went into the house on this occasion. I stayed in the car. My Grandma and Grandpa had a tiny bulldog who just loved me. I had stayed in the car while my parents went into their house, and I saw him coming to greet me. But, my parents forgot to close the car door. Thinking fast, my eyes wide, he began slobbering all over me. The only thing I remember was, "How can I make him stop kissing me so I can breathe?" My first, creative idea was to make a pocket of air with my lips. I curled the top lip slightly over the bottom one so he couldn't get his tongue in my mouth. I survived for about fifteen minutes until my parents came back. It worked ... phew!

By this time, walking on my knees was getting harder, and I lost some strength. One night, while lying down on my bed, I tried to push my arm up toward the ceiling, but only my hand to my elbow rose toward the ceiling.

I thought, "Huh?" I was sure I was becoming my Dad. He would say, "It is what it is, move on. Don't miss today."

I was a big Mickey Mouse club fan. I had my Mickey Mouse ears, and would sit right in front of the television on the floor, cross legged, singing on the top of my lungs "M-I-C-K-E-Y M-O-U-S-E." I knew all of the songs for every day of the week, and my parents found it was hard to get me off the floor!

It was about time for me to start school, and so, my parents checked to see if I could go to kindergarten. But, I couldn't, because I lived in the county. I had to wait another year, and I would have to go to a special school in the city. We were lucky enough to live in Kenosha which had one of the few orthopedic schools in the nation, and the school had therapy as well as education. Nap time for all grades was a must! In 1951, there were a lot of students with polio (using cots instead of desks) in the classrooms, people with heart problems, cerebral palsy and a number of other disabilities. The school had ramps for people in wheelchairs as well as steps that people on crutches often preferred. Ramps were almost unheard of at that time. There were five classrooms organized by grades and ages and three therapeutic rooms set up for hydrotherapy, physical therapy and speech therapy. Everything sounded good to me, except naps.

Although it was another year before I could start school, the principal, Otto Steffenson, still talked to my parents about any special needs which they or I might have because of my disability. He also was involved in Easter Seals on the state level, and indicated that I might need a Hoyer lift to get me off the floor, or in and out of the tub. The lift was brought into my home at that time. I was beginning to use a stroller for distances, and was beginning to be "pushed around."

Though I thought the lift was great for getting me on and off the floor, I thought it served a much better purpose as a swing while I watched the Mickey Mouse Club! The lift never really worked for getting me in and out of the bathtub, because the balance was off. It would tip all over the place.

There was one more huge surprise before I started school. Mom and Dad told me Mom was going to have a baby! I thought Mom was just getting fluffy with her bigger tummy! We picked names before the baby was born, and I can't remember what name we picked for a boy, but Mom and Dad thought they'd better name the baby Susan if it was a girl since everyone thought that should have been my name. They were so happy she was coming, her middle name would be Joy!

~ 2 ~

Meeting Susan

The baby was about ready, and my Mom packed my bag so I would be ready to spend some time with my Grandma and Grandpa in town. I was excited. I saw the baby's crib in Mom and Dad's room, and I was a little disappointed that the baby would not be with me. If the baby was going to cry a lot, like I did, I knew I would be glad the baby wasn't in my room. A baby was like a doll to me. Come to think of it, I never really played with my dolls much even though I had a cradle, a rocking chair, changes of clothing, bottles and dolls, but dolls were heavy. I preferred my bubble blowing monkey, my steering wheel that kept the car on the road with a battery-operated moving path, a dollhouse with movable furniture, and board games like Candy Land and Chutes & Ladders.

Well, the new baby was born on July 25, 1952. Mom started having pain so Dad did not even go to work. At 7:00 a.m., Dad carried me to the car followed by Mom carrying our two suitcases! We drove over to my Grandparents in town first, and Dad carried me into the house while Mom carried my suitcase. My parents made it to the hospital about 7:30 a.m., and they just barely made it. Mom only had five labor pains (passing out between each one) before my sister was born at 8:15 a.m. This time Dad only missed two hours of work. Happily, he bought my Mom roses, gave her a kiss, and was back to work by 9:00 a.m. Mom always believed that the reason the baby came so fast was because, the day before, she weeded our whole garden!

My Dad picked me up in the car after he got home from work, and went to the hospital to see my Mom. She peeked out the hospital window and waved at me. That wave was important as this was the first time I would ever be staying away from home overnight. Actually, it was the only time I remembered not being with my parents at night as a child except for Easter Seals camp at age 12, and staying with Patty and her husband one night when I was 18.

It was so good to see Mom wave at me. I was a little bit scared, but now I knew that she was okay. Dad told me that I had a sister, Susan Joy! I could not see her now as I was not allowed in the hospital at that age, because of hospital rules. This was the norm across the country in those days. Mom would be gone about three days.

My visit with my Grandparents was a little bit different. I got to see my Grandmother comb her long hair that dropped, past her waist. I had never seen it down before. She braided it, wound the braids around her head, and pinned the braids in place on the top of her head.

When we went to bed, Grandma and I slept in Grandpa's room. The room was small with a dresser, a table with a lamp, and the bed. I remembered looking over at Grandma that first night while she slept. Her silhouette was kind of scary without being able to see the features of her face, with only the moonlight coming through the window. The clock I heard was the most memorable of all, because it kept me awake. The dining room had a mantle clock which "bonged" the number of hours "bonged" on the half-hour with one long "bong". I could hear this all night, was so much louder than it seemed during the day. But, I finally fell asleep.

The next morning, I was busy. The most fun was exploring Grandma's house. I could still walk on my knees a little, and used my little chair without the back as a walker to explore just everything I could.

In the morning, there was soupy oatmeal for breakfast in the kitchen nook that looked outside the window into her garden. My exploration began when I went into the pantry. There was a good variety of food and cookware in it. When I could reach only a few things, I moved to another room.

Next, I took a little stroll to the dining room that had a little table with a telephone on it. The telephone was the type where you picked up the handle to put it by your ear, and then spoke into a microphone on a stand. Two separate pieces made that phone work. This was nothing like the one we had at home. Both of the phones had numbers you had to dial by running the number you wanted around in a circle. I hated dialing "0's." Grandma had a huge table in the middle of the room that covered most of the space. There was a China cabinet with beautiful dishes, and another long, "dresser" with multiple drawers, as well as that noisy mantle clock sitting right in the middle on top of it. Of course, I looked in the all of the drawers, and found their wedding pictures, other pictures, tablecloths, napkins, and a set of real silverware, and yes, it was real silver, and heavy to lift! (Note: did you know you can take off tarnish from real silverware with toothpaste and a soft cloth)?

I moved to the living room where we usually played games, and saw a very small television with about an eight inch screen in a huge cabinet. There was a lot of different furniture around such as a cushy couch and some chairs, a table in front of the window and some end tables with lamps.

(Note: How different their television was compared to the one that my Grandfather with the mink had. It was a much bigger screen! Milton Berle was on his black and white TV walking around in a woman's dress the last time I was there. Did you know Mr. Berle was one of the first people on TV? He signed a contract for 50 years just to do his comedy routines? Of course, Milton was not on television for 50 years though! Television changed tremendously).

Then, it was time to investigate my Grandma's bedroom. She was combing her hair again when I walked into it, and I went into her closet. Wow! I found a door in the back of the closet which appeared to have two stairs. This was going to be worth checking out! Grandma opened the door for me, and I conquered those two stairs slowly. It was similar to a little attic. It was a tiny room with a tiny window, boxes of old treasures, a few shelves, some old dolls, etc. What a treasure! I definitely wanted to spend some time there.

Before I knew it, it was time to go home, and I was ready. I wanted to sleep in my own bed. Dad picked me up since Mom was home with the baby. I could not wait to meet Susan!

When we got home, Mom was in the bedroom with the baby. I kissed Mom, and then, Dad held me over the crib so I could see my new sister. She was sleeping. What? She had hair already? I waited 18 months to get mine! When Susan finally opened her eyes, they were blue! Is her name still going to be Susan? Is she really my sister?

BY THE GRACE OF GOD AND YOU
A Chair Does Not a Person Make

~ Starting School ~

My world had now changed. Susie and her crib moved into my room before the end of the year. She was fun to watch, play with and tease even at such an early age. She took a lot of Mom's time. I was not sure how Mom did it since I took so much time, too. Not only did Mom have to do all my personal care, but she had to get up, and turn me at night when I called. Fortunately, I had a lot more things coming up that I had to think about now.

My Grandfather with the mink bought my first wheelchair. It seemed much too big for me. I would always sit in my wheelchair with my legs crossed up onto the seat which made my first wheelchair tip backwards. This created a whole new way of falling and getting lumps on my head. I remembered these falls more than the walking falls, probably because I was older. We found out that the Everest & Jennings wheelchairs were the best with balance. I finally got one of those wheelchairs. By the time I started school, I could no longer walk on my knees. I was not using the stroller, but was using the wheelchair all of the time.

I was preparing to start school. When we first visited the school, the principal's secretary came out of the building to greet us. I thought she had such a cute little wiggle as well as a quiver in her voice. I found out later that Betty Anderson had cerebral palsy. What a great role model to meet first! Miss Betty brought out a little circular chair with wheels on it. It had no handles, no sides, just a back. They sat me on it to take me into the building. Mom and Miss Betty set up transportation to get me back and forth to school by a taxicab. (I could not take the bus as the bus did not go out to the County, and I could not get on and off the bus myself.) To go into the school building, there was a rainbow-shaped ramp on the east-side, and was just outside the physical therapy room. The therapy room had four cushioned tables surrounded by movable curtains to ensure privacy. This room was where I was to have some of my treatment. (My knees were already contracted, and needed to be stretched, and my left hand was formed into a hard fist.) From there, a little hallway divided the therapy and hydrotherapy rooms. There was a little offshoot room to the right that had larger bathrooms, and a place to change clothes. We went through this area to the hydrotherapy room where there was a big Hubbard tank shaped in the figure of an "8 "(no middle of course) with a stretcher attached to an electric lift above it. You could get on the stretcher from a cot outside the tank, be raised up, moved across the top of the Hubbard tank, and be lowered into the water. There was another smaller whirlpool where a person could sit on a seat. The room, itself, looked kind of cold and sterile.

As we toured the school, I also saw my first grade classroom. I had a lot of fun looking at rows of desks that had flip open tops for your school supplies. Underneath the windows, there were a lot of toys and a play area. I caught a glimpse of one of my favorite toys-to-be in that room—a huge dollhouse with a real staircase, a lot of furniture, and doors that opened and closed! What a dream house!

From my classroom, we went down the hallway towards the office. On each side of that hallway were cots where all students took naps after lunch hour. The school office was small. Maybe there was room for two visitors, and it was the same for the principal's office. No discipline problems here, or the space would be bigger! I was ready to start school.

A few days later, I was picked up by a cab. The driver lifted me into the cab, and we were off to school. Yes, the school did have the driver put me on that same circular chair with

12

wheels. I was assigned to the third row of desks from the window, and was second to the back of the room. The teacher lifted me in my desk chair. I looked around to see some students who were already there, and watched others as they came into the classroom.

Barbara came in with a little bit of bounce with one leg shorter than the other. Another person had a limp as well as an arm that was tight to his chest, and another child would sometimes fall to the floor. I found out, later, that he had epilepsy. One person came into the room in a wheelchair. Marilyn had polio, and sat behind me. Randy had a hole in his heart, but I couldn't see it! Everyone was so different, yet so alike. Louise was a person that was most interesting to me. She had big braces on her legs. I didn't know how she could move with them. She also used a walker, and a helmet so she would not hurt her head if she fell. Sometimes, Louise would really get going with her walker, and would hit the wall. That was how she earned her nickname, "Crash." (We loved her, and gave her the nickname with complete affection).

Before noon, I had to go to the bathroom. The lady who helped in physical therapy came to get me. Her name was Mrs. Zigner. She was a large lady with a boxy figure, and short, permed brown hair that looked a little coarse. Mrs. Zigner put me on my circular chair, and pulled the chair backwards from my classroom into the bathrooms between the hydrotherapy and physical therapy rooms. It was lonely in there, but it was the closest bathroom to my first-grade classroom. She left me alone a while, and came back to take me to the lunchroom on time.

I hadn't been to the lunchroom before. The room was all the way down the main hallway, past the office (which was in the middle of the building), and all the way at the end of the other end of the building. About five of my classmates sat with me at the same table. There was a bell that went off. (I found out it was a couple of chimed sounds hit with a stick on a miniature xylophone of four keys, and struck from low to high). We said a short prayer that was led by the teacher in the highest grades. He was the only man teacher in the school, and his name was Mr. Dietrich. I was always kind of afraid of him. He was always very professional and immaculate, and I never did see him smile much.

Now what was I going to have to eat? On that day, we were having ground beef and gravy over mashed potatoes with green beans, red Jell-0 with fruit, milk, and a cookie. I had a chance to talk with some of my new friends. I learned what they liked, and didn't like, to eat. This was important for later in case I didn't like to eat something, and we would trade each other for our favorite foods. I was the only person that liked rutabaga, so I would have a lot of that in the future.

I also had a chance to look around the lunchroom. I saw some of the fourth graders, like Mary, who had that cute little wiggle like Miss Betty and trouble speaking. She used a baby buggy to get around which aided her balance. I thought that was interesting as it was the same concept as when I used my little chair without the back to help me balance on my knees. Susan was on a cot, because she had polio. Billy, who I found out later, also had polio, but he had no movement from his shoulder to his hands. Another boy, Marshall, was in Mr. Dietrich's room. He looked like he was 7 foot tall on his crutches. No one looked famous (except for Marshall because he was so handsome!), but I heard that one of the daughters' of a person, who was on the Arthur Godfrey TV show, once went to my school.

BY THE GRACE OF GOD AND YOU
A Chair Does Not a Person Make

We left the dining room when we heard the xylophone chime backwards (high note to low note). Nap time! We went to sleep on cots in the hall. (I didn't think anyone really slept, but it was a good break for the staff). The custodians, Greg and Gino, had the responsibility of getting us on and off the cots. Gino bore most of that responsibility. Once in a while, Gino would twirl us around in circles in his arms. I didn't remember anybody having done that to me before, and it made us laugh. After rest hour, we would go back to our classroom.

At the end of the school day, we would pack up what we needed, and left our classroom to wait for our cabs to take us home. There were usually five to seven people in my cab going to the south side of town. Sometimes, they had cabs with a couple extra seats in them between the back and front seats in order to fit everyone inside.

By the end of the first week of school, we would have our therapy schedules also. Someone always seemed to be missing from a class here, or there, a couple of times a week. By the second week of school, I began hydrotherapy in the Hubbard tank. I enjoyed that a lot with the water as hot as I could get it. Mrs. Perkins would come in to stretch my legs while I was in the tank. Mrs. Fischer would help me transfer to the stretcher to dress and undress me. I had a couple of chances to try the whirlpool, but I always felt as if I was going to fall down in the water. Stretching my legs hurt me more when I was on the tables in the physical therapy room, so I ended up with only hydrotherapy.

One day, at the end of that second week, Mrs. Zigner had forgotten I was in the bathroom, and I was late for lunch. She came back to get me about 15 minutes before our lunch hour was over. Eating fast, I stuffed my coleslaw in my milk carton. I never liked coleslaw anyway, and still don't even to this day! Mrs. Zigner felt bad about forgetting me, so she gave me a cute, paper doll cutout book, later discovering that she gave these to several of the students. I thought that was so nice, unless she forgot all of those students in the bathroom, too! She never forgot me in the bathroom again, but I got some more paper doll books anyway.

Some of the activities in first grade were fun. Miss Druse, whom we always hoped would marry our first grade cab driver, Tony, gave us new words to learn every day. She would make a ladder on the board with the new words on it, and we would have to try to verbally climb up the ladder by reading the words. One of our first exercises was to be placed into teams of two to draw the outline of the other person on butcher paper. I'm not quite sure what the purpose was, but I did realize how tall I was compared to the others. It was also interesting to be on the floor without a rug, and the fun I had working with another person.

About one month into school every year, a clinic was provided where we saw an orthopedic doctor who would help monitor our progress. He seemed to always want to put braces on people, or provide a surgery to straighten out their back.

Mom always protected me during those times as she told him, "No braces, no cutting. With Carol's diagnosis, it will not help her strength. She doesn't need to go through any more than she has to at this point."

The doctor wasn't very happy, but Mom, she always won. I was glad. The school even tried to schedule her with two different doctors. She still won! After a few years, I didn't even have to go to clinic anymore, although I continued to go to hydrotherapy.

Orthopedic School always had fun events. Magicians would come in and perform. The Shriners took the whole school to the circus once a year. The police took us to a Milwaukee

Brewers ballgame, and at that time, the team was called the Braves, and our parents had a chance to go to these events, also.

From first through third grade, we would go to an all-girl's school called Kemper Hall. It was a scary old, huge building that used to house nuns. No parents were there! Making it even more scary, students from our school would go to Kemper on a night close to Christmas by taxis. A different girl from the school would be assigned to each of us individually. We would be taken across a dark room, around a lot of corners, and to an open, freight elevator door. Once upstairs, we would go into a room where there was a huge Christmas tree with a lot of presents under it. We would sing songs, get a treat, and then gifts were passed out. I got a beautiful dress that fit! A doll and some games were there, too. Ronnie was really lucky. The girl that took care of him was Roy Rogers' daughter. He got a cowboy hat and toy guns with a holster. It was fun!

By the time spring came, I was using a very old wheelchair that they must have found in the school's attic. It had a very high back. I used to have to sit very far forward in the chair in order to push the big wheels which were in the front. And, naturally, someone came along, and grabbed the back of the chair pulling it backwards. It was the first time I fell out of the wheelchair.

Another student had a crush on me. While we waited for the cab to go home, he would push me behind the school where there was a huge hill going straight down into Washington Bowl, especially known for its bike racing. I was scared, because the student had seizures, and would make me watch him play on the monkey bars. Sometimes he'd fall. I was always afraid that he would hurt himself, and the taxi driver wouldn't know where we were. I could not push myself over the grass to help him if it did happen. After a few days of this, I had a plan. I never told anyone, but I would try to push myself to the secretary's office to visit with Miss Betty until my taxi came. It worked. Most of the time, Miss Betty would see me before, and pushed me there. The student wasn't in our school for very long. Not sure what ever happened to him.

The only other thing I remembered about the first grade was that I was in the newspaper for the first time with Eddie. The article showed the Women's Bowler Association from whom we had received wheelchairs for use in the school. Eddie was a cute third-grader who happened to have Spina Bifida which is an open spine. His legs could not bend, so they were straight out in front of him, even if there were no foot rest. By the time he was a little older, Eddie could tip his chair on its hind wheels and go down stairs without assistance. He now was in the classroom "upstairs".

The biggest difference about first and second grades was that it was upstairs with a l-o-n-g 15° ramp that accessed Mrs. Strange's classroom. (Legal grades of ramps are now 5°). Mrs. Strange was an older, regal looking lady with white hair. She was kind, and quiet. I didn't remember a bathroom upstairs; there was just a long, skinny classroom on one end, a long, skinny physical therapy room on other end, and a big room full of cots in the center. The cots were used for rest hour. It was a lot darker upstairs, so I would often sneak my hand onto Louise's cot, and try to scratch out a tune with my fingernail for her to guess what it was. She guessed the right tune a few times, but I wasn't very good at it. I was sure that all the scratching sounded alike! I would whisper something funny to Louise, and she would burst out laughing. I didn't mean to get her in trouble, but it did. I told her she had to laugh more quietly. (To this day, when I laugh, I make no sound, but tears will be streaming from my eyes, and down my face when I am really laughing hard.)

One day, I was very surprised when Randy passed me a note in second-grade.

It read: "I love you, do you love me? Yes, or No. Check one." What was this about? He was a friend. Marilyn was sitting next to me. I asked her what she would do. She said, "Check no." So I did!

Then, she told me, "If that was me, I would have written 'yes' all over the paper!" Thus, my first relationship ended.

I had a routine of going to the bathroom after lunch, but one day I just could not hold it. I was waiting to get pushed out of the lunchroom. I could not wait, so I went in my pants. I felt so bad that I made myself sick. I asked to go home. Mom noticed my pants were wet when I got there. I didn't know if anyone else knew. She said not to worry about it, and tell the truth. She suggested I go to the bathroom before lunch, so that I wouldn't have to try to wait. I started planning my bathroom times at a very early age!

Mom also worked on straightening my hand that was in a fist. Every night, she would place my hand on a pillow so that it would begin flattening out. At first, it hurt, but I did not notice it after a while. In about six months, it was a lot easier to move my left hand around. I could open and close my left hand which wasn't frozen into a fist now.

In third grade, I still had Mrs. Strange. The school seemed to be doing things differently. Every six month, or so, they would weigh us. It was an interesting process. Someone would take us, individually, into a room where a regular doctor scale stood. Of course, many of us could not stand on it, so they would place a wide board on it, then a chair, and, finally, one of us on the chair. Once, it appeared that I had gained too much weight, and they were angry at me until they realized that they had forgotten to subtract the board and the chair's weight from my total weight. I was always conscious of my weight after that. With my back now curved, my rib would hit my hip on my right side giving me no waist at all. I always felt like I looked fat even when I did not weigh much.

Another new thing was started after every lunch hour. I would have to go to the kitchen which was right next to the lunchroom with my physical therapist. The kitchen ladies with their hair-nets and white uniforms were all cleaning up the area. Mrs. Perkins would warm up some tomato juice on the stove, and add a powder that my Muscular Dystrophy doctor had recommended for me. Once it melted into the juice, Mrs. Perkins would hold it up for me to drink. (By this time, I was using an edge of the table to help me push my arms to my head for eating and drinking. Without the table, I could not hold a drink by myself.) The medicine tasted a little bitter, but it wasn't bad. Mrs. Perkins tried it, and didn't like it at all! (She was not a good example to follow to teach a child how to take medication)! I took this every day for a year, or more. It was loaded with Vitamin E to see if it would help my muscles. Vitamin E combined with this powder, was associated with strengthening muscles in Muscular Dystrophy. It is also known as a "sex vitamin". I never really noticed my muscles getting stronger. Apparently, the Vitamin E didn't make me stronger, but it did have a side effect. I began to develop a chest, and started my period during the summer I was 9 ½.

The Orthopedic School had not touched on the subject of puberty until the middle of fourth grade, so this development in my life was a surprise to me! Our family was coming back from vacation in Florida when I found out what "growing up" meant. We stopped at the last motel before we got home. I was lifted onto the toilet, and saw some spotting in my underwear. I got a little scared. I think my Mom was surprised, too.

Mom just stated, "Oh, that's nothing. It's normal. You probably will be getting that every month now."

I responded, "What?"

She explained, "You are just becoming a woman."

I thought, "*What?? At 9 1/2? Huh! Okay.*" This was how I learned to accept everything that happened in my life. Don't panic! Get an explanation and roll with it!

This year, too, Louise also had a new therapist, Mr. Olufs. He seemed very young, and had a lot of energy. He finally noticed that Louise's braces were much too heavy for her, and worked with her to get rid of them. She started walking on her own with saddle shoes that next year, and she lost her nickname, "Crash"!

I also learned about Louise's speech therapy. I understood her speech better than ever before. She had problems with words that started with vowels as those are the only sounds that come out through the air in your throat. She could say words like "honor" without a thought, but she struggled to verbalize the word "on".

I would sometimes tease Louise in the lunchroom, and take a drip of water or milk with my straw, and flip it at her. Louise would do the same thing to me, but she would get caught. I wasn't always the angel people thought I was!

Fourth grade was back downstairs. Miss Grasser was our teacher now. She was a very beautiful, younger woman who had lost the use of her left arm/hand which was curled tight, and held next to her body. She seemed to have no problems in the classroom because of her disability. Again, being the little matchmakers my classmates and I were, we were always hoping that Mr. Dietrich and Miss Grasser would get together. That never happened.

Also, in the fourth grade, we started to go to a different place for our Christmas dinner. The Elks Club was nice, roomy and inviting, but three things were very different.

- We had our party at noon, not at night.
- Our previous school Christmas dinners were always with young females. Now we were with older men.
- How was I going to ask for help cutting my meat, or doing the other things with which I needed help?
- I'd never been at a formal dinner before. First, there was soup (very good). Then, salad and bread (good, too). What I did not realize was that there was more food coming. It was chicken à la King. I thought, "Huh, what was chicken à al king?" I tried it. Now I knew. I didn't like it. I was very glad I was full, BUT chicken à la King did not have to be cut! (I found out from the kids in the higher grades that the meal was always the same, so I learned to like it!)

The year I was in fourth grade was also an election year! Eisenhower was running for Presidential re-election. (Gee, I'm old.) Our class went through the whole process of an election. I wrote out about 30 ballots for our classroom which consisted of both fourth and

17

fifth graders. I had trouble with spelling Eisenhower at first, but not after writing all of those ballots out! Another student was given the responsibility of making a ballot box. Still another had to count the ballots. Eisenhower won both elections—in the classroom and in the United States. The coming summer, my parents had a trip planned to Washington DC. My sister would have been about five, and I was about 10 1/2 years-old. We went to the White House and both my sister, and I were frisked! Let me tell you a little more about that later after I backtrack to tell you what was happening at home during these school's years.

~ 3 ~

Growing Up

Susan was called "Susie". She was crawling around on my bed by the time she was one year-old. I would play with her, tease her, and feed her. By the time she was four, she had heard us say to her enough times:

"Don't let Carol fall on you, or you would be just a little grease spot!"

She was afraid to crawl around me too fast, or climb on me as she thought that I would fall over on her.

After years of hearing this, Susie said that the first time I did fall on her, "I just could not believe that I survived. I wasn't a grease spot!"

She wanted me to fall on her again and again just to see what would happen. That's my sister!

Susie always knew that Mom had to help me with everything, and that I took a lot of her time. She never seemed like she was jealous, nor would she complain. Only once did I remember Susie feeling that she needed to seek a little attention. Mom had come into the room at night to turn me.

Susie asked, "Mom, would you turn me, too?"

Mom didn't say anything. She just went over and turned Susie too! That satisfied her.

Susie did complain to Mom about my teasing her. She would always sit as close to me as she could to make it easy for me to reach her.

She would say, "Mom, Carol is tickling me."

Mom would say, "Just move away!"

Susie would say, "Oh, I never thought of that!"

Susie was always good about sharing the excitement of Christmas with me. On Christmas Day, we would both wake up early - earlier than our parents did. She would go into the living room, and peek underneath the tree. Susie would run back in the bedroom, and tell me exactly what she saw. She would not touch anything, but would let me know if anything was unwrapped, or if Santa had eaten all the cookies! Then, she would wait patiently with me until our parents woke up, so that I could out of bed and get dressed. Well, maybe we weren't too patient. We were making as much noise as we could without being too obvious! Our parents would get up, and we would all open everything together.

We always had a huge tree, and were always afraid that it was going to be too short. Dad would go with Mom to get the tree, hold it up next to him, and Mom would choose one that was about four-feet taller than he was. By the time the tree was in the house and in the stand, two feet would have to be cut off the top to snugly tuck it into the corner. We tied it to a curtain rod, so that it could not topple over onto the floor. And, we had a little tree for someone else! We would all help. My job was to string some of the popcorn and put the tinsel on the branches of the tree that I could reach. It was always a lot of fun until the dog would come by wagging his tail and knotting all of the tinsel that I put on the tree!

There were times we would have babysitters, too. Sometimes I liked babysitters better than I liked my Dad taking care of us, because I could never wake him up if he went to sleep. Patty, one of our babysitters, stayed a lot with me even though she was only two years older than me.

Her cousin, Diane, would come over, too. We would make fudge, or play games.

My parents never went out much, and if they did, it was usually for bowling, because my Mother was on a weekly team on Mondays, while my Father's team met on Fridays.

Before the age of nine, I often had some bad, re-occurring dreams - and they were in color! The way I handled these dreams was by remembering them each night - before I would go to sleep. I would look around my room in the dark, and have one dream that I would remember by my bed, one by the window, one by the closet, one by the television, and one on Susie's wall. The dreams stopped after I began doing this, but at least, I never walked in my dreams. I was usually on a cart close to the ground pushing fast with my hand, or maybe I just never saw my body.

But, even in my dreams, I had questions.

"How can people stand to walk with all that bouncing up and down, back and forth, on opposite feet? When I'm riding in my wheelchair, my view of the world seems smooth."

Dad liked to do a lot of traveling, and we would go with him. While he liked to travel, my Mom liked coming home. Susie and I would sing in the back seat about anything at all, and we would sing about "the bumpy road, the bumpy road, the bump, bump, bumpy road", or the "smooth road, the smooth road." We would look for license plates from each state, play car bingo, or exercise by putting my fingers on the top of Susie's toes. She would lift up her leg, but my fingers would fall before her leg grew too tired to move.

For about 20 years in row, my parents would visit their friends, the Holtans, in Boulder Junction. Mo Holtan owed four factories, so when Dad became a supervisor in charge of two of the three Johnson Motors buildings in Waukegan, Illinois, he met Mo Holtan.

They had a guesthouse that they made accessible for me with a portable ramp. They had seven children, one was Susie's age, and one was mine. There seemed to be something going on different every summer. Susie enjoyed being in the Musky Parade. I enjoyed riding in a convertible. All of us enjoyed the cookouts including lobster on the grill. (Dad always teased us that he was sad that he ever introduced us to lobster when we were young, because it became expensive when we got older, but we always celebrated special occasions with lobster!) All of the Holtan's children loved to water-ski no matter their ages. They could water-ski on each other's shoulders, or barefoot. For many years, they put on a water show at either Trout Lake or in Minocqua. One year, when I was 16, I even shared my measles with them! Another year when I was 10, they had a pet skunk named Petunia! Mo, their Father, and the entire family were always good to me.

For about 15 years, we also spent a week in June at a resort in Bena, Minnesota which was a town of about 500 people (2010 census showed it is now 116 people). Dad met Kelly, who shared this vacation home with us, through his job too. There were three cabins for different families if needed, and a Lodge where a lady named "Em" cooked all of our food. Chuck would take my Dad, or my Mom and Dad, fishing. I would play for hours on a labyrinth, or with the kittens, they always seemed to have. Susie was around either playing outside, or with me and the care-takers' daughter, Ruthie.

In general, it was very relaxing except for the very first year when there were thousands of inch long fish flies. They scared me to death, and I could not knock them off myself easily. At least they didn't bite like mosquitoes!

This place was owned by a decal company connected with the salesman my Dad worked with named Kelly. The most unusual experience I had on these vacations was in the lodge. It was pouring rain outside. I was watching it out of the window over the dining room table. My sister turned my wheelchair around for some reason. I was now looking in the opposite direction to the opposite window across the lounging area. It wasn't raining at all on that side of the building.

My sister had a bad experience though when she went wading in the lake. She saw her first bloodsuckers. Susie felt that one was going to jump right out of the lake at her as she ran away from it through the water in what appeared to be slow motion. Ruthie told her not to worry. Even if the leech had latched itself onto her, all Susie would have to do was put salt on it to kill it.

Dad ended up with several weeks of vacation a year—maybe four. Two weeks a year, he could take his vacations whenever he wanted, but the other two weeks had to be taken when the plant was closed during the last two weeks of July.

At the end of the third grade, we took our first long family trip to Florida. On the way to Florida, we saw tobacco drying in Kentucky, Nashville's Grand Old Opry, Lookout Mountain's summit in Tennessee, picked a piece of cotton (very prickly and scratchy in the "pod") in Georgia, and saw oranges growing on the trees in Florida. (Oranges are brownish, but a gas is used to give them the orange color). We went to Silver Springs, Florida, and had fun on a glass bottom boat. I thought for sure I would fall forward into the glass bottom of that boat. I could see myself swimming with the fish below, and even being eaten by them! Cypress Gardens was a beautiful place where we saw Esther Williams' swimming pool. It was in the shape of Florida! At the Parrot Jungle, Mom and Dad put a parrot on my head, and one on each of my arms. I was okay until I saw that the parrot's tongue was bigger than my finger! (I could've done without this stop).

We stayed for a week at a place in West Palm Beach where the rooms had kitchenettes. Susie and Dad, in particular, enjoyed the swimming pool. Mom was not too much for water. Neither she, nor Dad, could swim. Dad was brave enough to jump off the diving board, and do a frog swim, or breaststroke, until he reached the shallow end of pool where he could stand on the bottom! Susie was just four years old, so she used a life jacket. I wasn't ready to try it, yet. I enjoyed looking at the salamanders (as long as they weren't coming toward me).

We would talk a lot to the owners of the motel who had written a book about their experiences taking a small cruiser by themselves through Chesapeake Bay and down to West Palm Beach. It was a fascinating and funny story. I still remembered one of the excerpts where the non-experienced captains were waving at people on the shore giving them three beeps with their horn. They did not know that their pattern of honking was a signaling distress (SOS) causing everyone that was waving to wonder what the problem was. Later, when these new shipmates came closer to the docks, they needed that SOS signal since they didn't know how to stop the boat! Someone yelled, "Throw the motors in reverse."

That helped!

Dad also took all of us deep-sea fishing on the Atlantic Ocean. I found the waves on the ocean to be too difficult for me to handle. I was sitting in a comfortable chair inside the fishing boat's cabin trying to press my feet against the floor when a wave almost threw me out of the chair! I needed a safety belt. But, Dad caught a huge tuna of about 40 pounds, and cooked it on the grill at the motel sharing it with everyone there!

Come to think of it, a safety belt would've been very helpful when Mom was learning to drive. Every time she came to a stop sign, she would hit the brakes. I would always sit with my feet crossed underneath me on the seat of the car, and right after we got to the stop sign, I would end up with my head on the floor and my bottom in the air! I hated riding with my Mom at that time! My sister never seemed to have that problem! Mo found out about my seatbelt problem, and put one in the backseat of her car for me. It was not required at that time, but it really helped.

A safety belt would've also helped when our family would go asparagus hunting. Even though we would go along the County roads slowly, I was afraid to say, "There is some asparagus!" since as soon as I would say it, the brakes were slammed. It didn't matter who pointed it out. The brakes were pushed. I really liked looking for asparagus, but finding it was scary. Since we were going slower, landing on the floor was not as bad.

We often went for rides on the weekends, and we would get ice cream cones, or hot fudge sundaes at a drive-in, two of which were Dutch Maid or the Spot. Besides our rides in the County, we would drive by the lakes, especially Lake Michigan. I always thought the waves out in the distance were palm trees in Hawaii. Not only was I looking in the wrong direction, but I still had a lot of geography to learn! We also followed the shoreline on the south side of town where Boxer, Joe Louis, trained for a Chicago fight, and saw how that building was battered by the waves. Joe had lived in the basement of that mansion to get away from the Chicago hubbub.

The next year, we went to Florida again, and to the same resort. There were two big differences on this trip. One was that Dad went sail fishing by himself. We all stayed back and, of course, this time, he caught a sailfish instead of a tuna! It took him a couple hours to pull it into the boat. It was 7'2" long. The captain of the boat wanted to know if he wanted to have it stuffed. Dad asked the cost, but he knew we didn't even have a wall that long to hang it on! He said to cut the line, and let it go. But, he did receive a certificate proving that he caught it.

The second thing that was different was the route. We went to Washington DC first, and stayed at the Mayflower Hotel. We walked a lot of places. I particularly liked the Smithsonian Institute, and seeing all of the inaugural gowns that the first ladies wore as well as Mrs. Lincoln's mourning pin.

We walked to the White House. There was a huge, long line of people when we got there. (It is not like today where a person is usually asked to call their congressional representative to get tickets to tours of up to 10 people at a time). We proceeded to the back of the line which was more than a block long, and Dad was pushing me. Susie and Mom were a little behind us. We almost got to the back of the line when a tour guide, who had been following, caught up with us. She invited us to the front of the line (that's one of the positives of being in a wheelchair), and walked us all the way back up to the entrance.

We met two people there that took us into the White House. There was a very steep ramp going up three steps at about a 45° angle! At only 10 years-old, the angle still made it difficult to get up that ramp! Two Secret Service men took us over to an area by a telephone.

They called the President and asked, "Sir, are you using your elevator at this time? May we use it for a visitor?" (I was excited because I knew the President was there as the flag was flying on top of the building). The voice on the other end was President Eisenhower! He said, "That would be fine."

Security talked to my parents, and told them they could not go with me, but Susie could go if she wanted. My parents agreed. Before we left Mom and Dad, Susie and I were frisked to make sure we had no weapons. We both giggled. We had an opportunity to go through some of the areas that the public never saw. The elevator had been put in for FDR, since he was the only president that had a disability, and needed the elevator for access. As a side note, it was amazing that there was only one public picture ever taken of Roosevelt in his wheelchair. His radio fireside chats did not indicate that he was in a wheelchair. Most of the people felt that Franklin would not have become president, or maintained his presidency if people would have seen his chair!

The hallways were beautiful with pictures, lighting, etc. When we got to the elevator, it opened into a rather small area that had mirrors on all sides from the middle of the walls of the elevator to the top. The mirrors made the space look much bigger than it was. We went up one floor where we rejoined our parents. We got to see several rooms. The White House rooms looked fairly small to me even though I knew a lot of important people had been in them. Areas were roped off, and the two men explained a little bit about the different areas before the rest of the tourists entered. When we left, we left through the front door. Dad was able to tip the wheelchair back, and took me down the front stairs.

At home, Mom was always there if I needed help. During the summers, the neighbor kids would come over to play Monopoly in my garage. Sometimes this game would go on for weeks at a time. Different neighbors would sit in, but I was always one of the partners. Getting to the garage, actually, getting me in and out of the house, was getting difficult for my Mom due to a couple of steps. Dad made a portable wooden ramp to help with that so Mom would not have to pull me up the two back porch steps anymore. On the front porch, Dad had spoken to Kelly about building a ramp. Kelly had contacts with different companies, so he had a metal ramp made for me with high sides that were about four to six inches high so I would not fall off. That ramp is still solid today, except for one of the bottom corners that my Dad sliced off with the lawnmower.

My Dad was a racecar driver with any lawnmower. He never took time to turn the lawnmower around, he would just push it all the way to the front of the yard (we had a half-acre), move the lawnmower over slightly, and walked backwards to the end of the lot doing the same movement over and over again. Mom would get mad because he always would mow some of her flowers down. Patty's parents, Jimmie (Gertrude) and Denny, used to love watching Dad mow the lawn because he did it so fast. They got a kick out of it. One day, while pulling the lawnmower backwards, Dad did not notice a hole in a bed sheet hanging on the clothesline. The hole was hooked over the handle of his mower. The sheet just ripped right off the clothesline, but Dad just kept going!

At Halloween, Patty and another neighbor, Elaine, put on my Mom's bridesmaids dresses to take me trick-or-treating. I was dressed in my Mom's bridal dress, and we were carrying some of 'Grandma's with the kitties' gladiolas, which were too big for us, so we kept dropping them, because were too big for us. After Mom took some pictures, the girls pushed me in my stroller across the street to the store. Since the store's driveway was full of gravel, I fell forward out of my stroller. Patty put me back into my stroller. We went home without any candy. Patty did bring me some candy later. (Until I was 18 years old, it seemed like there was a rule that I had to fall out of my wheelchair at least once a year)! After that, I played it safe every Halloween. I would sit by the front door with Mom, and helped pass out the candy instead of going around the neighborhood collecting it. Yes, of course I dressed up when I passed out the candy!

Uncle Al's family was growing at the same time. Eight of his 10 children were already born. David was my age with Billy a year younger than me, followed by Stanley, Barb, Tommy, Karen, Jeff, and Jimmy, with Vanessa and Mary not yet been born. Their family would come over, sometimes unannounced, and Mom would whip up some tuna salad, baked beans, and more, for everyone to eat. The kids would play outside, or watch the home movies that my Dad had made. We had many picnics on every occasion possible. Everyone always seemed to have a lot of fun playing Badminton, croquet, baseball, and especially eating! I was particularly good at eating, and still am!

At Christmas time, Mom would find out everyone's size, and make all of my cousins' new pajamas. Mom used to make all of my clothing, too! Stanley was the only one with a disability called "Down's Syndrome". He had problems learning and getting along.

In 1956, my Grandma in town died. I was nine, and Susie was four. I remembered the telephone ringing late at night, and I heard my Mom send my Dad to their house. Grandma had been mad for a week, because the mantel clock that was in the dining room had been stopping at 10:30 p.m. each night, and would have to wind it up every morning! Dad got to the house about 10:15 p.m. Grandma had been very weak and sick. Dad held her in his arms, and told Grandpa to call the ambulance. He could hear blood gurgling in her throat, from an aneurysm. She was pronounced dead at 10:30 p.m., the same time her mantel clock stopped ticking every night! This was the first time I had to go to a wake and a funeral. Dad was pretty strong. But, Susie kept telling Grandma to wake up, and she couldn't understand why she wouldn't open her eyes. It was comforting seeing everyone at the wake, but I didn't like seeing Grandma lying in the coffin. All I could see from my wheelchair was her closed eyes and her nose.

After Grandma's death, and for about eight years, Grandpa in town took care of their house, but came to our house every night for dinner. (He spent some time living at Uncle Al's too). When Susie started St. Luke's School, he would be the one that would pick her up every day to bring her home after first stopping at Grandpa's favorite bar. She would always get candy or chips, and Grandpa would get a beer or two. (He loved his beer and seemed to drink more now, and drank about two cases of beer a week along with a bottle of whiskey). He never seemed drunk, but he was lonely. He would always get the definitions of his words mixed up, and as Grandpa would say, "It is hot outside today. That humility is really high out there."

While eating, Grandpa would make sure that he would push all of the food dishes away from him and in front of my Dad's place at the dinner table. He always wanted a lot of room to eat. Dad would feel squashed.

Grandpa fell, and broke both of his wrists, and was able to get to the telephone and dialed my Mom for help. When she got there, she asked how he could dial the telephone, because his wrist must have been hurting really bad.

Grandpa said, "Oh, they don't hurt," while twirling both of his hands around in a circle, they just wobbled all over the place! We figured the alcohol must've helped him! He was always a teaser with a twinkle in his eye!

Susie went to Victory School two blocks from our house for her first one and a half years of school. Susie and my parents felt that she was not learning anything new. Dad always wanted her to go to a parochial school as he did, so she was transferred to St. Luke's for most of her second year of education. Grandpa took her to St. Luke's school until my Mom obtained her driver's license. She was really upset when, right before Christmas that year, the teacher told the class there was no Santa Claus! St. Luke's was a member of the Wisconsin Synod. This Synod was very strict, and did not want children believing in anything but Christ. Susie felt bad because the kindergartners were in her classroom, and she cried and cried.

One of the things that I always used to love doing was sitting at the end of our driveway with no sides on my wheelchair, and my feet curled up in my lap. I would pretend that I had a baby in my buggy, seeing if I could fool anybody that drove by me. When it would rain, there was this perfect puddle at the end of the cement driveway that I would take a stick, and poke it into the gravel. Sometimes I would find worms, and give them a ride on the stick, or a bath in the puddle. Once, my Grandpa in town was backing his car out of our driveway. I realized that he didn't see me sitting yards behind his car. I yelled at him to stop, but he didn't hear me. I braced myself so that I would not fall out of my chair, and I was ready for his car to hit me. Fortunately, Grandpa only drove two miles per hour. He felt the contact with my chair. He stopped. There was no damage done, but it was a little scary!

Speaking of scary, Susie, at the age of four and five, had her own muscle-building program. Any time you would look for her, she was hanging on Mom and Dad's bedpost at the bottom of the bed. She would put her hands backwards and lift herself up so her feet would dangle. She would do this for hours, day after day, year after year until she would have to bend her knees, because her feet would no longer hang free. She became physically very strong. When Susie was about nine years-old (I was about 14 years-old), she insisted on lifting me from my twin bed to her twin bed (about five feet apart). She was so skinny and little!

She said, "Hush up! I am going to do this!"

Mom was outside in the garden and Dad was at work, so I knew she was going to win on this one. She put her left arm under my head and right arm under my knees, lifted me, and spun me in a half circle to her bed!

She exclaimed, "That was easy!"

She quickly returned me to my bed. I think we never told Mom!

Although she sounded like a go-getter, Susie was the only young kid I knew that would ask to go to bed. She was always tired before her bedtime, and would ask, "Mom, can't I go to bed yet?"

BY THE GRACE OF GOD AND YOU
A Chair Does Not a Person Make

The Telethons made me realize that my disability was hard on my parents in many ways—physically, emotionally, financially, and taking time away from Susie, and their own marital relationship. Susie wasn't too much help, either, because for a while, she seemed like she was going to be just like me. Every time Susie would go outdoors, she would barely have time to play before she got hurt, and came back crying. She fell on stones, bloodied her knees, got scrapes, cuts, and had to have stitches in her forehead!

Despite all of the stress that we put our parents through, I only remembered them fighting one time. I didn't know what the fight was about, but Dad packed a suitcase, and then, never left. Apparently, my Mom was very sick at the time. Moms are never allowed to be sick. Dad was impatient with having to do something out of the ordinary.

My sister remembered Mom saying, "If you leave now, when I am so sick, don't ever bother coming back!"

Another time, Dad was impatient with me. He was putting me into the car, and my shoe fell off. I was afraid of my Dad, but I decided to try to make him laugh by saying, "Catastrophe! Catastrophe!" It worked. He laughed, and put my shoe back on!

Mom always stood her ground with Dad, and she had a lot of energy! She always helped in the PTA at Orthopedic School, and at Home League through the Salvation Army. She even started a Girl Scout group at the Orthopedic School, and was its leader for a couple of years.

Our family attended St. Luke's Church in Kenosha and would go to church every Sunday. Dad was the church's treasurer. The church had about 20 stairs to get inside, so Mom thought that I could go to the Salvation Army (with only two steps) where Patty and Buddy went. (Patty could pull me up those two steps by herself.) Our pastor at St. Luke's did not like that idea because the Wisconsin Synod did not allow anyone to worship with people of different faiths. They did not even want you to be a Girl Scout, because you were pledging allegiance with different people. To me, St. Luke's Church had an image of a more angry and punishing God where the Salvation Army had a loving God! The Salvation Army never really baptized, only dedicated babies to God, because "the Captains" knew that the Army was the door to a different church a person would eventually choose.

Anyway, when I was about seven, my Mother told the pastor that I would be joining the Salvation Army Girl Scouts—the Sunbeams. Mom felt this was important, as it would give me an opportunity to be around more people and be involved in more activities. As a side note: the Salvation Army was the first to offer wheelchair assistance that would work for me. St. Luke's was more concerned that my Dad was not tithing, because of all the medical bills. Dad was befuddled trying to do the right thing. Unfortunately, St. Luke's was not helpful, but Dad never lost faith in the church. We were members until my sister got married in 1973. At this time, we transferred to St. Mary's Lutheran Church, and it was very accessible.

I took my job of being a Sunbeam very seriously. I worked very hard to get all the badges that I could! First, there was Mrs. Anderson, an older member of the Salvation Army that lived two doors down from me. She had a difficult time walking, but only had a very small, two-inch step into her house. I could get in her house very easily by someone just tipping my wheelchair back. She taught me how to cook. I think we started with potatoes, and I didn't peel them. I think I prepared and cooked them better than my Mom did when she started making potatoes.

She told me, "I boiled the potatoes with forks in them as I was told that you had to stick a fork in them to know when they were done."

We made potatoes, green beans and hamburger, and ate it for lunch! I had earned my cooking badge! I set the table with its proper settings after Patty showed me how to set a table correctly. Patty also taught me how to read a songbook, since people would be singing in church, and quite frankly, I had no clue how to follow along! It seemed so easy when she showed me how to read it!

Mom put all of the encyclopedias (that Dad thought we would never use) upright on a card table in the living room. I started working on the rest of my badges. Most of the information, I could get straight from the encyclopedias. I could slide an individual book toward me, lay it down in front of me, turn the pages, get the information I needed, leverage the book back up, and slide it back into place. (To make sure that the books didn't tip over, Mom used my baby shoe bookends that were bronzed when I was a kid).

I finished badge after badge until finally, I had only two to finish. I was stuck on these, because one was a swimming badge. In order to get permission, I was required to write out all of the arms, legs and hand movements, and, other than the Hubbard Tank, I never really swam in water. I had to identify the different swimming strokes, and include an explanation on how to do them. I passed.

The second badge that I had difficulty with was a nature walk where I had to identify, and get the leaves of so many different kinds of trees. I drew pictures of the trees and their leaves. Then, Mom and Dad took me to the park where we found an oak tree, an elm tree, a birch tree, etc. We took a leaf from each one. The leaves that I didn't find, Mrs. Anderson had! I taped them on some paper, and turned in all of my work. Again, I passed!

I was now a Commissioner Sunbeam at 10 years old, having passed every badge! There was a ceremony in the new Salvation Army building downtown which now had eight steps. It might as well have been 20! I returned to St. Luke's Church to complete my confirmation classes. The pastor came to my house to give me lessons before I completed my Commissioner Sunbeam work.

I used to be scared to death of feathers—yes, feathers! My Dad bought a bunch of chickens, and chopped off their heads in the backyard. The hens would flop around for a while, with feathers and blood flying. (I was shocked when I found out that feathers were in my pillow, and when the feathers poked out of the pillow, I was afraid too). It took me a while to get over that fear, but I understood—the feather wasn't alive. I should have been afraid of the bird. When I was in fourth grade, my Dad bought more chickens. I helped with them this time while Mom put the decapitated hens in a pot of boiling water so the feathers would be easier to remove. I helped pull the pinfeathers out so we could eat the chickens later. The most interesting part was removing their insides. We would often find eggs before their shell was fully formed.

During this time in my life, we had a parakeet instead of a dog. The parakeet was very. It could say, "Pretty Bird" (that was his or her name since we never really knew its sex), and could mock our whistles. One day, I came home from school.

Mom said, "You will never believe what happened to me today. I was in the living room dusting, and I heard you calling me. I knew you were at school. I went into the bedroom. The bird was sitting on my lampshade saying, 'Mom, Mom, Mom…'"

Now, in addition to everything else, Mom had to sort out who was really calling her! After about four years, the bird had other problems. Susie and a friend were playing, and ran into my parents' bedroom with the bird flying behind them. The bird was crushed as the door closed, and the bird lost its eye. When it was older, it developed first one, and then a second, tumor on its breast. The tumors became very heavy, and the bird kept falling off its perch. One day the bird was very wobbly, and it looked as if it had a stroke. Mom put a drop of whiskey in its water, and the bird perked up for a while. The family knew he was suffering too much, but Mom would not let Dad kill the bird at home. We all piled into the car, took it down to Waukegan, where we had originally bought it, and had it gassed. After that, we tried fish— guppies and angelfish along with a snail who loved to lay a lot of eggs on the side of the glass tank.

During these years of my life, the family also started getting involved with the Muscular Dystrophy telethon, and Patty and Buddy would get excited collecting from the neighbors. Our family would go to the telephone banks and take pledges. We did this yearly until 1999, and only missed two years! I could take the telephone calls, and write the information, but I could never press my pen hard enough to make my writing show through to the copy of the pledges. Someone else would do that for me, usually Mom. By the time I was eight years old, I had watched the telethon enough to know that my life expectancy was about 15 years. I was starting to understand what that meant for me and for my sister. Muscular Dystrophy was passed onto the male child, but the gene that carried it went to the females. My sister's children could get Muscular Dystrophy. Susie was tested, and was not a carrier.

MDA sent a lot of newsletters giving out information, contests, and lists of people who wanted pen pals. In fourth grade, I liked these newsletters much better than the *Weekly Readers* that we received from the school. One of the newsletters had a poem contest in 1959. I submitted a poem. It read:

I've never entered a contest before,
So I'm quite excited you see!
I'm sure it won't be a great big chore,
Especially if the winner is me!

I thought it sounded cute. It was fun to enter the contest, but I was surprised when I won. I don't remember the prize, but it was published in the next newsletter.

From two other newsletters, I picked up a pen pal address from Washington State and one from Indiana. Both of the people had Muscular Dystrophy. Joan, in Washington, was about a year older than I was. I had my Mom read my first letter to her. In so many words, Mom verbalized, "It was boring!" I liked to try to write long letters, but fill them up with jokes that weren't very funny. So, Mom helped me write a more interesting letter with all the things that we had seen in Washington DC including being frisked. Joan was bedridden. I was happy when she wrote back saying it was the most interesting letter she had received! That made me feel good as she commented, "It was like you were right there talking with me." We wrote back and forth a few months. The next letter I received was from her Mother. She was sad to tell me that Joan passed away. I never really got to know her. Look how she touched my life!

My second pen pal was Christian. The funny thing was that I read the name as Christine. I thought I was writing to a girl for about three years until I got a letter from Leah. She wrote, "You have been writing to my brother. I was hoping that you would be interested in writing to me, too." At first, I panicked. I wondered if I talked about something stupid like my period, but she reassured me that he always enjoyed my letters. I asked her to give him my apologies, but afterward, I only wrote to her. Christian and Leah were from an Amish family. I had no idea what that meant. Christian (Chris) was older than I was, and he was in a wheelchair, because he had Muscular Dystrophy. Leah was still walking, but using a lot of energy. Her walk was very labored. Chris drove a buckboard with horses pulling it. (There must have been a ramp or a level platform for him to get on with his wheelchair.) Leah did a lot of the canning and housework. Their Dad was the blacksmith and the coffin maker of their Indiana community.

All of the men had long beards and mustaches. The women all wore long dresses and bonnets on their head. Because of their beliefs, they had no electricity and nothing cushy, except for their bed. Because they were not allowed to marry outside of their community, there were a lot of people with Muscular Dystrophy (M.D.) in their area. On one of our trips, we asked prior permission to stop and meet them. It was good to see to whom I had been writing. We had a difficult time finding them because almost everyone in the community had the last name of Schwartz. Their middle initial identified the families, and that is how we got the address and directions to their home. We traveled deep into a rural area, passing several people in horse drawn buggies, and went through a covered bridge. Their house was very nice and practical.

Several years later (maybe when I was 30), I had received a letter from Leah indicating that she had met a man of a different faith. She wanted to marry him, but had to choose between him and her Amish community. She chose to marry, but the community gave her a funeral. She was not allowed to be with or speak to anyone there. After she moved, I did not hear from her again. I have often thought of her. I know, by the time she married, Leah was in a wheelchair. This was, sadly, a different type of death to me.

I also was involved with Easter Seals at this time receiving some equipment as well as being the Kenosha poster child one year. In the summers when I was eleven and twelve, I started to go to Easter Seals camp. Those are the years that I missed going to the Holtans in Boulder Junction. I did not like the camp when I was a kid in adult sessions, so I skipped going during my teen years. I loved the visiting, people, scavenger hunts, campfires, singing, dances, and Indian ceremonials. I hated the spiders (which I could not brush off), cold June nights, trying to get someone to move me at night, and being sick when I got home. Barbara, from school, went with me, and had beds next to each other, so, I often had to wake her up at night to get someone to help me.

The camp was 400 acres of woodlands in the Wisconsin Dells. It had a swimming pool, a boys' dorm, and a girls' dorm, which, at the time, consisted of two long rooms of twenty-two beds, and toilets in between those two rooms. There was a dining hall, a nurses' station, an office, and a very special place called the Castle. The Castle was a summer home in the shape of the Castle with the beautiful fireplace, piano, space for a hundred wheelchairs, and a beautiful view of the sunset on top of a hill looking down towards the Dells. The land was donated by the Uphams to Easter Seals for the purpose of a camp for people with physical disabilities. Everything has become more and more accessible on the hill, and now there are more paved paths through the rest of the property with up to seven campsite areas along with a respite camp, providing 24-hour care during the summer and several weekends during the rest of the year.

The Indian dancers from the Dells, and our counselors, performed a war dance before going on "the warpath". One of our counselors was of Indian heritage. Afterward, we had a campfire where about ten or twelve of us were going to sleep outside the building at the Black Hawk campsite. It was very cold, so we all stayed by the campfire as long as possible. We heard a noise, and saw movement among the trees. An Indian warrior appeared with war paint and a shrieking war cry. He stopped our singing group, and pointed his bow and arrow at us, but eventually, he went away. It was staged, but I thought that I was going to die at the time! The counselors put us on the floor in the Black Hawk building, because it was too cold outside to sleep. I saw many spider webs, and thought about those most of the night. The Indian was totally pushed out of my mind, because those webs were terrifying - where were those spiders?

Larry, another boy from Orthopedic School, was at camp with us. There was to be a last night dance, and he had to have a date! Larry could walk, but he had little control of his body, especially his hands and arms from cerebral palsy. Larry and I decided to go to the dance together, and we had a good time. He could really swing my wheelchair around to the music! We figured out that our date was somehow a set-up when we ended up as a couple on the royal court! But, not King and Queen, thank goodness! (FYI: Larry later took up smoking. I heard that he almost set his friend's house on fire when he lost control of his hand, and a cigarette hit the curtain. His cigarette would flip up, and often land in unusual places).

It seemed as if every time I went to camp, I would wake up at least one or two nights during the two-week session, in those long dorm rooms, and see something flying over my head. I knew that it was a bat, but I didn't want to scare anyone. If I would see the counselor go past the door, I would call her, and tell her about the bat, because I knew the campers would be scared. Usually, the counselor was not that much help, because she was just as afraid as the campers were. The counselor would say, "Don't worry." Then, she would see it, scream, and wake everyone up. It was always a no-win situation!

In general, I was always very impressed with the counselors. They threw their hearts into helping the campers have fun. The campers always impressed me, because this was where I learned how to succeed by watching others try and succeed. I tried miniature golf. I could not lift the golf club, so the counselor had me try a badminton racket. I could not hit the golf ball far. We tried a Ping-Pong ball instead, and that's how I was able to play miniature golf! By this time, I could no longer wheel my own wheelchair.

It was at camp that I realized how I accommodated my limitations. When I brushed my teeth, I never moved my hands, only my head. I was starting to get my arms in place by grabbing my index finger with my mouth and swinging my elbow into place so that I could reach my head, feed myself, comb my hair, and brush my teeth. My index fingers built up big calluses, just like my knees when I used to walk on them. Once my hands were in place, I would bump my chin against my thumb to push my hands (with arms in the form of a teepee lying against my mouth) away from my face to reach something in front of me. Of course, I opened all bottles of makeup with my teeth! At some point, I also stopped pointing with my fingers, and pointed with my eyes. Although, people would still watch my fingers, and get confused!

When my parents picked me up from the Dells, Mom was a little upset that I didn't get homesick, but I was very sick. Every time I did get sick, I had a cough for at least three weeks. (I couldn't cough, and I often choked until I vomited. The same thing happened with blowing my nose. I could never blow hard enough to get the mucus out, so I always just picked it. Yuck! You have to do what you have to do!) I just hated that Mom would always make me wear a blanket around my legs. She insisted that it would help stop me from getting sick. I started thinking about how I could talk Mom out of that blanket!

~ 4 ~

Finishing Orthopedic School

When I returned home from camp the second year, I had a cold. I opened my eyes one morning to let Mom know I was ready to get up, and found my eyes were pasted shut! I panicked. Mom comforted me saying, "That's nothing. It is just your cold. You can see." She put warm water on my eyes to wipe them clean. Thus, I began learning never to panic, and developed two steps to prevent it. First, I thought about what was happening. Second, I would decide what I was going to do next.

It was time to start fifth grade, but I still had a cough causing me to miss another two weeks of the school year. Our fifth grade class was going to be quite large, so, we were placed in Mr. Dietrich's room. When I was in Miss Grasser's room, I had sat in my wheelchair diagonally to the desk, and did my work on top of it. This year, I was sitting in the back of the room at a table I shared with Ruth to do my work. I was a little upset when I did my makeup homework. After doing about 90 pages of math, with only 7 math answers wrong, I received a "B." I didn't think that was fair, do you? I don't remember the grades on my other homework, but I really liked math, because it was so easy for me.

Mr. Dietrich gave a lot of homework which I had never had in the past, but I learned to like him. Although one day, I had the hiccups with one very loud hiccup, and Mr. Dietrich looked at me hard. It scared me half to death! No more hiccups ever in that class!

Mom and Dad would make me do all my homework right after supper. If I was stuck, they would help me. I loved math, but I hated long division. Those problems took so long! I loved listening in class and watching what was written on the board. That was the way I learned best. I always tried to shy away whenever I read aloud, and while I was a slow reader, I was an excellent student, and earned good grades.

In fifth grade, more students arrived like Kathy who had a kidney problem, and was very thin. Mark (not sure what problem he had since we never really talked about each other's disabilities), Charles (I always thought we looked alike, and could've been brother and sister), and Kenny who made the class interesting. I think Kenny had a heart problem, but I know for a while, he stole my heart! I also learned how to study, got rid of that blanket I always had on my legs when I was outside, and became a little less shy. For the sixth-grade, Miss Grasser had left, and the class was moved into Mrs. Hess's room. One of the special things going on that year was a play! The name of it escapes me, but the theme revolved around the importance of math. Kenny and I had the leads. He was to strangle me with a telephone cord. I did fine, but struggled to get my hand up to my neck before he wrapped the cord around it, so I could look like I was struggling with being choked, instead of looking like I was struggling with my hand! The best part of that play was a commercial break where everyone sang something similar to this:

"Get Slurpo's Slippery Syrup soon, and then you will discover your teeth fall out, your hair turns white, and you never will never recover!"

Mrs. Hess also let us play games by separating us into teams. One of these games was throwing an eraser into the garbage can with a correct answer. Every basket got so many points. In another game, we looked up words in the dictionary that we didn't know. Mrs. Hess's favorite word was "superfluous." I always remembered that word!

A school newsletter, the Orthopedic Flash, had a special article playing on people's names. For mine, Mrs. Hess wrote, "If Carol was only a Hymn instead of a Carol". Another person's last name was Burger. Mrs. Hess wrote, "If Burger was only a sandwich instead of a burger." I thought that was very clever.

In sixth grade, we gave out Valentines. We usually did that every year, but this year was special to me. Kenny had given one to everyone in class. Small wallet size Valentines that were very sarcastic and funny! I saw a lot of people's cards, and I thought, "I wonder what I will get from him." It didn't take long to get mine as the teacher passed them out. It read, "You are smart, loyal, cute, good… and so is my dog!" Personally, I thought that was much more flattering than the ones that other people got. I kept it for about four years in my wallet.

Mrs. Melville, across the street from Marilyn, boarded two classmates, Susan and Diane, in her home. I had a chance to socialize with the girls during the school year. Susan was from Paddock Lake, and I think Diane was from Lake Geneva. Marilyn had a neighborhood play in her garage, and my Mom took me over to watch it, because it was outside. It was fun! It wasn't easy for me to go to other people's homes, because of the stairs.

Mom was very active in the PTA as I mentioned before. She knew the staff and the Mothers of the students at school. She sometimes would say that she felt bad, because the only time that people would recognize her was when she was pushing my wheelchair. Whenever there was a special event, she would help. They used to have a lot of card parties in those days, and played cards, or Bunko (similar to Yatzee with dice) for fundraisers. I learned a lot of card games early as my "Grandparents with the kitties" would come over every Saturday night and play canasta or pinochle for hours. My "Grandparents with the mink" liked to play, too, but Grandpa was much more serious about his cards, and far too serious for my Mom to play with at times. Personally, I liked it, because I would learn a lot of strategy from his comments.

My Dad liked Pinochle and Sheepshead. I learned how to play Sheepshead when we visited the Holtans. Mo Holtan was very serious about that game, and that's where I learned a lot from him. Mo liked playing for money, too, which made me learn the game a lot quicker if I wanted to survive!

Whenever I asked Susie for something when she was small, I would turn it into a game. For instance, if I was hungry for breakfast, and wanted a piece of toast, I would improvise by saying, "Let's play Car hop! Could I have a piece of toast please?" It would've worked really well except Susie liked very lightly toasted bread! So, I would complain, and send it back to the cook who was Susie. I grumbled, "I wanted toast! I did not want warm dry bread!" Good thing I usually did not order toast!

When Susie and I were left alone together for a while, Susie would love to clean, and rearrange the furniture. Unfortunately, Mom usually didn't like our efforts, so everything had to be put back in its place! Mom did like the cleaning since my wheelchair always brought so much dirt in the house (now-a-days more so than ever) that we were embarrassed if anyone walked with white socks on our rug! Their socks weren't white anymore!

Around this time, I started two scrapbooks—one of Elvis, but the bigger one was of Ben Casey, Vince Edwards who played a doctor on a TV show of the same name. I had his picture on my pillowcases, and his doctor shirt with its opened top button by the neck!

The Chicago Cubs were also very close to my heart. Louise was a big Cubs fan, too! The day before each baseball opening season, she would pack a little overnight bag, come home with me in my taxi, and we would skip school to watch the game on TV! Of course, people knew we were doing this (the suitcase was a big clue), but it was so much fun! Louise and I had time to try to bake a cake for my Mom, but when Louise mixed the batter, it spattered onto the walls! Mom would never let us make a cake again!

Louise always needed a special spoon to eat. We would take one of our spoons, bend it down, and twist the scoop part forward. She was eating with the spoon when Cub's player, Ernie Banks, hit a homerun. She flipped everything on her spoon onto the wall! Her homer was quite a distance, too! After Louise would leave, my Dad would always end up with Louise's bent spoon!

My friend, Kathy, had so much energy, we would help each other with math and, work on some projects together. She was the lead singer in the commercial for our play as well. I noticed that she became very pale towards the end of the sixth-grade, and began missing a lot of school. Mom told me she was very sick. I didn't understand what that exactly meant until she died a month later from kidney failure. Mom went to the wake. She thought I needed to know what happened, so she decided to tell me the details of what happened. Kathy's body was swollen, because her kidneys did not work any more, and they could not eliminate the water from her system. The urine was coming out of her pores, and there was a bad odor. Kathy knew she was dying. She thanked her parents for all they had done, and her pain ended.

Dennis, who was in the fourth grade while I was in the sixth, passed away shortly after Kathy. I never heard the details of what happened to him.

In seventh and eighth grades, we went back to Mr. Dietrich's room. While in the seventh grade, and I didn't know how Randy did it, but he convinced Mr. Dietrich to allow him to put up mistletoe at Christmas. Kenny pushed me under it, and held my head so Randy could kiss me. Life was mixed up. It would've been better if Kenny would have kissed me!

In the eighth grade, two students in Mr. Dietrich's room were always chosen to host special members of the community/school system for the Orthopedic School's Thanksgiving dinner. Kenny and I were voted as host and hostess. My big chance! While we were writing out the invitations, Kenny (who was teased as being teacher's pet) said something about Mr. Dietrich indicating that we would make a good couple at the Thanksgiving dinner. I was embarrassed. I didn't know if I blushed. I just smiled, and finished my work, and didn't say a word! Unfortunately, my big chance never came to be, because I was very sick for Thanksgiving. Absent again!

That was Kenny's last year at school. He went to another school. It was also the last year for Ronnie, too. He died from a complication due to his Muscular Dystrophy.

I stopped responding to death. It was just the fulfillment of life to me, but most of the people had been so young! I had Muscular Dystrophy, too. What did that mean to me? I wasn't going to think about it. I was never afraid of death, only the pain of dying. Many students were being integrated into their community schools. Marilyn, Vicki, Mark, Kenny, Susan, Ruth, Eddie and many others left.

August 11 of that summer, my cab driver for many years, Eddie Garlow took my parents, and me to a Cubs game against the Braves in Milwaukee. It was his way of celebrating, because he would no longer be my cab driver. The schools were now changing to bus transportation with wheelchair lifts. We had seats in the fourth row near the Braves dugout. Eddie carried me to my seat. The Cubs' Jack Curtis, and the Braves' Warren Spahn, pitched a pitchers' duel with both having given up six hits. Each side gave up one run, but the Cubs also gave up an unearned run. At the last out, everyone stood up, and went crazy! This was Spahn's 300th win. Eddie jumped up, too, to see what was happening, and he quickly ducked down, and whispered in my ear, "Warren is throwing kisses to the crowd, and we don't want any of those kisses. We are Cubs fans!" I thought it was a very considerate thing for him to do, since I could not see a thing.

Ninth-grade went very fast. The students that were not mainstreamed were all in Mr. Dietrich's room, but we changed schools to an Orthopedic Wing in the new, Jane Vernon School on the south side, and it was very close to my house.

The new custodian, Mike, looked just like Ben Casey. I didn't mind that at all! We still had all of our therapies. Bonnie was still there (who had been accidentally shot in the spine by her brother leaving her paraplegic). I admired everything she could do. She could take complete care of herself. Larry, Jimmy, Frankie (his kidneys were starting to get worse), and Les (who was on crutches, and so smart that he skipped a grade) were in 7th grade. Barbara, Roy (who had a brain tumor), Betty (bad kidneys), Louise, and I made up the ninth grade.

Vernon students were taken by bus back and forth from school to home, and vice versa. The bus company took out several seats in the back, and put in tie downs for the wheelchairs. When the bus would turn the corner, sometimes, my chair would tip backwards and my head hit the window. Once, my brakes were not on, because the safety belt had not clicked. When turning the corner, my wheelchair rolled forward to the other side of the bus, and I fell out of my wheelchair. I broke every blood vessel in my face. I looked pretty bad for a few weeks.

Tim was back in Orthopedic School for therapy. He actually went to high school, and rode the bus home with us every night. Tim was in a wheelchair, now. He came to the Orthopedic School Wing just for therapies in the afternoon, about three times a week. He was cute and funny. I had already forgotten about Kenny. I had therapy right after Tim in the Hubbard Tank, so I had a chance to see, and talk to him often. Mrs. Ruffalo, a bright redheaded assistant who helped in the water therapy room, helped me keep updated on him. I told Tim that I was going to be a Mother just to get his attention! Actually, I was a Mother to my guppy's 32 babies! (Remember: Tim used to go to Orthopedic School when I was in first grade, and he was in fourth! I really paid no attention to him at that time. He was too old at the time). Sometime in February, I had Tim sign my autograph book. He signed it while he was on the bus, so the signature was a little shaky. He wrote, "Best wishes, _____, Tim." I could not figure out what he had written. It looked like it could have been "love." I didn't think he would write that. You know how overly analytical girls could be. I was a daydreamer, too. It didn't look like it could be any other word! I never saw him again after that. I never knew what was happening to him. I didn't know he was only one grade ahead of me. He must've been sick a lot.

Mrs. Perkins was still giving me therapy. She was taking care of Tim, but never said anything about him. I was excited when I found out that her husband went with Admiral Byrd and shared those adventures in Antarctica. I thought that was amazing!

The school hired a new teacher, Mrs. Rogers, for us in 10th grade. There were only four of us in class now—Roy, Betty, Louise, and me. Mrs. Rogers was a very good math teacher, and I learned most of my algebra from her. For English, she played a lot of Scrabble with us. She got really mad at me once. She inadvertently took her turn before mine. I was having a very difficult time finding a place to put a word on the Scrabble board, and finally, used the space that she was going to use. She got very angry at me, and things were never the same after that. I'm not sure why.

At one point, I was tested to see if I could go to public high school. The principal spoke with my Mom, and my Mom spoke to Mr. Stoker at Bradford High School (the first free high school east of the Mississippi). Most people at Orthopedic School had been mainstreamed into regular classes. That's what they wanted to do with me, now. Before I knew anything that was going on, Mom spoke with Mr. Stoker.

He stated, "I don't think she could handle a full day at our school. I don't want to see her fail."

Apparently, he had the input of Mrs. Rogers.

"Carol is breathing hard by the end of the day, and she cannot handle high school."

My Mother said, "Let her try." She had not noticed that I was particularly tired. "If she fails, she fails. We won't know until she tries."

I always thought people learned more from their mistakes than their successes. I also thought people made progress when they made the mistakes farther apart. The real problem was the worry of what would happen if I had to go to the bathroom. There was no one to help at high school. I had already trained my body to go to the bathroom in the morning, and then when I got home at 3 p.m. I was completing a full day of school. (At 15 years old, I was already getting up at 5 a.m., so my Dad could help my Mom get me out of bed. He left for work about 5:30 a.m.) Another problem was the stairs leading into the high school. It was decided that I would take a full load of classes in half a day. I would be home by noon. The bus driver, George Alfredson, would take me up and down the stairs in my wheelchair, since he was also doing the same with Ed. Because George had no help, I decided to wear a safety belt tying me to the chair. One time, I would have slid out of the chair onto cement steps when I was tipped forward if I hadn't had the belt. Mr. Stoker still did not want me to go to high school, but he agreed. In 11th grade, I would start Bradford High School as a junior.

Before I started high school, we took a trip to California. Mo thought that it would be better for me if we had air conditioning, and he put a system in our car. On the vacation, the air-conditioning really helped when driving across the desert from Las Vegas, Nevada, to California. We always left on our vacations at about 5 a.m. to get through Chicago, before traffic crowded the streets. That meant we had to get up at 3 a.m. to get started. Susie always fell asleep fairly early on the trip. As we drove west, we saw the Rocky Mountains as we approached Denver. At first, we thought we were seeing clouds because they were so high—

not the case. We went to the top of Pike's Peak where the air was so thin on top that I even got weak in my knees, and I didn't even stand! We crossed the Royal Gorge, and I was put in my wheelchair. I could feel the bridge sway in the wind as I was pushed across a 2000 feet drop! We could see the ground through spaced boards on the bridge! I didn't vomit though, but I thought about it! We saw the Painted Desert, Petrified Forest, Grand Canyon, Hoover Dam, and Lake Mead. In Vegas, we stopped at a Lamplighter Motel for the night. Susie and I were too young to gamble yet. We were lucky enough to see a crowd in front of our motel after lunch that was waiting for Elvis Presley to go by as he was filming *Viva Las Vegas.* We were not lucky enough to see him, though. Next, we visited my Aunt Pearl (one of "Grandpa's in town" 12 other siblings), and Uncle Bob (a retired salesman from Jockey International). We went to Disneyland, Knott's Berry Farm, a Hollywood Wax Museum, Grauman's Chinese Theatre, Dodger Stadium, Pasadena Boulevard's Rose Parade Route, and the Rose Bowl. I seemed to be allergic to either the smog, or the sun in Southern California, because I had welts under the skin on my arms.

After a five-day visit with my aunt and uncle, who had grapefruit and poinsettias growing in their backyard, we headed north along the Pacific coast to see the Sequoias, but somehow, we missed the turn, and never got to see them. We crossed over the Golden Gate Bridge and back, saw Alcatraz, and ate lobster on Fisherman's Wharf. Dad was always a fast walker, and he and Susie moved far ahead of Mom on the Wharf even though he was pushing my wheelchair. Mom was fast, too, but she didn't want him to get too far ahead of her, because it can be dangerous if people don't stick together. What happened going across the Golden Gate Bridge was funny too. Just like in the movies, as we started across the bridge, the person on the radio said, "and today, this is what happened to Buster Crabb (the first Tarzan)…" As we crossed the bridge, the radio frequencies stopped the radio from working. Just as we were driving off on the other side of the bridge, the man on the radio said, "…and that's what happened to Buster Crabb today!" We never did find out what happened to Buster Crabb that day, but we all laughed.

Because I was getting bigger and heavier, we started planning our vacations a little differently, making sure that the motels had restaurants and no steps. We would plan what we would do the next day so that Dad would not have to lift me out of the car so often. I even started using the bed pan in the backseat of the car to accommodate.

(Incidentally, I never was a picky eater. I would try anything except raw celery! When I would bite into it, I would just get sick! Mom finally told me that I ate five stalks one day when I was three years old. I vomited all over the place. I never remembered eating that celery, but my brain somehow remembered that I didn't like it. I still cannot eat it!)

I enjoyed everything I got to see, and did not feel bad at all that I did not get to see the inside of the Rose Bowl, because I never had been a football fan. I was also very glad I never had to get out of the car in San Francisco with those dangerous steep roads and sidewalks on multiple hills. I didn't know how anyone in a wheelchair could function in that city. Heck, I didn't know how the cars made it up the hills, or even continued going forward after having to stop at a stop light/sign. I could barely move myself, feeling as if I was actually lying down on the back of my seat.

BY THE GRACE OF GOD AND YOU
A Chair Does Not a Person Make

On the way back home, we saw Reno, Lake Tahoe, and Virginia City. Virginia City was particularly interesting since that city used to be called Ely. We discovered later that my "Grandpa in town's" Father had started the first bakery there, and had a silver mine, before he came back to Wisconsin to help with the family farm. We decided to make our own, "self-guided tour" around Virginia City, since there were some old interesting slot machines. A person sat in the lap of the life-size cowboy, or dancehall girl figures, and the slot lever was, e.g., a gun or a hand one pulled down to make the slot machine work. In the barroom was a bigger than life-size picture of a lady whose dress was made out of silver dollars. In another store, there was a souvenir shop where you could make your own newspaper headlines, print them, and take them home as a souvenir. Our headline read, "Ken Schaufel falls off barstool, breaks arm." We thought "Grandpa in town" would get a kick out of that. The only thing that made Virginia City difficult to get around was the sidewalk. It was made out of logs so the wheelchair bumped up and down over every one of them. I really liked the rustic effect of the sidewalk, but the ride over them? Not so much!

We drove along the Salt Flats next. It was a perfect day, and they were a beautiful sight! The sky was a bright blue, and its color reflected on the couple inches of water that was lying on top of all the salt. The scene stretched for almost 100 miles on a flat terrain in front of us. Around us were mountains, and a road stretching straight down the middle of the scene across those 100 miles. There was a sign, somewhere, that read "fill up your gas tank. Next station 75 miles." We did see some salt removers. The next stop was Salt Lake City where we were able to catch the Mormon Tabernacle choir singing. I stayed in the car, but could hear the voices. Beautiful, just beautiful!

We drove through the Tetons, Yosemite Park and Yellowstone. I loved Yellowstone, especially Old Faithful, and, of course, I loved shopping at the stores! You can still depend on Old Faithful today to blow on a regular basis! Dad stepped out of the car to take a movie of a grizzly bear we had seen sitting in a stream, but when that bear stood up, Dad's movie ended with him running back to the car!

The next to last stop on our way home was Mt. Rushmore in the Black Hills of South Dakota. Very impressive!

When we returned home, one of our angelfish was missing! We found it about four months later. It was a skeleton on the floor behind the fish bowl. We asked the pet store clerk what might have happened, and he said, "Maybe, when you were gone, the temperature in the room became hot, and the fish became uncomfortable, and jumped out of the bowl." His explanation made me feel better. I thought maybe it was suicide! The other fish were okay.

Before I started high school, I got a new manual wheelchair with a commode seat in it. It really made things easier at home. If I would have to go to the bathroom at school, my Mother could bring the pan to slide on rails under the wheelchair, and assist me in the nurse's office if I had an emergency. All I needed was a regular chair to put my legs on, lean forward, pull out the hard seat underneath me, pull my pants down, be sat back up and go. It was great! It was much easier than having to transfer to a toilet. I could not do any of this process myself, but the best thing was NO LIFTING! Other people could help with the bathroom with just short verbal directions. Although I was now prepared for a bathroom emergency, none occurred throughout high school.

38

Occasionally, Mom and Dad would feel comfortable enough to take a day off and go fishing while Susie and I were at school. They rented a boat, one of these times, to go out on the water near Wilmot Dam. Dad was casting his fishing rod, and the fishhook caught my Mom right through the eyelid. Luckily, it did not scratch her eyeball at all! She was acting feisty, and held the hook by the fishing line away from her eye all the way back to shore. They went into a bait shop, and the owner got the pliers, cut off the end of the hook allowing it to slide out of her eyelid. Mom just fainted!

On a more serious note, my Mother got a phone call sometime during this same year, from a prominent man whose son was just diagnosed with Muscular Dystrophy. He did not know what to do, and was afraid to love his son, because of all the hurt and fear he felt. Mom shared the phone call with me, because she wanted me to know that she had felt many of those things also. When the doctors diagnosed me at the age of four, they suggested that I be put in a home. A lot of parents end up in divorce, because of the pressure of the disability, and all the care that was needed. Sometimes, the other children needed to go without other things, because of financial costs, or additional attention that the disabled sibling may need.

Mom and I had a good talk about her feelings. It was hard when the doctor told her I had Muscular Dystrophy, and was probably going to die by the age of 15. She loved me, but she didn't want to hurt when I died. I understood that feeling, since many of my friends had died already. For a while, Mom admitted that she didn't touch me as much. I never really thought about how a parent might feel before this. I started feeling angry, because the child doesn't know why a parent might feel this way. I did not understand when I was smaller, but I was aware that something was different. The discussion helped me put things into perspective.

I had to write something down as a result of that phone call. I tried to write my feelings from a boy's point of view, because the man's child was a boy, but that didn't work. I finally wrote this poem in an hour and a half trying to show what a child might be experiencing. At 16 years old, I wrote this poem:

BY THE GRACE OF GOD AND YOU
A Chair Does Not a Person Make

SOMETHING'S WRONG

I went to the doctor yesterday.
 Mommy and Daddy were there.
The doctor was testing my muscles,
 And Mommy was saying a prayer.

When the phone rang this morning,
 Mommy's eyes became red.
I left the room so quickly
 Cause I thought someone was dead!

Later, I asked Dad, "What happened?"
 And he held me, oh, so tight!
I felt a tear on my shoulder
 And said, "Daddy, it'll be alright!"

Things went well for quite a while,
 Though I saw the doctor more.
I loved his gentle manner.
 "Your age?" "I'm only four."

His smile was always huge,
 The biggest I've ever seen!
And so many tears I'd seen lately—
 Why, when the earth's so green?

Grampa's eyes were always tearful
 As he looked at me lovingly.
I walked with him more slowly.
 Was it he, or was it me?

Something's wrong I know.
 How come I move so slow?

Why do they stop talking
 Each time I enter the room?
What is worry? What is death?
 Why do they spread such gloom?

"Mommy, why can't I go up stairs,
 Like I did before?"
"Mommy, why are your eyes so red?
 Please don't cry anymore."

"Can I have a wheelchair,
 All my very own!?
All the kids will envy me,
 And want one in their home!"

Something's wrong, I feel.
 I just broke a wheel!

About the chair, Mom,
 It is a lot of fun,
But how can I play,
 With friends who do not come?

I cannot get to their house.
 What do you suggest?
They have so many steps,
 I don't want to be a pest.

How can I meet more people,
 If I just can't get out?
What about the M.D. camps
 Mr. Lewis talks about?

Something is wrong,
 I need it, and I know.
 Oh, Mom, please let me go!

Well, I went and I did it,
 Though Mother was quite scared.
I camped out, swam, rode horseback,
 And anything I dared!

I felt as though I was "with it".
 I let out a relieving sigh.
Oh, the counselors, friends and staff,
 And I even met a guy.

Reflecting, as I'm older,
 I see the struggle clear.
Not being accepted for myself,
 Was my biggest fear.

A chair does not a person make,
 Nor a brace, a man.
It's not what a person "cannot do",
 It is what a person "can".

Please, just let me feel
 Like I belong
Though I am weak
 And you are strong.

Something's wrong—
 I know it is true,
But I'll never be afraid
 By the Grace of God and you.

Carol Ann Schaufel

~ 5 ~

~ Starting High School ~

It was the summer before I started at Bradford High School. Patty came over to show me her yearbook, and to give me some pointers. As I thumbed through the pages, I saw that Tim had died. It was a surprise and a shock, but I kept everything inside showing no emotion. Was this the way the rest of my life would be? I made a conscious decision that there would be no more close friends for me, but I needed to remember that. I was hurting again! I gave Patty some money, so she could buy a yearbook for me. It was the only picture I had of him.

Diane met me at the north side of the Bradford building the day I started high school. She took me to my locker, and we opened it up. A board was attached to the arms of my wheelchair so that I could use it as a table. I piled supplies and books on it that I would need throughout the day, and Diane took me to my first class. Outside, I had to be carried up the steps, but inside there was a freight elevator with which I became very familiar. Diane had picked up my key for the elevator, and we were on our way!

My first stop was Latin class. My teachers already knew that I would be leaving five minutes early to get to my next class. I asked the person next to me, whoever that might be, if he/she could take me to my next room, and how that would work. No one refused, and they all became friends. I was pretty shy so that was a hard thing for me to ask others for help. Mom always said that I was her responsibility, and I shouldn't bother others. I had seen other people with disabilities who asked for too much too often. I never minded when people asked me for help, but I really had to work in order to ask others for help. My next class was Geometry, followed by American History. My last class of the day was American Literature, and then we were back to the locker, and the freight elevator to get to the north door. I made it through my first day! I loved all my classes, especially Latin and Geometry! I enjoyed the socialization, passing notes in the hall, talking with classmates, and I even went to a football game (much too cold for me). I never really liked the library, because I could not reach things, nor skim through them. I always had to depend on someone else to find books, or articles. (I wished there would have been Internet back then!). I became used to the freight elevator, and had opportunities to use many of those in my lifetime. While I was in high school, I passed all my classes with all A's in every quarter, except for the first quarter, where I received one B in art.

I remembered one, specific day the most during that first year - Friday, November 22. I barely returned home from school, and was sitting in the living room about to begin my homework. Mrs. Falcon, Harley's Mother, was talking with my Mother. (Mrs. Falcon regularly brought us eggs from her farm). There was a news bulletin on TV, and all three of us watched stunned just like the rest of the world!

"President Kennedy has been shot."

It was very scary. Everyone felt so vulnerable, including me. It was as if the world stopped spinning. Then, the news said, *"President Kennedy died. He was assassinated."*

BY THE GRACE OF GOD AND YOU
A Chair Does Not a Person Make

We continually watched television, all weekend long, taking in all the developments. One thing never made sense to me. Why, when Kennedy got shot in the back of the head, would Mrs. Kennedy be climbing on the back of the limousine to get part of the President's skull? With the power of the gun used, wouldn't the piece of his head have gone forward towards the driver? I could never put the pieces together. Many are still wondering who really shot him. (The investigation of the case was sealed for 25 years).

Another thing I noted in high school was that every person seemed to be so self-conscious of the way they looked. I heard "my nose is too big," or "my neck is too long," etc. When my body was distorted, there wasn't much I could do. I couldn't remember anyone at Camp nor at Orthopedic School that didn't accept people just for who they were. I had seen people with burns on their faces, or faces that were "tilted" by a birth defect with one eye being on the cheek. I always saw the person underneath. That is where I thought the real beauty was. The only thing that really bothered me, one day, was when I had to be carried down some stairs, because the elevator wasn't working. I thought, "Oh, what are people going to think of me when they see the commode opening in the bottom of my chair?" It was covered with a seat. Well, I guess everybody has something they worry about.

On Christmas morning of that year, Mom noticed I was very disappointed, because I thought we were going to get a dog. She laid her coat on the couch where I was sitting in my wheelchair, and all of a sudden I saw the sleeve move. Out of the sleeve came this tiny, black puppy who was a combination of Heinz 57 varieties, but mostly Cocker and Terrier with white paws! No, we did not call her Boots, but "I always liked Mo Holtan's dog, a copper colored Labrador whose name was Penny. Our Penny had a black coat, about forty pounds when she was grown, and we had chosen her name to honor Mo's dog. She would drag Susie, and all the kids in the neighborhood, on a sled in the winter. But, not for her own fun! She was just mad at the rope attached, and ran the sled all the way around the yard. She protected me, too, even from friends.

Ronnie's parents came over, one day, when Mom and Dad were not home. Ronnie's Dad tried to help me with something I was doing, but the dog stood between him and me, and would not let him touch me.

Even when Penny was playing with me on my lap, she got excited, and shared her excitement by giving me a bloody nose that lasted for at least half an hour. My first and only bloody nose!

"Grandpa in town", and Penny became friends too. They would even take naps together lying on the bed in Mom and Dad's room. Penny would lay on the floor next to him. One day, I looked into Grandpa's eyes. They had such a twinkle, and were so very watery blue. I had a strange feeling that something was going to happen, and he died the next month.

I can't remember Grandpa's funeral, but I remembered the day he died. Mom was walking around the corner from my bedroom to the living room. She almost tripped, because she felt something tugging on her skirt. She looked around to see what caused the tug, but she couldn't see anything. She looked at Penny who was lying on the floor next to Mom's bed, crying. She encouraged the dog to come by her, but Penny would not move, and continued crying. A half-hour later, the telephone rang. Grandpa had passed away about 45 minutes prior to the call. After the call, the dog was fine. It was like she knew before Mom. Grandpa died on Dad's birthday, Friday the 13th.

The second year of high school consisted of a second year of Latin, Bookkeeping, Senior English (mostly writing), and Art. My classes were in the afternoon this year, but not because of my disability. Because the whole school was on double shifts. The students that were to graduate from Bradford High School went in the morning. Those who were going to be going to Tremper High School went in the afternoon.

Somehow, I had caught up in grade level with Eddie (the person I had my picture taken with in first grade when we got our new wheelchairs). We rode the bus together back and forth to school. I got to know him much better. In January, the new school opened, so my classes were, again, held in the mornings. Throughout high school, though, my health was much better - even *after* talking my Mom out of the blanket that she always wanted to put on my legs!

With the new school came different, but the same, problems. This time, instead of a freight elevator, there was a very small elevator. I had to take my pedals off of my wheelchair to get into it so the door would close. I wished the elevator had more room inside. You could never fit two wheelchairs inside of it. Sometimes, we would have to wait for someone else who was there first to get to the floor they were going.

The second problem: Stairs. About three led down into the art room. The teacher assigned two male students to carry me in my wheelchair up and down those steps. I felt embarrassed. I did not expect to find these steps inside the building. The students didn't seem to mind, but I felt it wasn't fair to those who had to carry me.

In addition, the fire drills at Bradford must have been in the afternoons, because I didn't remember having participated in any of them. At Tremper, I was involved in two drills. We could never make it out of the building on time, especially if I was upstairs. When we would get back to the classroom, the teacher would say to the person pushing me that we would've lost our lives in that fire. Know that if there was a real fire, I was not to worry. The teacher and the students would help me down those stairs.

The last problem was that there was no flat entrance for the Lyceum programs. So, if Eddie and I had to attend, the only place we could go was on stage behind the curtain. I can't tell you if there were any problems with the bathrooms since I never used them. I knew there was one in the nurse's room that people in chairs could use.

After the first semester, my history teacher from the previous year found me, and thought that I should take a test on the U.S. Constitution. I did do that, and came out fourth in the city. The top three would go on to a state test for scholarships. I knew two of the others who passed in the top three. They both shared that the state tests was very involved, comparing one part of the Constitution to the next. The teacher was happy that I took the test, but most of my studying had been done the previous year. One very sad note was that this teacher, Mr. Gebhart, caught the bad flu that was going around that year, and passed away. He was in his early 40s. He made history so interesting.

I had an excellent English teacher that year also. He was a little on the dramatic side, but very effective. I had to do a research paper, which really prepared me for college. It seemed to take me forever to get it done. I don't even remember the topic. This teacher was involved with one of my orthopedic schoolmates the following year named Phil who had Muscular Dystrophy, and had worked really hard on his research paper. He was hospitalized from a bad cold, and passed away. The teacher took this really hard as the Mother brought the research paper to the teacher after Phil died saying, "He worked so hard on this paper. I had to turn it in for him." The teacher did not know what to do, and could not even bring himself to read it. (Side note: The teacher developed schizophrenia later in life, and became homeless. He passed away recently.)

Then, a little miracle came along called Craig in February! I became a godmother to my godmother's grandson. It was a very special day! What a treasure!

Roy, another one of my classmates from Orthopedic School, was going through a very hard time that year. He was so sick from his brain tumor, and had such horrible headaches that he was taken out of school. By May of our senior year, he passed away. He was always so good-natured, and patient. I always was teasing him about his middle name, Lambert. I used to say, "Laaammbert" as I "baa"ed like a lamb.

My school counselor had referred me to the Division of Vocational Rehabilitation (DVR). A Mr. Biandi came to my house, and gave me an application for services. DVR assisted persons with disabilities who wanted to get into the job market. He gave me an IQ test, saying that I did extremely well.

I met with Gene Giordano who would be helping me go to college at the University of Wisconsin, Kenosha Campus, and later, it was renamed Parkside. In high school, I earned only one B in Art for the first quarter based on some watercolor paintings, but otherwise, I made all A's. Even though Gene talked about accommodations, I never really asked for any. I should've asked for a half sheet of paper, because I could not really reach to the corners of the artwork. Just like I did with other things, wherever my hand fell on the paper was where I started a test, a form, or whatever I was doing.

There was one watercolor painting I particularly remembered. It was of a man walking through the forest. (Just like at camp, I always loved being on the path in the middle of the woods). I was not expecting the colors to run as blurry and dark as they did. I decided to make it an "at dusk" painting to make the darkness make sense. The man on the picture was fairly small in the scheme of things. I thought it was a good picture, but after looking at it, it seemed very depressing and lonely. Mom seemed concerned that I was depressed as well as the other people that looked at it. I could see why they thought that, but it definitely wasn't what was happening. All of my socializing was at school. The neighborhood kids were older, and I couldn't go inside anyone's house, because of the steps. The parents of some of the friends I had didn't want their child to come over, and bother my parents all the time. Maybe I was lonely, but I never really felt alone. I always kept myself busy doing something with my hands, or my mind. Like on trips, I would try to spot a license plate from each state, or recall as many cities as I could through the state we were traveling. I would look out the window, and find something that started with each letter of the alphabet. I would take the letters on the car license, and discover a word that had those letters in order, but throughout the word: WKA would be awkward.

BY THE GRACE OF GOD AND YOU
A Chair Does Not a Person Make

On a school-wide basis, I graduated 15th out of 500 students. DVR thought I could make it through college. I didn't remember taking the SAT test, but I guess I did. My school counselor must've also suggested my name for a scholarship, because I received a $500 award from the AFL-CIO to begin college, which I used for transportation. DVR was going to pay tuition and books.

Meanwhile, Louise was taking high school classes through the teachers at the Vernon Orthopedic School Wing. As the time came for both of us to graduate, we found out we would be together at graduation, along with Eddie. But, we were all there—in alphabetical order, of course. Louise and I were both worried about crossing that stage where we would get our diploma, because there were stairs. However, the principal handed the diplomas to us in front of the stage. Our biggest worry was trying to flip our tassels from one side of our mortarboard to the other. I'm just glad someone was pushing me at that time.

At my house, things became complicated, because Mom had three different graduation parties for me. All the people would not fit in our house at one time, and because Mom's parents were divorced. We had to have three different parties. One party was with Uncle Al's family, another with friends/neighbors, and another with other relatives. I received money that I put away for transportation to go to college. I especially enjoyed a tiny, two foot long plug-in organ from Uncle Al. I started learning how to read music. I could play it pretty well. It had no foot pedal to push, and I only had to use my right hand. About 18 months later, I got a big organ. Frankie, my schoolmate at Orthopedic School, came over to give me pointers on the playing. He played an accordion in a band. As he was teaching me, he would say, "Just a minute." He would lie down on his side on the organ bench pretending that the organ was his accordion, so he could put his fingers on the right keys! He always made me laugh.

The family took another trip this summer to Niagara Falls. Again, we got up at 3 o'clock in the morning, and were on the road by 5 a.m. I enjoyed seeing a lot of sunrises. Now, I was sitting in the front seat instead of the back as it was easier for my Dad to get me in and out of the car. We always chose cars very carefully, so there was a lot of room in the trunk for the wheelchair as well as suitcases. It was always nice to find a trunk that had a flat surface into the opening as the wheelchair could then slide in and out of the trunk more easily than if it went down into a deep space, and needed to be lifted out.

This time, we were traveling through Detroit, and went through the long tunnel between Michigan and Canada. Canada was interesting. When we stopped for lunch, I ordered a hamburger and french fries. I was surprised when the waitress brought a bottle of vinegar to sprinkle over the fries. I think the waitress was just as surprised when I asked for ketchup for my fries instead! The vinegar, to me, tasted just like extra salt. It was good, but I liked the ketchup better.

Niagara Falls from the Canadian side was very beautiful! You can't really see the falls from the American side, and get the full effect. I was surprised with the thunderous noise of the water rushing over the falls, and in the distance, its misty spray was sent along the sidewalk in front of us. The days we were there were sunny and warm, so that spray felt good!

In truth, I was more impressed with the Horseshoe Falls which were right next to Niagara Falls. I could get very close to the water running over the top edge. The semi-circled water plunged 165 feet into the Niagara River below. It was hypnotizing. We found a place that we could go underneath the Horseshoe Falls, so we decided to be adventuresome. We had to go down an elevator, and then three steps. We had to put on a raincoat to go the rest of the way. There was a rocky, cave-like path underneath the falls which led to three openings. The farthest was solid water plunging down in front of us. The next opening was covered with the rapidly moving water covering two thirds of the view. Through the third opening, we stepped onto a watered-down deck where you could look up at the hundred-plus feet falls with water coming down close to us. We were definitely shouting to hear one another talk, and getting hit with the falls' spray the whole time. This was the most vivid memory I have ever had.

That night, we ate on the top floor of a restaurant, and watched the lights change to different colors on the falls. Of course, we had lobster, but it was kind of a surprise, because it was the whole lobster, not just the tail! The lobster's eyes made me feel guilty, and it was the first time I saw the green stuff inside of them! Yuck!

The next day, we took a tour of the museum that had information on all the people that tried to go over Niagara Falls in a barrel, or other types of containers. Not too many made it alive, but one person that did was an old maid schoolteacher who seemed to just have a small gash by her eye. There was also a boat tour we could have taken on the Niagara River. The boat was called *The Maid of the Mist*, but that looked hard to get onto with my chair, so we skipped the boat.

On the way back home, we were lucky enough to find a motel that happened to have a trampoline! Dad was the first to try it, and was bouncing really high until he figured out that he did not know how to stop bouncing. We were all laughing even though we knew it was a little dangerous. Dad finally figured out how to stop—mainly by trial and error. Then, Susie joined him on the trampoline. They also found out that they couldn't jump up and down together! If one person was up, the other person was down. Mom and I were laughing so hard that we had tears in our eyes, and could barely take a movie of them jumping. For me, a lot of things looked like they were more fun to watch than to do.

~ 6 ~

Entering college

Now that I was ready for college, how was I going to get there? City buses were not accessible, and Mom could not lift me. I was now responsible for getting myself there. Susie was only 13. Dad had to work. Ed was still driving for the Cab Company, and came to the rescue in more ways than one. He not only picked me up every time I had to go to school that first semester, but helped pull me out of bed. I was totally ready when he came! He would grab my wrists from under my arms, and my Mom would take my knees. They would slide me sideways into my wheelchair which was easy since the side could be removed. Susie was happy to see Ed again, too! When Susie was little, she would always jump up on a box in the utility room, and give him a hug just before he would take me to school! I really never liked it when Ed teased me. He would take the one handle of my wheelchair, shake it, and say, "Jell-O." At that time, I was about 115 pounds, and I just didn't think it was funny!

To pay for the cab, I painted about two thousand Sweetheart Soaps in gold on the intricate design around the top of the bar. I would then paste a picture from a greeting card like a flower, butterfly, or dog in the center of the soap. Then, Mom would dip the top half of the soap in hot, clear wax. The wax would allow the top of the bar to go untouched while the bottom could be lathered. Many people bought the soap to put on their bathroom sinks. We would buy the bar for about 8¢, and sell it for 50¢. This was really my first job. I also had a couple of other craft projects, since I could not get a job in the community without much movement.

The University of Wisconsin in Kenosha (UWK) was a two-year school, and my first day was confusing. There was no elevator in the school, and I had a chemistry lab class on the second floor. The school arranged for some young men to carry me up and down the stairs.

Most of my classes were on the first floor, but because of the lab equipment, the class couldn't be changed to an accessible room. I had not seen Kenny since the eighth grade, and he was in my Psychology class. I never really liked psychology, because everyone I knew, were not considered "normal" by the book's definition. I liked sociology better. "Normal" never had any meaning to me. As a child, I got things done, and not in the same way everybody else did. I knew a lot of people that thought they were "normal," i.e., without a disability, but I knew in my heart that it was not the case. I guess "normal" was a relative word that was based upon an individual's own point of view. For example, it was "normal" for me to panic if I had to go to the bathroom, and no one was around the house to help. That was probably not a "normal" reaction for most people, but it was for me!

In my French class, I asked the person next to me if he could push me to the next class, because he was in it, too.

When I asked his name, he told me, "Brother Fred."

He was young, and had no collar.

I asked him, "Brother?"

"Yes, you know, a monk. I'm studying to be a priest. I am at St. Benedict's Abbey," he explained to me.

Since I was Lutheran, and had little contact with Catholics, I learned a lot from him. He was at least 6'4", tall, and very skinny, and from Buffalo, New York - close to the location of Niagara Falls! He was always a very compassionate person, and he became one of my best friends! He always promised he would officiate at my wedding one day! My friends Jodi, Thelma, and Mary (who lived next door to Diane) became Fred's good friends, too. The five of us got together, and started an Inter-Varsity Christian Fellowship group. It was very interesting how different people, and different religions, interpreted the different versions of the same Bible. It was also surprising to me how similar the Koran and Mormon Books carried similar messages, but with different messengers. In general, most people look at the differences in religious beliefs. I was always fascinated with the similarities.

We always had a lot of fun when the group was together. Jodi had some brothers who could carry me up into her house, so we usually met there, or at my house. Whenever I started laughing, I would laugh so hard, tears would come from my eyes. Jodi would always bring a box of Kleenex along whenever we would get together, partially as a joke, and partially, so they would be prepared!

Thelma was in my chemistry lab, and the lab teacher was Mr. Tamborino. Thelma was very tall, about six feet. I never really knew how tall I was as I would measure my heel to my knee, my knee to my hip, my hip to my head, and added the numbers. Of course I never got the same answer even though I could add. I was somewhere between 4'9" and 5'1." It depended on how much I stretched, and straightened my back. I basically just chose the number 4'10" as an average, and kept it, because a couple of my friends were midgets. At that height, I could be a member of the *Little People of America*. I liked their beautiful "Cinderella Shoes" catalogs that were adult shoes for small people. I am still most comfortable with a size 5 1/2. Of course, I did not use high heels as my ankles were also contracted. High heels would look like the heels were poking holes in the opposite leg. As another side note, Millie, one of my older friends who was a midget, told me that when the *Wizard of Oz* was filmed, the directors had a hard time, because most of the little people had never been with other little people. They were so fascinated with each other, the directors had to round them up from the cornfields! Isn't it surprising that this movie was finished at all?

Thelma and I would be doing our lab work together. If something had to be cooled, she would hold it above my head. I would tip my head up and blow at my target. I was good at bending the glass tubes and helping with directions. Once, we just could not get an assignment right! We were supposed to mix two chemicals to get a blue solution, but when we did it, the solution always turned green. We asked Mr. Tamborino for help. He said that we were mixing it right. Yet, even with his help we produced green again? Neither of us was very good in chemistry! We passed chemistry with good grades. It was just the lab that caused problems!

I met some other people that liked to play chess. We started a small group, and played chess between classes.

UWK also had a choir. I joined that for one semester. My voice was okay, but it always was somewhere between soprano and alto. For sure, I wasn't a base or tenor. It was fun though. Our concert was good, just some rough spots in two or three places. The most fun was when some of the group went to a nursing home to sing for Christmas. The nursing home had two floors though, and we were caroling through the hallways. Thelma and I had to use the elevator, so we were always a little bit behind!

When I got home from the caroling, my Mom said, "While you were gone, the church came caroling for the shut-in at our house." She didn't know how to tell them that I wasn't there, because *I was out caroling* at the nursing home. It was an embarrassing Moment for me too. I guess I never saw myself as a shut-in. I don't think that the church thought I would be out caroling either.

My English teacher was Mrs. Shanahan. The first thing that I wrote for her was something pretty idealistic about the hopes and dreams of a bride and groom from a wedding I had just attended. She really broke the essay apart. "Realistically, what problems did they even have during the wedding day and what they would be facing in the future?" she asked. She was a very good teacher, but I would tease her about being negative at times. I even asked her what her favorite color was.

She asked, "What do you think it is?"

I teasingly replied, "Black?"

She laughed and expressed, "Really, it is white."

That was a shock, and a different answer than what I was expecting!

By the end of my first semester, Eddie's boss at the taxi company told him that I was taking too much time to transport. The cab company was losing time and money! Ed could not take me back and forth to school anymore. We were back to the same problem. I did not know if I would be going to school the second semester.

One of my friends from high school, who used to push me from class to class, had a boyfriend who was also going to UWK. His name was Ulf. I had met him a couple of times. He was very nice, and a little quiet. Another friend, Mary, shared this transportation problem with him. He was in a group called the Circle K Club. Unknown to us, Ulf spoke with the group, and six different men volunteered to take me back and forth to school for my classes. A miracle!

It was a little different, because the only person that had lifted me before was my Dad. I could only wear dresses, jumpers, and skirts. Mom was still making my clothing through the first year of college. I didn't know if my underwear was showing when I was lifted. I was happy when slacks and sweatpants came into fashion. Most of the guys were pretty big so they lifted me easily. Terry's car had one problem that I remembered; we were riding along smoothly in his car with two other passengers when all of a sudden the car started jerking and died! We ran out of gas. The two other men in the car pushed the car towards the gas station, which fortunately was not very far. It was an eventful semester! Just as an extra note…Terry had a Mother who was an author, Eva Merow. I didn't discover this until years later. She summarized books such as Black *Beauty,* into 63 page books for young readers. She was part of the reason I am writing this book.

Before the fall semester started, and thanks to the MDA, my family found a hydraulic lift that sat on top of a vehicle. I would sit on a thick canvas cloth, and an attached a back support was hooked up, and then, hooked both together. All of this was attached to a bar that was at the top of the car with a device that looked like a clothing hanger with metal chains on two sides. Once we were sure that all the hooks were securely in their holes, I would be pumped up with a movable, hydraulic handle, and lifted off of the chair. Once I was free, Mom, or whoever was helping me, would back my wheelchair out from under me, and push me into the car. A knob then was turned to lower me onto the seat. We had a light wheelchair (20 pounds) by then that could be folded, and then slid in and out of the trunk easily. In any car, about all you could see of me was my eyes to the top of my head through the passenger window.

Mom became the person who took me to school every day. She did a good job, and did not seem to mind it too much - except for on very snowy and slippery days, because we had to go up a big hill at the back of the college to get to the main floor. There was only one day that was so icy that we could not make it up that darn hill!

The car lift helped Dad, too, because he had a couple of hernias. One was when he had his first job at a restaurant just out of high school, so getting me in and out of the car became difficult for him. Sometimes, I felt like a sack of potatoes being tossed into the car—nothing personal, just a necessity.

I started doing some volunteer work after Mom could take me back and forth. Right next to the college was a nursing home. I knew some people from Orthopedic School that lived there. Chuck, who painted beautifully with his mouth, was a quadriplegic, and about seven years older than I. He did a pen-point of Gov. Knowles, and painted beautiful scenic pictures.

I met with many of the residents, and one was deaf. I knew some sign language so I would visit with her for a while. I would visit the nursing home at least once, or twice, a month to see everyone. I also, learned the basics of grade 1 Braille. (Grade 1 has no shortcuts, and words are fully spelled. Now they call it "non-contracted Braille"). I bought a slate (a metal object the width of a piece of paper filled with rows of small cells covering 1/4 to 1/3 of a standard size paper), and stylus (a ball like object with a rounded poker underneath to form dots in the individual cell backings which had two columns of three dots each). The slate was hinged, and opened for you to clamp a piece of thicker Braille paper to imprint a dotted message. After learning which combination of dots to punch in one cell for every letter of the alphabet, and each number, I mailed short notes to some of the nursing home residents who could read it. I did not do Braille for very long, however, since I could not punch through the light cardboard type paper with just my hand. I needed to use my chin to make the dot combinations correctly. No matter how short the note, I had a sore, and sometimes a bruised, chin.

The first semester of my second year of college was very busy. I had decided to go into speech therapy. My speech teacher was very good. When I gave my first speech, I became really nervous, so nervous that I could not remember anything. Even my notes seemed foreign. The teacher let me start over again, and I did just fine. I gained a lot of confidence that day, even though I wouldn't want to live through that day again.

Two of my former classmates from Orthopedic School, Betty and Frankie, had been very sick from kidney problems. Both of them were looking at surgery. Betty was given a 50%

better chance than Frank on survival. Betty had her kidney transplant first. One thing after another seemed to go wrong for her. A nurse got her feet stuck in Betty's tubing, and the tubes were pulled out of her body. Another nurse brought Betty some medication. Betty did not know what it was, so she wanted to wait. The nurse insisted that she drink it. Betty did, but found out later that the medicine was a cream for a rash she was supposed to rub on her body. Betty passed away.

Frankie had been going to college like me, but had missed a lot of days. DVR was helping him as well, but he had to talk DVR into continuing to help him, since he wasn't progressing with his degree fast enough. He finally had a kidney transplant. Frankie did great! I think he got his transplant from a 10-year-old girl, so he always teased that he did not know which bathroom to use! DVR continued to support him. He became a music teacher, and principal of schools in Racine. He has become the longest living transplant recipient in history. I was proud to know him even though he did once throw an icy snowball that hit my eye, and left me almost blind for a half-hour! Kids!

At the end of the fall semester, my parents and I took a trip to Madison to interview with a Professor Minifee who was head of the speech therapy department. He did not say too much to me while I was there, but he did send me to a different person in DVR's Madison office.

When I spoke to the man at Madison DVR, he shared that the professor did not think I could do the job. He thought I couldn't reach a person's mouth to help form a word. I needed to know much more about a speech therapist's job. I felt really bad, and wanted to cry. Why wasn't the Professor honest with me while I was there, and why couldn't he discuss it with me? This was one time when biting my tongue failed me. I cried anyway. The rehab counselor handed me a box of Kleenex. I put my hand up on the side of my chair with my mouth to reach it. Just as I was about to reach it, he put the box a little farther away. He stated, "See, this is what the professor meant." I was not ready to deal with any of this. I was ready to leave. My parents left with me.

A few days later, I had a letter in my mail from the professor saying, "Who do you think you are—some kind of giant killer? Look at yourself, you are a quadriplegic. You can't....." The letter went on for two pages. This made me angry. I spoke with my speech teacher, Ms. Sovich. She really thought I could do the job. We started working together. I started checking out some things in the school system seeing how the speech therapists worked. I visited some of the schools and therapists. I found out that not all schools were accessible, but the therapists thought I could do the job. I was starting to get angry again and... Ms. Sovich died in a car accident.

I started to think that maybe God had different plans for me. I began thinking maybe there wasn't a God at all. Ms. Sovich was the 15th person who had died that I felt close to before I was 20. I was lying in bed one night thinking, "I am 93 years old. What have I done with my life? What can I look back on?" And with the pain I had been having in my stomach— was I the next one to die? I leaned forward with my foot kicked into my stomach every night so I could sleep.

BY THE GRACE OF GOD AND YOU
A Chair Does Not a Person Make

I realized I was testing God for a while. All of the deaths were getting to me. There was no ride to school when Ed came back into my life. That could've been a coincidence. Next, Ed couldn't take me to school anymore. Ulf was there to help, and then, Ulf had a different schedule, and he asked the Circle K Club to be involved. Next was the car lift, Professor Minifee, Ms. Sovish's death. So many ups and downs! I didn't know what was going to happen after that.

I asked for one undeniable proof so that I would know God was there. I was watching one of my favorite TV shows. The telephone rang. Mom seemed to be talking a long time. I was ready for the channel to be changed (no remotes back then), because my soap opera was on TV. I could not turn off the show, *Double Exposure*, so I watched the show while I was waiting. They had a new contestant with some very unusual facial features. I had had a dream the night before, and remembered that face even when I woke up that morning. Now, I am seeing the face on TV? That must be another coincidence.

The internist had told my Mother, "The pains Carol is having in her stomach are from being depressed and feeling sorry for herself." My pains had been off and on for a year! Mom told the doctor that I wasn't depressed. She did not think that was the right diagnosis.

I started vomiting my way to the hospital, and had to have surgery. It was a kidney stone, but since I had such a curvature in my spine, my specialist doctor did not want to do surgery. Dr. Richards was an excellent doctor, and about five years prior, he had been stretching my bladder opening, because it was so small. The last time I went, I thought that was enough. I didn't want to go through it again, and I didn't. Dr. Richards didn't feel that he could do the surgery, but there was a new doctor in his office - Dr. Frazier who had just come from Bethesda Hospital in Maryland.

A lot of things were going wrong when I went into the hospital. No one could find my veins, or my pulse. Dr. Frazier did say it was a good thing that the kidney stone was in my left kidney, or it would have been much harder to reach. The nurse came in to shave my lower stomach the night before surgery. I was getting very nervous, because unlike most of my friends, I had never been in the hospital for surgery.

I made my final deal with God since the surgery was going to be in the morning. I prayed for two things: That I would not be afraid, and that Ulf would come for the surgery. I hadn't even seen Ulf in over a semester, and had no idea what he was doing. I promised if these two things happened, I would never doubt Him again. I shared this with no one for many years.

In the morning, Mom was with me, and the nurse gave me a shot which made me sleepy. Then, the nurse pushed me into a very cold looking room. She slid me on a hard table, turned me on my side, prepared my IV, and left the room saying, "I'll be back in a minute." As I was lying there, I felt what seemed to be a warm hand way down on the left bottom side of my back. I opened my eyes, but no one was there. The touch was very comforting. I wasn't scared anymore. The nurse and doctor came back into the room, and were ready to start the IV. I was told to start counting backwards from 10. "10, 9, 8..."

I woke up in the recovery room. I stayed there a while, just remembering how good the warmed up blankets felt. In about a half-hour, they took me to my room. Mom was there with the doctor. My surgery was exactly where I felt the warm hand on my back, and bandages covered the shaved spot. The only problem that the doctor had was that my skin was very thin where he had to stitch the incision. He ended up using chicken-wire instead of regular stitches to give the area the support it needed to heal.

The doctor left, and Mom said, "Guess who was here while you were having surgery?" I had no idea.

"Ulf," she told me.

I asked, "How did he know that I was here?"

She did not know, but that he came just as I was going into surgery, and had left for work right after I was put into recovery. Before I zonked out, I prayed to myself.

"Thank you God!" And, I kept my promise of never doubting Him again. I don't even remember worrying about anything after that!

Later, I found out how Ulf had known about the surgery. Mary had called Jodi, and told her that I was to have surgery the next morning. Jodi was doing her internship in nursing at St. Mary's Hospital in Racine. Neither Jodi, nor Ulf, knew that the other knew me, but Jodi was his passenger riding back and forth to work every day. The day of the surgery, they had another rider who rode with them on occasion. That day, the rider got up and her tire was flat (imagine that!), so she called Ulf for the ride. Jodi thought for sure the rider knew me, but she didn't. When Jodi said my name, Ulf turned off the radio, and asked her, "Who?" Jodi said my name again. He asked for details, took off of work, and was there to sit with my Mom while I had surgery. It was a one in a million chance for any of these things to have occurred. Prayer answered!

A couple hours after surgery, I felt like sitting up. Mom on one side, and the nurse on the other, helped me to sit. I had never felt that kind of pain before. I had them stop every second or two. Then, as soon as I sat up, I was as white as a ghost. I asked to be laid right back down again! They laid me back down just as slow as when they helped me sit! I think the third day was the hardest. I also told the doctor which pill I could not take, because it made me nauseated. He was surprised that I knew which pill it was. However, I did find that the more I moved, the less pain I had, and I was out of the hospital in a few days.

Dr. Frazier brought in my kidney stone which was the size of the end of my Mother's finger, and looked like it had spikes on it. My Mom took the stone to the internist.

Angrily, she told him, "Remember the pain that you said was in my daughter's head? Here's the kidney stone that caused it!"

I was surprised at all the cards and flowers I received. One of the cards I received was from the kids at college. It was a lunch bag that was folded in half. The front of the bag read: *I bought a card to help you get well, but darn it all I lost the thing!* On the inside it read: *So, here's the bag it came in.* The bag was stuffed with notes from everyone—teachers, friends and strangers.

I always wanted to tell Ulf the story, so that he would know what he had done for my life. About six years later, I heard a knock on the door about seven o'clock in the morning on a warm, summer Saturday. Mom went to the door, and asked him to wait on the closed-in porch. Mom came into my room to let me know that he was there, so helped me dress, and run a brush through my hair, before I went out to talk with him.

Ulf was sitting on the glider, and it was good to see him! He had married a girl from Puerto Rico, and they were visiting his Mom who lived in apartments about five blocks from my house. He was out jogging, and recognized the house, so he decided to take a chance, and knocked on our door.

He asked, "I hope I'm not dropping in too early."

I just told him, "I'm glad you don't go jogging at 5 a.m."

We laughed. Then, we talked for a while. I had a chance to share what happened the day I had my kidney stone surgery, and how he fit into that. I was so happy he now knew!

It was quite some time, before I returned to school. Mary and Thelma had been planning to go to school in Madison to help me with attendant care.

Thelma was in my Zoology class with me in a previous semester. We had to pith a frog, and did not do it right. I thought of how much the frog felt the pain. We had a lot of piglets that gave their life for us in that class as well.

When I returned to school, we were in Anatomy. I wasn't sure this was the class I wanted. After my surgery, I knew I had to drop some classes, so anatomy was definitely the first class I dropped. I did not know how I could have completed the makeup work in a lab class. I had to drop two classes, but I kept two classes in which I knew I could make up the work.

The rest of the semester, I had to decide what I was going to do with my life. I decided to give up fighting for something that I knew I was not supposed to do. God seemed to be batting me over the head not to be a speech therapist. I wasn't sure that I wanted to do speech therapy anymore, anyway. I knew Math was very easy for me, but I had only taken Trigonometry and beginning Calculus at UWK.

"You can do Calculus in your head, but can't balance a checkbook?" Dad used to tease me.

Carthage College had a four-year program in Kenosha that I could complete while commuting from home. (NOTE: Mary decided to go to school locally. Thelma ended up with a medical problem called Crohns' Disease which caused many problems for her during that time. She wouldn't have been able to take care of me. God's plan worked better for all of us. PS: Both friends got married and were very happy.)

I knew that I could get a degree in Math, but what would I do with that degree? Carthage had a teaching program, but could I teach? No one ever told me I couldn't be what I wanted to be until the Madison professor. My parents never asked me questions. It was just assumed that I would work. No Schaufel had ever earned a college degree before me, and I had a long way to go. What good would a degree be if I couldn't work? I just decided to leave it to God, and do whatever I had to do along the way. It had been a good ride so far!

During the spring break, I did not have to study. Our family decided we wanted to go back to Washington DC. We stayed at the Mayflower Hotel, again, as it was easier to walk to places. We toured the Mint where they printed paper money, but no "samples" were given to us! The process was fascinating—blank, large sheets of paper were put into machines which printed the money on both sides. When the sheets came out of the printer, a person would flip through the large sheets, like fanning through the pages of the book to make a little motion picture. If there were any mistakes, they would be taken out, and destroyed. The final step was to cut the huge sheets into individual dollar bills.

As we walked back to the hotel, Dad was pushing me when he heard an African American man say, "You ain't seen nothing yet, Whitey!" Dad took the statement seriously. We left the city the next morning. The next evening was the 1968 race riots in Washington DC.

It was scary to think we were that close to being involved in the riots, but it was even sadder to think individuals felt discriminated against so much that it would come to that point. Everyone should have equal rights and equal opportunity. My Mom or Dad never said anything bad about anyone of a different culture or color. My Uncle Al, after his experience in Asia, could not even eat rice, because it reminded him of his war experience. When I was about five years-old, I do remember my Mom answering a question when I saw black people for the first time.

When we were going through Chicago, I asked.

"How come the people's skin is so dark?"

Mom responded, "Because they are made of chocolate."

I thought how cool would that be! I loved chocolate. I knew that they were not made of chocolate! But, I was never afraid of people that looked different after that. People were people!

At the end of the semester, for the first time at U.W. Kenosha, and for the second year in a row, I received the Peter Antaramian Award for "scholastic achievement and character". My parents were very proud of the awards, and I was on the honor roll carrying a full class load. My parents had sacrificed a lot to help with my success, besides the daily personal care I required. Susie, too, had been a lifesaver on many occasions.

I had one residual condition from my surgery, and it was a partial loss of hair on the very top of my head. The sides and back of my hair were still thick. One of the medical staff had mentioned that the hair loss was probably from an overdose of anesthetic. I have no idea if this was true, but I did have the hair loss. (Grandpa with the mink used to kill the mink with an overdose of the anesthetic. I guess I was lucky just to lose some hair)! I started wearing wiglets, and eventually, full-size wigs. This saved a lot of time as all someone had to do was wash my hair as need, and then just throw on my wig which I could comb by myself except for the back. Kmart used to sell a lot of wigs which were perfect for me as well as being a good price.

People would say, "Where did you get such beautiful hair?"

I would always say, "Kmart."

It was a good conversation starter! No one really knew I wore a wig. Mom started using one, too, and told me that I should just start saying, "Thank you" when people complimented my hair. I did not really care if people knew, and the wigs helped so much. They gave me an instant professional look as well as being an energy and time saver. What a blessing that my hair was thin!

Susie had two good friends in the neighborhood—Trish who lived across the street and Jimmie's baby girl who was ten years Buddy's junior, Carolyn. Susie was old enough to help me with the bathroom once in a while, now. At one point, I got stuck between the wheelchair and the stool I leaned on.

When this happened I just said, "Let me think a minute," so I could figure out what to do next and not fall.

Susie responded, "While you're thinking a minute I am going to go get Trish or Carolyn for help!"

She made it back in time! I was saved!

On the other hand, Dad and Denny, Jimmie's husband, had a call from Trish's babysitter one night. The babysitter was getting very sleepy, and saw smoke in the air so she called for help to check it out. Dad and Denny took a flashlight to the house across the street immediately, and found a gas leak. Everyone was evacuated from the house, and they turned off the gas. Trish and Debbie were already asleep. Good save in the nick of time!

Susie and Carolyn were always together even though they were about five years apart. I was truly surprised that Jimmie and Denny even let them be together, because Susie always had bad ideas such as grabbing pliers to pull out Carolyn's loose tooth. Once they were playing baseball, and Susie hit the ball straight into Carolyn's nose. It was broken. Carolyn cried, "I'm not pretty anymore!"

~ 7 ~

Transferring to Carthage

At Carthage, a Lutheran college, the first person I met was Dr. Munson. He told me I had to take two Bible classes in which I would study both the Old Testament and New Testament. I needed to read it at that time, too. I lost credits transferring from Parkside, and added a few more classes so that, within five years, I could graduate with a Bachelor degree as a teacher. I didn't think that taking 4.5 years to finish my degree too long while including the extra classes taken, making up two I dropped the previous semester, making up credits for my major, as well as taking one class in summer school! And, I did *not like* taking classes in summer. It's partially the reason I chose the occupation of teaching, because I loved the idea of not working in the summer! Since my major was going to be mathematics, and my minor in sociology, my degree would be a Bachelors of Arts, or a B.A. My Mom was glad I would have a B.A. behind my name instead of B.S. (for Bachelors of Science) for obvious reasons! My major and minor were the opposite of each other. My major, was very systematic and exact. Math produced an exact answer(s) for any problem. My minor could give you some possibilities of what an individual might do in a certain situation, but no exact answers at all. People just have too many variables! (That's what I love about people) My major and minor allowed me to use opposite sides of my brain, which was not a usual combination of subjects. Instead, most people like to use either the left, or right, side of the brain.

Dr. Munson's office was unique, because I noticed that there was a big, three-foot high, plant in a bed pan placed in the corner of his office behind his desk! Since I used bedpans all the time, it made me smile and more "comfortable." Dr. Munson also told me that I had to take another IQ test. I felt like I was starting career training all over.

This was the first time I registered for school by myself. At UWK, my Mom, or Mr. Kuegel always did it for me. Since computers were almost non-existent, I paced from table to table in order to sign up for the classes I wanted. Fortunately, I already had almost two years of college behind me, and only one class was filled that I needed. So, I took another math class, since I knew I was going to have to take some of my basics with advanced math classes. I would have to take at least two math classes a semester to be able to make up the major credits that I needed. I decided upon Linear Algebra and Calculus. It was a little hard, but with help, I'd make it. My math advisor and teacher, Miss Konsin, did not know I was taking "basics with advanced classes" until the end of the last semester, when I received my first, and only D grade slip in Linear Algebra, which was a six-week possible failure warning. (Linear Algebra was a math class that not only had the three dimensions of a cube, but the fourth dimension of time with an infinite number of other dimensions where things could move around in space). Miss Konsin wanted me to frame that little pink slip, as a reminder that everything wasn't easy for me! My final grade in Linear Algebra was an "A-". At UWK, I only had one class that was difficult, because the geography teacher had a French accent. I could never tell what he was saying. He would talk about the "swimps" (swamps) and the "minire" (manure). It was so complicated. We all read the whole textbook, but his tests were usually locations of the vineyards in France. It was my one, and only, "C" in college.

Carthage had elevators inside the two main buildings where I had classes. They did put a ramp going straight up the stairs at a very steep angle on the outside of the main building, but snow, or ice, made going up that ramp very difficult. Otherwise, I could get into the building by going into the underground garage behind the building. Mom and I would often use a designated parking stall in the basement for a few minutes hoping to get into my wheelchair, and up to my first class before someone needed the space. Mom could have never pushed me up that front ramp, and it reminded me of the one at the White House, which was much shorter.

The year that I started at Carthage, there were two other students using wheelchairs, as well as the librarian who was having health issues. The library/auditorium building had a flat entrance, but if anyone needed to get to the second floor, the only elevator was through the library. And, there was always a locked door between the library and the classrooms, and I needed a key in order to pass through it. I tried to schedule all my classes in one building to make things easier, or I would schedule my Tuesday and Thursday classes in one building, and my Monday, Wednesday and Friday classes in the other. Side note: Studies on accessibility for disabled persons was in its infancy.

Carthage had a beautiful campus. In the main building, once I was up the steep ramp, there was a beautiful, open view of Lake Michigan, and I felt as if I was on an ocean cruise. A spiral staircase was off a little to the right and to the left where a reception/welcoming desk was located, and then the bookstore. There was also a student lounge just to the left of the first-floor door just past the reception desk. On the second floor, there was a Civil War Museum off to the side, which has since moved to a full building in downtown Kenosha. Classrooms and offices covered the rest of the building, including a floor between the main floor and the basement. The basement had the mailroom, and a parking garage. I spent a lot of time in the lounge between classes, and got to know several of the students, many who lived on campus. The dorms were about a block away on the south end. The two main buildings were right together on the north end of the campus.

Most of the commuting students spent some time in the student lounge. It became an easy place for me to hitch a ride to class. It was the time of the Vietnam War. Some of the students were avoiding the draft, and others were already veterans.

One of the students I had known from high school used to push me around campus, but since Jim rode a motorcycle, he would always make me wear his helmet when he pushed me. (I could not believe how heavy those helmets were! I could barely hold my head up. It didn't do much for my hair either)!

There was another group of students in the lounge that liked to play pinochle. One semester, I had to wait about two hours between classes, so I often played pinochle with them. I even decided to skip a class, once, so I could play just one more hour. That was a mistake, because my literature class had a surprise quiz! I told the teacher the truth. "I skipped class." I knew I couldn't make up the quiz, but she indicated that everyone could drop one quiz grade during the semester anyway for their final grade, and I learned a valuable lesson!

When I had to study during the school day, I liked to sit in front of the huge windows looking out over Lake Michigan. I always thought how lucky we were to be able to watch the sunrise over this huge body of water that was ever changing in color and emotion. It could look dark, dreary, and depressingly cold, or be a light blue calm. Occasionally, especially with cloudy skies, the lake would carry multiple colors through different parts of its waves from a teal blue to an almost white glimmer. I felt fortunate to be born on this side of the sun watching a sunrise, because it felt more optimistic to me than if I was watching a sunset. I enjoyed thinking of positive things. I always thought of what I had to do rather than thinking about what I had done. In truth, both the sunrise and sunset are just as beautiful, including the sunrise and sunset of each of our lives!

I made good grades, but I was a very slow reader. Mom liked reading, so she often read several of my novels to me. In my other classes, I would often buy a textbook with underlined words, so that I felt like I had a head start on my classes. I always asked other students what types of tests teachers gave. Some gave tests from the texts, some from notes. Some even took information from under the pictures in the books. It made studying a lot easier and manageable. I found that if I was in class, I did not have to study as hard.

The one textbook that I particularly enjoyed was my 20th Century History class where the book not only covered history, but all cultural changes, mishaps, and scandalous incidents. It was a very interesting book! You almost wanted to get a cup of tea, and sit down to read the book - not that I wasn't sitting down already!

In dealing with my advanced math classes, I had an opportunity to meet some of the foreign exchange students. Helen was from China who came to my house a couple of times, and cooked us some authentic Chinese meals. It was the first time I had ever had them. Specifically, I enjoyed sweet-and-sour pork, and an egg, pork, and onion mix which was similar to Egg Foo Yung without the gravy. Mom, Dad, Susie, and I loved it all, even though the kitchen was quite a disaster. It seemed like Helen needed to use every pot and pan we had. But she was a good friend, a good student, and excellent cook!

Toshi was from Japan. He was in my first advanced math class, and came to the house to help me with math. When he heard that Helen had been there, he wanted a home cooked meal, too. His meal was more expensive, and had more food with which we were unfamiliar. Such as huge mushrooms that tasted like cardboard to me. He mostly used one frying pan on our table to cook a teriyaki and onion mix. The meat seemed tougher, and it's possible the onions were leeks. It was a good experience though. He sent me a letter after he graduated, and went back to Japan.

He had written, "I am so happy to be home. I had raw fish for breakfast!" And, as I read his letter, I thought, "I am so happy that I didn't have to eat raw fish for breakfast!"

A couple of new friends from the card games and classes would assist me throughout the day if I had to go to a different class, the bookstore, or to the bathroom. In a period of about two months, I had my body trained to go from whenever I got up in the morning to when I got home. I also regimented my drinking to help me plan better, and this kept me from having ask for less personal assistance. It was nice when people knew what I needed, and just helped without having to ask, e.g., shifting the right book onto the top of the pile in front of me for my next class. I tried not to be demanding like some people with disabilities that expected the help, were ungrateful, or assuming. People have their own lives, and their schedules that changed as much as mine did. Whenever a person might be absent, it could cause a mini crisis with having to change things, or check if I could depend on someone else for that day.

In the middle of my junior year, I was encouraged to take my GRE testing (Graduate Record Exam) in case I ever wanted to go to graduate school, but I certainly wasn't thinking about it! I would be happy just to get a job when it was time! I was only thinking that it was a good idea to take the test. Whenever I thought, "That will never happen to me," well, they did! My motto became "complete whatever you can today, because you do not know what tomorrow will bring", so I would always have my papers done early knowing that something would come along at the last minute to stop me. I did not do well on the reading aspect of the GRE, because I really did not have a very big vocabulary, but I felt I did excellent on the math portion with 70% correct even though I had yet to take the great majority of the needed math classes.

On spring break, I read, and studied, a lot of my Bible class work on the way back and forth to Texas where my family was visiting Dad's Air Corps friend who used to live in Port Washington. On the trip down, there was a gas war. Gas was $.25 a gallon! We made our way through many miles of the King Ranch where I saw several dead armadillos. Our friends lived in Brownsville, Texas, close to the very tip of San Padre Island where Fran took us out on his fishing boat. We caught no fish that day, but there was a lobster teasing us by crawling up the fishing line, then deciding to let go, and drop into the water at the very last second! We were all already drooling!

We also took side trips to Reynosa and Matamoros, Mexico, which are both fairly close to Brownsville. The money exchanges were very interesting. Looking in stores, something that costs $30 here might be marked 240 pesos, or more.

The driving in Mexico was crazy. Where were the stop signs, or stop lights? It was amazing there were not more accidents, and many cars sported dents and scratches! If there was an accident, our friend, Fran, told us that people just left their cars, or everyone would go to jail when the police came. The marketplaces were very interesting. We bartered for the price of an item, and we saw a lot of fresh meat out in the hot sun. It was definitely a different culture. Dad saw a little boy about six years old go into a bar, drink a shot of whiskey, and leave! Dad also tried what he thought was a carrot while we were eating lunch. He almost choked on it, as it was so spicy. He could not get a breath, and sweat was rolling off the back of his neck!

The next to last semester, I started student teaching. A few months before I started, I ordered my first motorized wheelchair for only about $600, and paid for it myself. It took a long time to get the wheelchair, so the chair barely made the first class that I taught. I observed five classes of about 30 people each at Tremper High School under the supervision of Mrs. Short for the first week. Mrs. Short was good enough to push me around for a few days until my wheelchair came. When it did come, Dad brought the wheelchair to school where I left it locked in the janitor's closet each night until the next morning. I had never been in a motorized chair before! What freedom! What responsibility! Driving the wheelchair myself, I realized how often people that pushed me had been pointing me in the wrong directions. They turned me away when speaking to another person, or directly facing me at a wall instead of what, or who, I would like to see. Once, I started driving my chair, I never stopped moving. I was always looking in a different direction - always turning! I would never sit still again!

Driving the motorized wheelchair was a responsibility, and took a lot of learning! The very first day I drove my wheelchair into the teacher's lounge, I had no idea that my chair was going to have a glide. I hit a table and spilled three teachers' coffees! Not a good first impression! I still needed help with the elevator to get upstairs, because I couldn't reach the buttons. Just as I turned into the classroom, I clipped the door with the end of my shoe, and it flew off into the room. A student by the name of Peady put it back on my foot. I found out later that Peady's Father was one of the men who built Easter Seals' Camp Wawbeek, and I saw her quite a few times during the rest of my life! It took a while to practice, and learn all my turning distances, gliding and backing up, especially in the crowded high school hallways where I tried to miss people's toes!

My Dad started bringing the wheelchair home on weekends so we would go to the Southridge Mall in Milwaukee to practice my driving. The chair was very heavy. He took it apart in pieces to put it into our station wagon, and then reassembled it. It was a job! I missed the motorized wheelchair at home a lot during the week. I decided that when I would get a teaching job, I would get a second chair, so I could have a motorized one both at home and work.

Mrs. Short gave me a lot of opportunities and information. Student teaching was fun. I'm not sure I was that good of a disciplinarian, but I think my chair fascinated the students, and it was just long enough to get a good control of my classroom. I used an overhead projector that was a little bit hard to reach. I knew then, if I was hired, I would need an overhead projector that could be lowered onto the table to give me more support for my arms. (Mo Holtan gave me a flat, portable overhead projector for graduation early, so I could try it out. He was a wonderful man).

The teaching and planning started getting easier. Soon, I was teaching all five classes! All the classes were Geometry. We were not too much into proofs yet, so I did not have to have a student write a lot on the blackboard for me. I prepared many overhead transparencies to flip on and off the projector in helping with my teaching as well as some direct writing and pointing.

One day, the principal of the school came in to see me teach, and evaluated how I was doing. Dr. Hosmanek was a very handsome, authoritative looking man who could own a room by walking into it. In other words, I was scared! Somehow, I got through it without dropping a transparency pen, or losing my shoe! Students were attentive, and participated. Upon completion of my student teaching, both Mrs. Short and Dr. Hosmanek gave me good reviews for my job placement file. (It also didn't hurt that Dr. Hosmanek became superintendent of Kenosha schools shortly thereafter).

For my last semester, I only had two classes, but I spent a lot of time at college. I had completed my job placement file, and started looking for jobs when Ms. Konsin told me the school was going to consider me for a part-time instructor position for two basic classes of

Algebra and Trigonometry, and also assisting with statistics for $1500 a semester. Ms. Konsin was going on a year's sabbatical leave to complete her doctorate. She was a good teacher, and I thought this opportunity would be an excellent chance to learn my equipment and strengths, before having to deal with the problem of discipline. I took the job! Ms. Konsin took me out to dinner at the Hobnob to celebrate my graduation, as well as to give me pointers on what to do on the job!

During the last semester, I also had a lot of time to practice with my electric wheelchair. I tried using about a two feet dowel to reach elevator buttons. It took a while, and several bruises, to get my timing right. Getting out of the elevator was easier. I just had to push the button, and position myself to get out of the door with the extra time of going up or down a floor. Pushing the button on the outside of the elevator was a problem only if the elevator was on the same floor as I was. Then I had to rush into it, and usually crushed my driving arm in the door. It was okay. I just learned to wear long sleeves to cover the bruises, and took advantage of anybody's offer to push buttons. I always hated when people pushed the elevator button if I had used all my energy to get my hand into position. They would push the button right before I touched it. Only once did I drop the stick inside of the elevator where I was trapped, and I was sure hoping someone would rescue me! I learned patience.

It was the first time many of the students had seen me on my motorized wheelchair, when a new student, who admired me, remarked about my chair.

"You are just like a princess on a throne," she said.

I know she meant it in a positive way, but I had a different train of thought.

"A princess is so distant from people, giving commands, telling people what to do." I never really wanted to be a princess only a person!

Graduation day was here - for both Susie and me! Susie graduated from high school, and I graduated from college with 3 weeks, each, of parties! The graduation ceremony was much different. We were in the Carthage Field house, and a stage crossed the front of the room with a ramp on each side which was set up so I entered and exited easily. Someone was to push me up and down, it was just too steep. Dad filmed a home movie during the ceremony. When they called my name, people stood up, and clapped. I thought that was nice. It brought a tear to my eye, but each of those graduating had done as much as I! Somehow, while driving with my right hand, I got that tassel around to the other side of my mortarboard, and took the "diploma" with my left hand. I was focused on turning my chair around, so that I could go down the other ramp backwards in order to avoid hitting a wall. By doing this, my hand pulled away from the controls, and the chair would stop.

~ 8 ~

Teaching at Carthage

Teaching at Carthage was a learning experience. I had Mo's portable overhead projector, Ms. Konsin's office space, and a program assistant, Norma, with whom I could consult when I was in trouble. The office was not in the main building, but in the library, so I had to contend with those locked doors on the second floor. Mom was still driving me back and forth to school, helping me get ready for the day, but I didn't need rides any longer, and she didn't have to push me.

I would get there early in the morning. One day, I was at my office doorway before anyone came, and couldn't believe what I saw! There was a little black snake that was creeping down the hallway past my door, and kept on wiggling north to south just outside the Zoology lab! I didn't think much of it, since he wasn't coming toward me. I rolled on down the hall to teach my first class, then returned. About 15 minutes, later I heard someone scream, and Norma went to find out what was wrong. The snake that I had told her about seeing that morning had found its way into the women's washroom. It had wound itself around the back of a throne, finding a victim to surprise! Since the snake had crawled out of its little tank, he was scooped up, and plopped back into it.

Two of the classes that I taught consisted of about 30 students. The Statistics class was very large—maybe 75 students. In such large classes, I began to wonder how I would handle cheating, and decided to deal with it when, and if it happened. People who cheated only cheated themselves, and when life became harder for them, they wouldn't be able to handle problems that were thrown their way.

Wisconsin weather caused a problem for a few days, and since my sister was driving, now, she would take me back and forth to work if needed. One day, there was a very bad ice storm. I usually never missed school, or work. Mom didn't want to drive, and Susie said that she would take the car around the block just to test the road conditions. When she came back, she snipped, "You are not going to work today! I barely made it to the corner and back. I had to drive with my door open to see anything!" And, it was my first missed work day.

Susie was in college, now, and continued her Spanish from high school. After two years at UWK, she got a job at Johnson Motors where our Dad worked. While she was in high school, she went steady with a boy named Ralph who lived in the neighborhood. Although I liked Ralph, they would not have made a good couple, because both of them were very accident prone. He almost knocked Susie out while he was swinging his arm to start a snowmobile, then, he knocked Susie right down, and gave her a black eye with his elbow. Another time, he was putting up a ceiling fan, and it fell, and chipped his tooth. He did let me trim his sideburns, once, and cut them too short for his taste! When Susie and Ralph broke up, he began dating Susie's friend. A few years later, I met his 200 pound, very friendly, St. Bernard who almost broke my leg while being friendly. Ralph, eventually, became an airplane mechanic.

BY THE GRACE OF GOD AND YOU
A Chair Does Not a Person Make

Carthage went very fast in 1971, and on June 11, 1971, my story, along with several other people with disabilities, was placed into the Washington DC Committee for the Handicapped DPI (Department of Public Instruction) booklet with a note from the executive secretary to me stating, "Your story is a joy. We admire you, and appreciate you. Wish we could be school kids again. We'd come to Kenosha."

The article read:

Miss Carol Schaufel has been in a wheelchair since she was four years old but she was able to pass a swimming test for her scout troop, the Sunbeams, even though she has Muscular Dystrophy and hasn't the strength or ability to exert the physical effort to swim. She did it by writing out all of the steps needed to swim like the position of arms and legs and how to breathe. Said she, "Wow, what a lot of writing that was."

It is the unusual determination of Carol Schaufel that makes her story worthy of being told so that others who are afflicted from this disease, which is incurable at the present, can take heart and get cracking at something they can do to make themselves happy and their lives useful.

Carol Schaufel lives in Kenosha, Wisconsin. She is a graduate of mathematics Magna Cum Laude (3.77 GPA) from Carthage College with a minor in sociology. Now she teaches at Carthage. Her education began in the Orthopedic School in Kenosha then onto Bradford and Tremper, two public high schools. In the fall of 1965 she started two years of college at the University of Wisconsin in Kenosha but later transferred to Carthage College.

Considering the fact that she is confined to a wheelchair and can pick up only one book at a time, her teaching abilities are remarkable. She cannot push a wheelchair so she has one that is propelled by electricity. Although she uses an overhead projector from her desk which projects what she writes in front of her onto a screen behind her, she also gets her students involved by having them do blackboard work that she cannot handle, having them open doors for her, and having them set up equipment too heavy for her to manage.

Miss Schaufel had first decided to go into speech therapy as a profession, but it was pointed out to her that there was much physical effort required and she had to give up that dream. In changing her schools from the University of Wisconsin to Carthage she changed her major to math. This presented some problems because it was necessary for her to learn the basics of her new major as well as to participate in the advanced classes simultaneously.

But, she made it.

She loves to travel and has been in 27 states, Canada and Mexico. She has also learned to write Braille and use basic sign language for the deaf.

Her success is due to her desire to help people and when it was suggested that she go into research, she declined and chose teaching because she loves people and wants to be with them and not separated as she would be by doing research.

During her teaching career she has learned a great philosophical truth, "that the first ones to offer their help were the ones people called 'longhairs' and troublemakers," and she

64

says further: "I thought I would have quite a bit of trouble getting a job because of the stories I had heard from other handicapped people, however, I found I didn't have half as much trouble finding a job as those of a 'normal' Carthage grad."

This was one of the first articles about me. Education concerning disabilities was still yet to be addressed. The article implied that I was "confined to a wheelchair", when in reality, the wheelchair set me free! I'm not bound to it, but I do depend upon it! The word "handicapped" actually comes from having a "handy cap" on the head, and was used for begging. A human is not a "disabled person", but is only a human with a disability, and everyone is a person first! They have changed the meanings of many words over the years. I, personally, never liked it when "challenged" was used, because my list of "challenges" would have been never-ending. I would be "vertically" challenged (short), "gravitationally" challenged (heavy), "physically" challenged (lack of strength), transportation challenged (couldn't drive), and other disagreeable terms. I really thought the word, "crippled", was distasteful. For me, that meant deformed.

Besides my teaching duties, Fred was ordained in June of 1971. My parents and I went to the ordination. When we got to him in line, he stepped down off the platform where he was standing, and gave us a Lutheran blessing. He always said that Lutherans were more Catholic than Catholics, in those days, and everything was in a state of change. It was good to see him again, because I hadn't seen him in about two years! It was a friendship that was important to me, and I wanted to keep.

I also worked on a committee for an Orthopedic School Alumni Reunion. Once we did all the work for the reunion, we also kept all of the names and addresses to start a social group for people with disabilities—a place where they could socialize, swim, or play cards.

This article was in the *Kenosha News* to give more background:

June 12, 1971 *Orthopedic Alumni Reunion First in 61 Year History*
organized by Louise Cooper, Dorothy Orth, Harriet Bardosy, Roberta Hall, Larry Roach, and Carol Schaufel.

Alumni Association hopes to arrange social gatherings such as splash parties, card parties and other kinds of recreational evenings for those who need special facilities-history was noted and provided by Mrs. Arthur BEMIS who attended the former open-air school in 1915 as one of its first students and who is the oldest known living alumnus.

The school had its beginnings under a tent at the Frank school, closing at Christmas time and reopening in the spring. The pupils included some who had been discharged from tuberculosis sanitaria and who attended the open-air school as a halfway measure before attending regular school. All were Eskimo-like and were wrapped in blankets, with heated stones at their feet. Kenosha "won" its open-air school in a contest conducted by the Wisconsin Anti-Tuberculosis Society. According to Mrs. BEMIS' research, the society offered equipment for such a school in a city of 15,000 population or larger that sold the most Christmas Seals.

Mrs. Mary D Bradford, then superintendent of schools, directed the local school children's participation, and Kenosha won the contest. The school was then moved to second floor quarters in the DEWEY building on 57th St. In the next few years, the school moved to the Bain School and later to the Washington Junior High School property.

The word Orthopedic became attached to the name of the Open-Air School in the middle 1920s, when the city learned it had 155 children who needed such a school if they were to get an education. The Orthopedic Open-Air School was dedicated in 1929 in the new location near the Jefferson School (above Washington Bowl). It remained there until it was housed in the wing of the Jane Vernon School in 1961.

When we were starting to track down former alumni of the orthopedic school, I met a feisty 10-year-old girl, named Denise, who worked on the project with us. She was small in stature, and used a walker very slowly due to her cerebral palsy. She was as smart as a whip, and helped out with a lot of work. To this day, she does a lot of work behind the scenes for different people and organizations. Her smiling face, and positive demeanor, inspired me. We would meet to go over some of the records and names. We found an old orthopedic school scrapbook. It was a lot of fun. Many of the students had passed away, but the party included well over 100 people. There were still some people we never found, and we were wondered what happened to them. Randy was one of these, and I knew that he had joined the service. Louise heard from his Mother only once during the years.

My sister, Susie, and I, also planned another party this year, since it was my parents' 25th wedding anniversary! Ralph's parents owned the Starlite Tavern down the street from our house, and we rented their banquet room for the party. We started our party plans, and planned for about 125 people! Mom wanted to make most of the food, and her friends helped her! She thought the whole thing would cost about $35, but it totaled about $800 when all was said and done! We hired my school friend, Frankie's band. For some reason, he started giggling when the band played *Take the Ribbons from Her Hair.* He was laughing so hard he couldn't sing which spread to the dancers who were laughing so hard they couldn't dance! One of my Dad's coworkers provided the centerpiece which was made out of $25 worth of quarters, having a huge heart around the number 25 with a semicircular staircase made of quarters also. We bought an oil painting as a gift for the living room! Everyone danced, even after the band stopped playing. I think it was my friend Les from camp that took a movie at the event. After everything was over, Mom and Toots (Diane's Mom) were still dancing the polka! Janie, my Mom's closest friend, made Mom her favorite Italian anise cookies. I'm sure Mom probably ate them while she was dancing that last dance!

That year, the Muscular Dystrophy Association discovered that a combination of chiffon margarine and safflower oil helped mice with Muscular Dystrophy to regain some muscle strength. So, for the first time, I went to an MDA doctor in Madison. Dr. Peters was an excellent doctor. He took some tests by sticking needles into my muscles and into my nerves. He wanted to take a muscle sample out of the back of my ankle for some testing, but Mom asked me if I really wanted to do that while we were waiting for the needle test results. She said, "The test might give you a specific diagnosis, since there are several disabilities under the umbrella of Muscular Dystrophy, but it won't change your situation." I decided that I didn't want to get the test. I did not want the pain of healing when I had not been healing that fast.

The doctor reported, as expected, that my limitations were more in my nerves than in my muscles. He explained.

"It acts a lot like polio, but polio cannot be contracted in the womb."

Another interesting fact was that intelligence seemed to come with my particular symptoms. It seemed to balance off with what the person can't do physically.

Mom kiddingly replied, "Dad was surprised because he thought your intelligence came from him!"

The doctor continued.

"Carol is not a good candidate for the treatment you are inquiring about, but a back brace might be helpful for her to give her lungs and heart more room to function."

I did not hear the part about the lungs and heart. I heard I would be taller, and have a figure! I wanted to try that.

We returned to Madison early one morning to get fitted for my brace. They set me on top of a small, tall stool on which it was hard to balance. The stool was under a swing-like device which they put under my chin to hoist me into the air. It straightened my back as much as possible until I was maybe 1/4 inch off of the stool. Then they put some type of gauze cloth on me, and plastered my body from the middle of my chest to my hips. It took about 20 minutes to dry, so I literally "hung around" until it did. My chin was a little numb. When we were done, I was sent home for three weeks, and returned, again, to try on the brace. It was definitely not as comfortable as the first time when I was hanging from my chin. It was a very hard material. From the minute I put it on, I had bruises. At home, I healed, and tried it again. It never worked for me. I had a very awkward figure with the brace, but it was mainly the bruising. It was the inability to drive my wheelchair from the angle in which I was sitting that made me decide to throw it away. Mom was happy, and thought it looked very grotesque. She hated looking at it. Maybe I would have fewer years on this earth, because of squashed lungs and heart, but at least I would be comfortable, and able to do more while I was here.

Health and life insurance were becoming my biggest problem. I was covered under my Dad's policy until I graduated from college. I never knew that funds were available for me through SSI, or even medical benefits, simply because I thought that I would be working. With the diagnosis of Muscular Dystrophy, health insurance was out of the question unless I had a job where there were more than 30 employees, and then, the insurance company did not ask questions about individuals. I was not covered under health insurance while I taught at Carthage, because it was part-time work.

Life insurance, on the other hand, was a whole other issue. The diagnosis gave me an automatic answer of "No" with the exception of Kemper Insurance who provided a scale of benefits. For instance, if I lived one year, I would get 20% of the value of the policy, two years 40%, three years, 50%, and so on until the 6th year, and I would get 100%.

When a person becomes an adult, a disability doesn't go away. Everything was so different, and things just became more difficult because I was bigger, taller, and heavier. It was a good thing I did not have to be lifted anymore. I still needed the care of a child, so it was often difficult to be seen as an adult. I was 22 years-old before I even began thinking of dating, curfews, and rebellion - something that most did at the ages of 14 to 16 years-old!

~ 9 ~

Easter Seals Camps

During those last three summers, I went back to Easter Seals Camp. This time, the camps helped me grow tremendously. I was not so afraid, and was more independent. I was in the 21, and older, adult group, and mid-July was much warmer. It was nice being in a place where I could help others as much as they would help me. Some of the campers couldn't write their own postcards. I could do that for some of them. Many had no speech, but would spell out a word using talking boards with an alphabet on sturdy paper, or a full sized wheelchair tray. But, if they couldn't do that, they would point to pictures. Mary, who was about three years ahead of me, was from Orthopedic School, and we became great friends! Mary who had cerebral palsy, and used the baby buggy for balance, no longer used it. Now, she wasn't even using a walker, or a quad cane (a cane with four feet on it). Her speech was cumbersome to understand, but her eyes, and behavior told everyone exactly what she was thinking. Together, we conjured up a lot of trouble! At one point, she got mad at me, and pushed my whole bed (and me) into the shower. She was laughing all the way thinking of her diabolical midnight plot! Fortunately, the counselor (personal care attendant) saved me before Mary turned the water on, or the bed would have been ruined! Mary and I would talk all night, or at least until 3:00 a.m. I crashed for four hours, before everyone got up to a recorded trumpet reveille on the loud speaker system.

The counselors were all college students, helping us have a good time, and they were same age as the Easter Seals campers. I sat at the table of a counselor named Les, who was a Jay Leno look-alike with lighter colored hair. He became a very good friend. Mary always used an apron as a bib, and a plate guard so food wouldn't fall off of her plate. Les would cut up her meat, and inconspicuously tie her to her dining chair with her apron. When Mary would stand up, she would take the whole chair with her, laughing hard, then shook her fist at him looking at her watch to indicate that she did not have time for this!

There were some great cookouts. The counselors would split up the work according to what the camper could do. I put the butter on the sliced potatoes, before they went onto the grill. For breakfast, we would have anything from French toast to omelets in a pan on the grill. Lunch might be hot dogs, hamburgers, grilled cheese, or brats. Dinners included hobo packs of hamburger, potatoes and carrots, or a pot of stew. Occasionally, a ketchup and mustard fight would ensue. No one cared what your disability was, but you sure weren't excluded from the fight!

Kool-Aid, cookies, and medications were also staples on our trips. If we were on an overnight, besides packing the food, we would pack sleeping bags, bed pans, or whatever we needed. We would be loaded onto a big, wooden ramped wagon which was towed by a tractor. The wagon could hold up to 12 people in wheelchairs along with about the same amount of people on the two side bench seats. For every six campers, there would be one, or two counselors, and it depended upon the specific care needs of the individuals. The outhouses, small and they stunk, caused the counselors the most problems, especially with the people that had little muscle control, or campers that needed two man-lifts. One camper, who had Cerebral palsy, was lifted off one of the two seated holes. During a front side, one man-lift—a standing up of the individual, and a turn into the wheelchair, a muscle spasm occurred, and flipped the camper's foot into the air causing his tennis shoe to fly off into the second hole—it is still there! No one was going to pull that shoe out of that hole!

We always had something to do. We would sing, share, play cards, participated in chess tournaments, and watched Indian ceremonials, which didn't scare me any more, heard the grand old Opry singers from the Wisconsin Dells, created amateur shows, participated in dances, and shopped, especially for the Dells' famous fudge. We also were alerted to kindling romances of both counselors, and campers, etc. Card playing was made possible for many by either a cardholder (a piece of wood that had slightly angled slits to hold cards), or an upside down box (where cards were held between the bottom and the cover). Some people used mouthsticks, and would flip out the right card, or someone would reach a card for them. The counselors usually had the job of shuffling and dealing because not many of us were good at that. Sheepshead is an old, complicated German/Wisconsin card game, and was my favorite. My favorite activities were sun-tanning, the pool, shopping, relaxing and eating, respectively.

Dances could become a little tricky too. About 20% of the campers were in wheelchairs at that time, and most of the wheelchairs were manual, while 80% of the campers could walk in some way with prosthetics, crutches, or walkers. Some needed no devices at all, but people had to push the chairs. (Progressively, more of the campers were using motorized wheelchairs, so now the camp has about 90% of the campers in motorized wheelchairs. More people also had more than one disability now). Some of the counselors were good at controlling the motorized wheelchairs at the same time they were dancing. Others would turn the motorized chairs into manual mode to push them around. I had one friend in a motorized wheelchair that could drive my electric chair at the same time he drove his. It really looked graceful and realistic, but it took a little practice! We would get eight of the motorized wheelchairs together, and we performed circle eight, as well as other fancy moves like the Shriners did with their miniature cars. Our only mistake was that we did it by the swimming pool, and we were afraid a new driver, Amos, would end up in the water.

My first time riding a horse was great. There was a ramp with a flat surface at the top, equal to the height of the horse, so it was like being slid (a two-man lift with one person in front and one in back) from the wheelchair to the horse. I was surprised that I could sit up pretty well on the horse. The director, Guy Wharton, sat behind me. Guy gave me the balance I needed, like sitting on a chair instead of a horse. It was a good experience. The next year, and the second horse I tried riding, was very heavy. My legs were spread so far apart, that I couldn't sit up at all. I just laid my head down on her. I bet the horse thought, "What in the heck is this! Someone tell her how to ride!" There were some things that were worth trying again and again, and others where once was enough. I should have stopped after the first horse.

BY THE GRACE OF GOD AND YOU
A Chair Does Not a Person Make

I loved the swimming pool—not that I looked very good in a swimming suit! The counselors found out that I could float, and it was probably, because my muscles couldn't tense up, and had fat in them. I could float anywhere. Someone could stand on top of me to get me on the bottom of the pool. When they would get off, I would come to the surface quickly, like a rocket launch. I would probably make a good lifesaver for someone someday. After two days in the water, I could hold my breath for three minutes, and "porpoise" my way, by moving my hips up and down, across the pool. I had two problems: I couldn't turnover by myself, so someone would have to watch when I started shaking my head to turn me over as breathing was important. I always had to have nose plugs as I couldn't keep the water out of my nose, or I would choke. If I would lie on my back, or use a snorkel while I was on my stomach, I could stay alone for long periods of time. If I tried to swim on my back, my spine curvature would make me go in circles.

There was a group of my friends that always sat on the steps in the shallow end of the pool. It was called *The Chicken Corner*. I would visit there once in a while, but most of the time, I liked the deep end of the pool, and since I could float, it didn't matter how much water was underneath me. Another favorite was exercising on the deep end ladder. Movement in the water was so much easier! (I always wanted to volunteer for a space mission—no gravity)!

Trying surface diving equipment in the pool was a little scary. It took a little time to get used to the breathing apparatus. Once I was under the water, it was fun, but I felt very isolated in that mask. It felt like I was in a different room where the air did not move freely.

The only thing I didn't try in the pool, was the canoe. Whenever there was a canoe trip set up for "real waters," staff would get up early in the morning to have the campers get the feel of the canoes at 6 a.m. Staff would put on campers' lifejackets, get them comfortable in the canoe, describe to the camper what would happen if the canoe tipped, and then tipped them out in the pool. The lifejackets would flip them on their backs, and counselors would come to get them.

I was always surprised at how much people with severe disabilities could do in the pool if they weren't afraid to try it. A camper named Steve, who had no voice, and difficulty straightening himself up, would slowly work his way out of his wheelchair to get out to the end of the diving board. He would slowly straighten, and dive into the pool. Most of the time, he had no problem, but the lifeguard was always watching. If he would get into trouble on the bottom of the pool, he would hold his pointer finger straight in the air (I mean water), so the lifeguard would come in after him. He had remarkable courage!

Another camper, who always astonished me, was Agatha. She was on crutches for balance, because her feet turned backwards. It made my feet hurt when looking at them.

The various accents of the Foreign Exchange counselors made it fun to speak to them. A flashlight was a "torch" for people from England, and "cookies" were biscuits. One girl from Australia was really embarrassed when the staff had to pass out bedtime "meds", because they were Kotex or tampons—something just not spoken about in front of men. I thought the funniest thing I came across was when my counselor from Japan was going to help me with the bathroom. I asked her to get the stool that I could lean on it to use the commode in my wheelchair. She was a medical student, and just didn't understand the word "stool". When I showed it to her, she busted out laughing. To her, "stool" was a feces specimen! The Easter Seals stores sold products made by people who had disabilities, and this made me think of one of those items. One item was a tiny, wooden stool, about a half-inch high, and placed into a miniature cylindrical, clear case that I bought, and gave to my doctor. It was called "a stool sample". And, now that I think about it, my doctor has not asked me for a stool sample since I gave it to him!

A lot of the previous campers visited the camp on Wednesdays, because they had started a social group named Wisconsin Wawbeek Associated Activities Club, which they named after the camp, or WWAAC for short. The group met twice a year. Once in the fall, when the members held a meeting, a banquet, and a dance in a hotel somewhere in the state of Wisconsin, and again, in the Spring for a business meeting which included choosing an individual for a personal achievement award, giving memorial funds to Easter Seals, and banquet details. A person by the name of Donnell signed me up as a member. I have attended banquets from that year until today.

At camp, you could be yourself. No one worried how they looked, or what others were thinking, because you were trying something that the majority of the world would think you couldn't, or shouldn't do. It was always like a little piece of heaven to many, including me, where anyone could go out alone into the forest, and feel safe. It was the first time I touched a tree! It seemed like there were no games. People just said what they meant. Getting inside everyone's thoughts, especially when they couldn't speak, was so interesting and heartwarming.

Steve, a counselor, became a good friend at camp. Before he was hired, he had no clue what people with disabilities could, and couldn't do. He was even surprised that he was going to have to assist with bathroom time. He just soaked up everything about every disability, and asked a lot of questions. He was the only counselor that I remembered who was never off, and who never took a break. He was always out there doing something!

As a special note about camp: I was always impressed by the directors of Easter Seals camps. I can't think of one of them that didn't get right in there, and work just as hard as all the staff with lifting, personal care, or whatever was needed.

Steve and Les became roommates in Milwaukee, and came down to visit me often. Sometimes we would go to places like the Sears Tower where people looked like ants from the 105th floor, or Chicago History Museum. Sometimes, we would go to a play in Milwaukee, or Chicago, and sometimes, my parents would go with us. We saw musicals with older stars such as Van Johnson in *Kismet*, Claudette Colbert in *Marriage-Go-Round*, and Leonard Nimoy in *The King and I*. Leonard split his pants dancing that day, and they came down a few times on New Year's Eve.

Steve became a physical therapist, and worked at the VA hospital in Milwaukee for a while. He would always shock me with some of the stories. Veterans were dying from lung cancer, but would continue smoking through their tracheotomies was just one of them. It reminded me, again, that I was not afraid of death, but I wasn't into the pain caused by the dying part. I was afraid of that!

Les wrote beautiful, long letters weekly that taught me a lot about him as well as myself. In person, Les was so funny, and the life of the party. He seemed to have no serious side. People could be so complicated! Both Steve and Les were very good friends. Les was the driver, and was how I learned to share in the cost of gas. There were a lot of things I would never have learned if someone had not explained things to me, since I had never had the experience personally. Les became a rehabilitation counselor, and he was a great influence for my future career.

June, a friend, was also at camp, again. She was in a motorized wheelchair with a disability under Muscular Dystrophy. I had been in a manual chair when I was in kids' session. Interestingly enough, she had a friend in California who wanted to become a teacher, but the DVR counselor in California said that it would be impossible. She became a speech therapist! How ironic. Her friend and I had the same disability, and the same limitations, yet we were lead in opposite directions from our original job goals. I started writing to June's friend for a while just to see how things were going. She really liked her job, and could do it.

I was happy I changed to teaching, and was excited to get out in the real world on my own. I felt my first year of teaching went really well. Miss Konsin was back so Carthage was out. I had an interview set up for the day after camp with the Kenosha Unified School District. I had one interview already with a small school system in Winthrop Harbor, Illinois. It was about six miles from my house, but it did not have a good feel. It wasn't a good match. I did not really try in that interview, but the interview gave me some ideas on how I would act in my next one.

~ 10 ~

Job Interviews and First Year

Mom was a great alarm on the morning of my interview, even though I was tired. For the last two weeks at camp, I slept about four hours a night. This was not a good way to go to a job interview. Mom dressed me, and put me into my chair by a new, sliding method, so that she could assist me out of bed by herself, and into my wheelchair. Mom took the side off my wheelchair, which was parallel to the bed, put my back towards the chair, placed the hard seat of my wheelchair halfway under me, and halfway onto the chair. She pulled me onto the chair with the seat, and spun me around. Then, we put the side of the wheelchair back on the chair. Getting up and ready to leave home took about one hour. I never ate breakfast.

I grabbed a copy of my completed resume. Unlike most people who presented resumes, I added something after the basics of name, address, and phone number. I put "uses motorized wheelchair, neuromuscular disease, and good health." I knew that being in a wheelchair would make me different. I wanted them to know that up front, because I did not want them to be surprised or uncomfortable. I had good references from within the school system, and now I had experience. I was tired from camp, but I was ready to go. After reading an article in a magazine for people with disabilities, I surmised there would be an interview question on my health, which I answered on my resume. I would need equipment to assist me for teaching including fire drills and safety information.

I was in the principal's office, waiting for Mr. Saksvig. Whenever I was nervous, like in a dentist's office, I would always yawn. When I was at the dentist's office, I would always remain in my wheelchair. I only took a painkiller - once - when he pulled my molar. I was just so tired, I knew that I had to fight it, or I would look disinterested in the job for which I was applying. Thank goodness, I didn't have to wait long!

A short time later, the principal came out of his office, and held out his hand to shake mine. I lifted up my left hand, since my right hand was driving. I didn't want Mr. Saksvig to feel awkward. He shook my hand, and he assured me that they had looked at the information from my placement file at Carthage, and was impressed. When I was student teaching, I think the principal may have spoken to him as well. In those days, there was no American's with Disabilities Act, so an interviewer could ask anything in terms of my disability. In consequence, I believed that if a person didn't know *how* I did a job, I wasn't going to *get* the job.

BY THE GRACE OF GOD AND YOU
A Chair Does Not a Person Make

Some of the questions I was asked:

Because I was in a wheelchair, was I going to be sick a lot?
What would I do in case of emergency?
How would I handle fire drills and discipline?
What accommodations would I need?
What would I do if I dropped a pencil?

I answered the questions as they were asked.

Was I going to be sick a lot?
I anticipated, "I am seldom sick. I do not anticipate missing days."

That was the wrong answer! That year was very different from my college years where I had not been sick at all. Kids carried, and spread, totally different germs to which I had never been exposed. I used all 10 of my sick days that first year, and probably could have used more. I even received a flu shot for the first time, but still had the flu twice! I lost 14 pounds in two weeks, and will never get a flu shot again!

How would I handle an emergency? I was so very tired, I couldn't think on my feet - or should I say "seat?"
I squinted, "Gee, what would you do in an emergency?"
Recovering, I told him "I don't think anyone knows what one would do in an emergency, but because I have to deal with so many little crises all the time, like not being able to reach something I need, I'm sure I would stay calm until everything was over, and then I would probably fall apart."

Mr. Saksvig asked the next question.

"How would you handle fire drills?"
I answered, "I would need a first-floor classroom. I would ask one student to close the windows, and everyone else to leave the classroom in single file, proceeding to the designated exit out of the building. The last student out of the classroom would be asked to turn off the light, and close the door."

"What accommodations would I need besides a first-floor classroom?"
I responded, "I would need an overhead projector cut into the center of the six foot table like there was in the dining hall."

Every teacher had access to an overhead projector, and the cost of the table was about $20. I thought the hardest thing to get would be the first-floor classroom.

"What would I do if I dropped a pencil?"

I thought that was an unusual question, but it probably came from my comment on "little crises."

I answered, "I understand there will be about 30 students in each classroom. I thought one of them could pick it up for me, but I could always keep several extra pencils on my desk as I would need to do the same thing with transparency pens."

The principal added "and how will you handle discipline?"

That was a tough question. I had handled classrooms before, but not junior high students.

I answered, "I would treat students with the respect that I would want them to give me in return. I would not discipline in front of the group. I would get the parent involved if appropriate, and try to find out what was causing the problem as sometimes the problem is not in the classroom."

After the principal was finished with his questions, he asked me if I had any questions. I asked some questions about the grade level, and the specific classes I would be teaching.

He told me, "I was thinking about that myself. In general, I think ninth grade would be the ideal grade for you to teach. This particular job opening is for seventh and eighth grades. I really want to hire you, not only because of your qualifications, but I know that Bullen is the perfect school for its accessibility. The only time you would have to go upstairs is for the library, or faculty meetings. I am 90% sure I will have a ninth grade opening in two, or three weeks, right before school starts. I would like to see you take that job instead of this one. In the seventh grade, the girls start liking boys, and in the eighth grade, the boys start liking girls. They are little harder to handle, and more squirrelly. By ninth grade, most everyone has made the decision to be good, or bad, and a lot of those who have chosen bad, you didn't see very often."

Personally, I was hoping for a high school position, but there really were no openings anticipated for several years. I agreed to wait. He indicated I would need to interview, again.

I was called a week before school started, interviewed again, and was offered the job. In the meantime, the principal was working on a first-floor classroom. One of the other math teachers agreed to move upstairs. I was all set to teach four "algebra 1" classes, algebra one was a general algebra class which was divided into two parts, and one was an eighth grade general math class. I would have 5 classes with about 150 students - 30 in each class.

~ Teaching Ninth Grade ~

When I began teaching at Bullen, it was in its third year of existence. We had about 20 busloads of students who came from the surrounding areas - farms, a poorer city area comprised of African Americans, and a trailer court across the street where many of the residents were Hispanic. By the time I started teaching, the school had calmed down. One of my early training sessions explained some of the differences in the cultural backgrounds. The things that stood out the most in my mind were the difference in personal space. Hispanic people always stood closer to people than white people. White people felt comfortable at a four-foot distance between one another, where a three-foot, or less distance, was more acceptable to African Americans and Hispanics.

Hispanics liked details of stories; whites liked the punch line, because they are always in a hurry. Many Hispanics were taught it was not respectable to look their elders in the eyes while whites felt the person must be lying if a person didn't look them in the eye. There were so many things to learn. Respect was so important. Just like with disabilities, I always knew people were people first.

I was excited about my first year teaching contract, and I signed for $9600. This was an okay salary for 1971. I did not have much time to become nervous, since I was to begin working a few days after I signed the paperwork. I was assigned a classroom that was right next to an exit which was great for fire drills! What could I anticipate? I had so much to learn, and so much to do before the first day.

I also discovered that the teacher, who had traded rooms with me so I could have a first-floor classroom, had a prosthetic leg. I don't remember how Phonzie lost his leg, but I know it was when he was very young. He used to play basketball with it. I thought it was cute when Phonzie told me was that when the students got mad at him, they would say, "I hope you get termites in your leg!"

Mom helped me set up my classroom, which was on the South side of the building. In the meantime, Dad brought my second wheelchair to school locking it in the janitor's closet which was located on the North side of the building, where there was a close place to park the car, so that I could enter the school easily. The bulletin board in the back of the room covered the same space as the four blackboards in the front of the room. I had a lot of bulletin boards, and we started with the back of the room. Across the top in the center of this huge bulletin board, I put, "Algebra Is a Language." Underneath this, I separated the space across the back of the room to include "THE WORDS" which were letters, and numbers, cut out from stencils. "THE PHRASES" were, "2x +5 and 6 – x. "PUNCTUATIONS" like parentheses and brackets. "THE VERBS," math signs like +,-, x and ÷. "THE SENTENCES" were completed with =, >, =, ≠, etc. altogether creating e.g. 2x +5 (6 - x) - 8= 7x - 3x +2 (3x - 2). The front blackboard had a strip across the top that was a bulletin board. I filled this bulletin board with a few palindromes. I used numbers, names, or sentences that read the same forward as backward like 21012, Otto, or "Step on no pets." I also checked to make sure I had enough books for each student. I received five class lists, and a gradebook, as well as paperwork for my lesson plans.

There was a staff meeting with over 70 people, and when it was over, I went back to my classroom. Wow, this was *my classroom*! Mom had finished the bulletin boards, so we walked outside for a break just to check out the exit close to my room. It was perfectly flat, and very easy to navigate. Going back into the building, however, I saw some graffiti on the door, and was obviously missed by the custodian. Of all the swear words on the door, there was one I did not know. I asked Mom what it meant.

"Mom, what does 'pussy' mean?"

No one was around, but she turned red, and whispered, "Sh! I'll tell you later!"

Have you ever heard of Murphy's Law? Like, 'the best laid plans get stuck in the copy machine" or "if there were three main events happening in a month, they would all fall on the same day and time?" Well, that was about to happen to me. In 1972, I was Vice President of a group called ABLE. All summer long, we collected signatures to get the "curb cuts", or ramped corners, bill passed. (More about this later.) We collected 9000 signatures in Kenosha! But, the date the bill was to be put before the Legislature was scheduled for the same day as my first day of teaching! I couldn't call in sick, yet I needed to be in Madison. I discussed this with my principal, and received verbal permission to go while a substitute teacher took over for me. I was already set for the first day, and had set up my seating charts, and a review test to find out my students basic skills, so the substitute would have no problem. It was a good thing I handled the situation right as our group, and others who joined us, were on all of the local television channels presenting the signatures, and the Bill passed!

The second day of school was really my first, I introduced myself in a serious, no-nonsense manner, which led to very few discipline problems that first year. While the students were correcting their test from the day before after a short review, I started memorizing the names on my seating charts, so when my third day came, I could at least call everybody by their first name without looking at the chart.

On one of the review tests, I noticed that one person could not subtract. To find out why, I watched her do a few problems. She was working from left to right instead of right to left. We corrected it, and she worked better for the rest of the year. Knowing my students better was important to me, so, I had them design a "Coat of Arms". Splitting a shield into four sections, I asked them to choose a picture, or words, and answer each of the following questions:

1. What is the most important thing in your life?
2. What would you do with $1 million?
3. Write three words that describe you.
4. What do you want out of life?

Of course, the pictures on their shields were varied. Some drew doves for peace. Some, pictures of their family. Some, a dollar sign. Some drew a marijuana leaf. It was most interesting how they described themselves. Some were very positive, and some negative. Lonely was not a description I expected to hear. This exercise was very helpful. I could see the students' artistic abilities and creativity, as well as the lack of foresight, or disinterest. For many, it was a good thing that neatness didn't count.

My wheelchair also helped keep discipline for the first few weeks. By the time the students got used to me, discipline was set. One student had even told me that her parents believed that "all people in wheelchairs were mentally retarded, so I had difficult time learning from you at first." Feedback from parents gave me an indication on the progress of teaching and learning with their son, or daughter. For most students, I thought I did okay, but there was always someone that you could not assist due to fear of the subject matter, lack of time, or disinterest in the subject. I told students that I would be calling their homes. I tried to call everyone that first year within the first few months to give parents a little feedback, to encourage a student to do better, e.g., how helpful the student was, or how much he/she was progressing. I tried not to make phone calls on difficult students, although I did send an occasional one to the office. I found that a few of the parents were working, or thought, "The child is in school. He/she is your problem now." That was always sad to me. It made me appreciate, even more, how great my parents were. Support at all ages was needed from parents.

I tried to do some things which would make math more interesting and relevant for students. When I was teaching averages, I asked the teachers to give me their weight and sex on a piece of paper, so that we could find the "average male" teacher, and "average female" teacher's weight in the school. I withheld all the names, although the students found it fun to try to guess whose weight was whose. The teachers thought it was fun to participate. The average weight of the winning teachers was shared. The names of the closest teacher to the average male and female weights were announced on the loudspeaker.

I decided to move my students to different seats every quarter. There were usually a few that needed to sit in the front, because of special vision, or hearing concerns. The second quarter each year, I would take a blank seating chart, tell the students how the desks were going to be numbered, and take a pair of different colored dice, and we would talk about the odds of students shaking the number 7 compared to the odds of shaking a number 2, or 12. The students stood along the wall, and one by one, I would shake the dice. Those with special needs shook one die for the first front row of seats. As the desks filled up, the person would have to continually shake in order to find an empty seat. When everyone was sitting again, I considered myself lucky, because there was only one time friends happen to be sitting together! If students complained about where they were sitting, I just told them that they shouldn't gamble! Remember, I lost once too—but my odds for 'winning' were better.

I tried to make things interesting by having students choose a share of stock from the Stock Market at the beginning of the year - one for each that the student thought would make the most money. At Christmas, the class would look at the stock to see who would have made the most money, and with some guesses on why that particular stock made money—what was happening in that season, or in the world.

When I was sick, I would have a cough and trouble talking. I would use the overhead projector, and not talk at all. I would write a problem, so students could see it on the screen behind me, and then, write a name for a specific student to come up, and solve the problem. If that person was right, I would draw a smiley face. If they were wrong, I would draw a sad face. If the next person was wrong, I would draw a mad face! If the next person was wrong, I would just draw a hangman! I wasn't sure if this was going to work, but thankfully, it did. The students were a little noisier, but engaged in learning! Students commented that I talked too fast. They told me I was easier to understand when I was sick and taking medication!

That first year of teaching went very smooth. I even had time to update the school's student handbook, adding a history on the person the school was named after, and the name origin of the city of Kenosha.

I also had a chance to go to a new teacher dinner that was held for the district in our community at the Elks club. I didn't think it would be a good idea to go with my parents, so my cousin Bill took me, instead. I was grateful for it, because I knew I was going to need some kind of help with eating. Bill had to take me up about six stairs.

My parents also drove me to a second social event that was at one of the new teacher's homes. I was always a very quiet person, and liked listening more than talking. Socializing wasn't easy for me. To my surprise, the party was in the basement, so I was carried down the stairs in my manual wheelchair, and it wasn't that bad. However, getting me *up the stairs* after everyone had been drinking was scary! Mike was strong and pretty stable, and took the front of the wheelchair. The vice principal, a little shorter and rounder, took the handlebars. Even though I was not heavy, then, it was still a struggle going up those stairs. My head fell back, and my wig slid off a little, but thank goodness, it did not fall off! We made it safely up the stairs, but it discouraged me from going to future parties. I never wanted anyone to lift my wheelchair, unless it was absolutely necessary. I would have felt awful if somebody was hurt. The manual chairs were probably 40 to 60 pounds, and a motorized chair was well over 230 pounds without me in it.

In morning homeroom, the one comment I always heard from students was "How come we have to say the Pledge of Allegiance?" *The National Anthem* was sung at football games, baseball games, etc., and every other sporting event. My take on it was: "Wasn't saying the Pledge of Allegiance easier than singing *The National Anthem?*" I also believed that the students needed to start thinking about the meaning of words.

When I had the second hour of the day off, and to keep busy, I would help MaryAnn in the office to alphabetize the absentee cards, so she could type up the list. After about four months of helping, Virginia, another lady who worked in the office, asked me to put something in a teacher's mailbox. I took the item to the mailboxes, and realized the box that I needed was on the very top, and there was no way I could reach it. My mail box was on the bottom. I took the mail back to her. Virginia was embarrassed, because she knew I couldn't reach it, but she was so used to me doing everything else that she forgot! I thought that was a compliment!

Mailboxes were little drawers. The first time I got my paycheck, I was so happy! For about three months after, I would forget when it was payday. What a surprise to find a check every two weeks in that drawer! I never had to budget, or handle any money before, but I did give my parents $25 per week which was all they wanted to help cover food.

The last hour of the day, the teachers had to choose a group activity to do with students. At different times during the year, I would have the coin club, sign language, or the ninth grade dance. I had saved pennies since I was a little kid, and even had some Indianhead pennies as well as some buffalo nickels. I had a friend, Edith, who was deaf and going blind. She started her first job at the age of 63. Edith got me interested in sign language. She was able to come to our club meetings once in a while. Our club even signed to an original song another student wrote for our amateur show.

At the end of every year, the ninth graders had an end-of-the-year dance. We would raise money by selling suckers, or having carwashes. At one of our carwashes, a huge garbage truck "sailed" past us. I giggled, because all the kids hid their signs until it truck passed. The driver saw that they hid the signs, and he laughed too! We would use our fundraising money for the decorations and music. It was a dedicated group!

I wasn't good in the sports arena, however! I did work the scoreboard and buzzer for one of the basketball games. I didn't mess up, but it was very stressful! Once they were even short of a track judge. Three of the other teachers worked stopwatches for the runners, but my job was to see whose hand or foot came out in front of the others in the close races. It was a much harder job than it sounded! I didn't want that responsibility again! I hope I called the winners right!

This is the letter I received from my principal after my first year of evaluations, and three years were evaluated to become permanently on staff.

June 20, 1972

Dear Carol,

Now that the year is over, I hope you will sit back and give yourself a well-deserved pat on the back. As a teacher new to Bullen staff and to the profession, you have certainly done a fine job.

Your concern for students and the way you became involved in various school projects certainly was appreciated by me. The hours that you put in the ninth grade party went a long way to make it the success it was. I only hope you will continue to keep up your efforts and enthusiasm in the years to come.

Your experiences this year as a first-year teacher will certainly help to make your next years' exciting and rewarding. I know I'm looking forward to many years of working with you here at Bullen.

Sincerely,
Robert Saksvig

~ 11 ~

Teaching Years

My second year wasn't as easy for a number of reasons.

First, the year started out with a teacher strike. Being a new teacher, I did not know what to do. I had gone to some of the union meetings, but I didn't know a lot about the process. I thought that unions were definitely needed, and I joined, but some of things on the table just looked like extra stuff for the purpose of bargaining. It was the same thing from the school district as well. At the union meeting, I felt pressured, like I was getting an exaggerated story, but many people were happy with the deal. Anyway, I decided to cross the picket line, because I was still on probation. Mom wasn't happy about it. She thought she would have flat tires, as well as other things might happen. Inside the building, there were not many students. I didn't remember teaching any math classes, but I did teach physical education—volleyball. The strike was over in about three days, and I did feel a little backlash from some of the staff, but at the time, I felt that I did the right thing.

The first day of real classes of year two, I was not as strict. Discipline was still pretty good, but I knew that I really did not like a totally silent classroom. I liked a little bit of a "learning noise." I liked to know that if the students didn't understand, they could, sometimes, learn from each other. I continued to give students responsibilities in the classroom like passing out papers, or writing on the board.

Once a year, I would take students to the library to look up some math facts. For instance, why is a Baker's dozen 13? What is a fathom? If we looked at the original definition of a "yard", and had two students come up to the front of the room—one with long arms (George) and one was shorter arms (Holly) –where would a customer get the better bargain buying eight yards of material? Would George, or Holly need to be the business owner?

I was very afraid that the students would find out what I couldn't do, and take advantage of me in the first year. Once I could get rid of that fear, I knew I could give them the responsibility for their own learning. The first thing I did, I thought was very good. The second thing I did was a very stupid way to do a good thing.

The day before Christmas break, students never get much done. I decided on that day I would sit down with the class, and let them ask anything they wanted to know. Every question from why my hair didn't grow, because I wore a wig, to if I could have children was thrown at me. I was sure that I could have children, but because of my back, I didn't know how much room that I would have for a baby to grow. We talked about my wheelchair, and how much it cost. My first two were about $600 and $900. I paid for them myself, but the next one was $6000, and insurance paid 80 %. Then, how fast could my chair go? I told them about 6 mph. I also answered questions on some other disabilities. How did a person who was deaf know when her baby was crying? Just like with the doorbells, or telephones or alarm clocks, the baby monitors had flashing lights—the harder the baby would cry, the faster the light would flicker. We talked about how some people in wheelchairs could stand, but not necessarily walk. Sometimes, we would look at differences between guide dogs, service dogs, and hearing dogs. So, I explained that dogs for the blind are named after the school that the dog came from such as Guide Dogs, Leader Dogs, and Seeing-Eye Dogs. Service dogs assisted people with physical disabilities. People, who are deaf, or hard of hearing, have hearing dogs that behaviorally let their master know that the phone was ringing, or someone was at the door. Students seldom asked questions about learning disabilities, or alcohol and drugs, but occasionally, they did.

After the sharing sessions, I would learn a lot about the students as well. One African American student had indicated that he never had any problems in school getting along with anyone, but he felt sad, because white students never asked him to come to their house or parties.

Another student had been involved with someone who stole cars.

I asked him, "If someone ever stole my car, I couldn't use buses, or cabs, to get back and forth to work. It would cause a lot of problems."

The student responded from his heart, "I would never steal anything with special equipment, or children's toys in it. I know how hard that would be."

I guess even some criminals have ethics!

Some of my students were fifteen, and already had a child. One of my white students had two. Some were pregnant. One, who was African American, was an excellent student, but committed suicide by shooting herself in the vagina. Nothing hurt me as much as her death. It seemed that white individuals looked at abortion more often than African Americans who never considered it, and the baby would become part of the family.

Another one, who always seemed to be seeking attention, attempted suicide. He wasn't getting the attention at school, or at home, that he needed. Some people saw him as a nuisance. I saw him as lonely.

Students had to deal with so much besides my subject matter. Sylvia was a very quiet student who was Hispanic. About the third month of school, I noted that her grades slipped from an A to an F in her work. She was always polite, and spoke with no accent. I found out that she did not understand English. How was the teacher supposed to know what the student needed if the teacher had never been told? How did I miss it?

Allowing questions to be asked of me seemed to help a lot of the students, and brought us all closer together. It took my fears away, too. One of the students used to try to shock me by turning his eyelids inside out, and asking me if I noticed anything different about him. Of course, I said, "No." This student asked me to arm wrestle one day, and I agreed. He put my arm on the desk as I requested, and plopped it into position.

James said, "Okay Ms. Schaufel, start pushing."

I responded, "I am pushing."

James was shocked, "Oh, Ms. Schaufel, you should never carry any money in your purse!"

He was afraid someone would take it from me!

I did do something very stupid, but turned out good. I asked students to keep folders, and their work in them. A student, at the end of the third quarter, had not done any homework. But, I knew she could do the work, but she handed me a folder full of paper that I had graded a B+. She had folded down the name of the student whose work it really was, and turned in the folder as her own. She had three quarters of F's, and knew that I saw the other person's name on papers. Both students should have gotten "F's." Instead, I gave the student that copied an "A" telling her that I knew she could get an A this quarter, she just had to get her paperwork in on time. She would at least pass the class with a D for the year. The other student's grade, I left as it was. Denise got an A that quarter as well as an award for the most improved student. She also helped other students along the way! What I hoped these students learned was that "If you cheat, you end up cheating yourself." Knowing where to find the answers, and figure things out, was really how you learned for a lifetime. It's not so much about today.

The third year I taught, I had three sets of twins. They could fool me for a while, but not for long. All were male. The brother of each set was in a different one of my classes. I could even tell them apart in the halls.

One year the English teacher in the next room bought a tarantula to give to the student who would improve his/her grade the most. I was very scared of spiders. This was a tarantula! I just knew that one of my students was going to win it. I had better start preparing. One day, I came around the corner, and saw a brown paper bag scrunched on the floor. I almost screamed. I thought it was the tarantula! Every morning after that, I forced myself to go into that English teacher's room, and watch that tarantula move around for about 10 minutes. I got to the point where I could at least tolerate it in its terrarium, that is. I was right! One of my students, Scott, won the tarantula, and I knew he would win it! Fortunately, his English class was after my math class so the tarantula was never in my classroom!

When spring came, another student brought in an albino spider, and held it right in front of my face. No problem! There was a snake too, but those were fine with me. This particular one was fine as it had no head! I had touched a Python before! Snakes feel soft.

At home, however, I was correcting papers while sitting on my bed. This little, bitty, jumping spider came near me. I was surprised by it, yet, I thought, "It is so much smaller than the tarantula at school!"

I hit it with my pencil case, and missed. I hit it a second time, and missed, again. I started getting nervous, and said to myself, "This is dumb. I am not that brave!" The spider made his way towards the end of the bed. No one was in the house. I knew the back door was open. What should I do? I had a rotary telephone which was always hard for me to dial, especially with a lot of big numbers in it like 7, 8, 9, and 0. I called Carolyn, Susie's friend next door, but it was busy. By this time, the spider was out of sight which was even worse than seeing where it was. Where would it turn up? I called the operator—at least it was only one number to dial—and I pleaded with her.

"Operator, this is an emergency. I have a disability, and the line I was calling was busy. Please dial it for me, and please break-in if you must."

"The line is not busy now, ma'am. I will connect you," the operator replied, and I thanked her.

Carolyn came over to my house in her pajamas! I told her what I needed. The spider was just about ready to appear by my knee, and she killed it!

"Is that all?" Carolyn asked. It took her less than a minute! She was my hero!

I made several good friends who were teachers. Merle was the typing teacher, and Bonnie and Rita taught math.

At times, the science teacher would check blood types. He always let me know ahead of time when this would be done. In the first three years, the students would stop me at the science door while I was on my breaks, and would ask me a question. While it was only finger prick, I just couldn't watch.

"Ms. Schaufel, can we check your blood type?"

I would always say "yes," but mean "no." It was difficult to take my blood, and the students would always have to go pretty deep with the lancer. I was type "O" every time!

Another, who taught cooking, had a mouse in her classroom, and it was getting into some of the foods. She asked the custodian to set a trap, but he didn't do it. So, she set the mousetrap, and caught a big, juicy mouse. The teacher put the mouse into a hot dog bun with ketchup and mustard, and left it, and a sarcastic note, for the custodian!

I had one student who was a very reliable student, Jeff, and one student, Mike, who was causing problems. Jeff stopped by every lunch hour. He would place my students' completed papers into the grade book for me, and I was thankful for the help. Then, for about a week, I noticed that my clock had a whole bunch of spit balls on it, but I had no idea who was "decorating" my clock. Eventually, I realized it was happening in my fifth hour class. The culprit was Mike who sat right in front of the clock. He took his pen apart, chewed up some paper, and used the pen's casing as a launcher. He hit the clock about 20 times an hour. End of the problem.

For whatever reason, several students kept calling me Mrs. Cooksie, who was an eighth grade teacher - and, African American! I told them, "Hey, just look at me! I do not look like Mrs. Cooksie! I am much shorter!" Obviously, of course, it was because I was sitting down!

I taught at Bullen for eight years with the opportunity to teach all different levels of classes, and a couple of classes which were not ninth grade. My Mom was a huge help, and stayed busy not only by driving me back and forth to work, but writing out my tests and quizzes every week, because I did not have enough pressure to write on the carbon paper to make it readable.

Often, I took students that other teachers found to be more difficult. One student was an African American student who was very smart, but his behavior problems kept him in the low math classes. I discovered that he could finish his work not only correct, but fast. I believed that his behavioral problems were created simply because he wasn't being challenged by the work in the lower math classes, so I transferred him into a beginning algebra class. He breezed through that class, so I decided to let him try the hard algebra class. That class was a little too much for him, so I sent him back to Algebra 1. We both got along well, and respected each other. One day I was having a bad day, and the class was noisy. I looked up to find that he was the one moving around. I called out his name, and told him, "If you don't want to be black AND blue, sit down!" I couldn't believe those words came out of my mouth. He smiled, sat down, and the class giggled. This was just one of two incidents I totally regret. I apologize!

In a similar situation, I told the class, "Sit down. You are acting like a bunch of wild Indians!"

Two of the students walked out. Why, I didn't know, but my students explained it to me.

"They are both Indian!"

I should have known better, when I considered their names. I always told people that they shouldn't "should on themselves", but in this case, I believe it was warranted! I'm sorry, Peggy and Terri.

I never was really angry at my students. When I knew they were doing something wrong, I'd say, "See me right after school!" The student(s) would come to my classroom, later, and I would forget why they were there! Fortunately, I did not do that very often. With discipline, I found that students would listen to me better when I was quiet. They probably weren't expecting it, or maybe, because other teachers yelled at them rather than asking them to do something differently.

My "evil" look would warn my students more than talking! For instance, I found a student sitting on the floor in front of his biology class. Although I didn't know who he was, I asked him to please go into his classroom, but he would not budge.

He uttered, "Make me"!

When I told him that I was going to slide him into his room, he still did not move, and refused to follow my request. Using my wheelchair, I gently slid him across the floor into his classroom.

On my way out, he jumped to his feet, and declared, "If you weren't a lady, I'd slug you!"

Returning to the room, I simply said, "Sit down."

Rumors began that I ran over disobedient students, and hurt them. The student, Robert, who started them was from a juvenile institution, and had instigated physical fights with teachers, and other students. I wasn't so sure what I did was such good idea, and about eight years later, I saw him at a rummage sale at his house!

He called me by name, told me who he was, and shared, "I am glad you are at my house to see that I turned out good! Wasn't I a trip in Junior High?" Miracles happen! And he was living right in my neighborhood!

While in school, one day, I saw that my motor was smoking. It had only done it once before, but I never knew what caused it. I had one of the students click the switch for the office, and the principal came down to the classroom, but the smoke had stopped by the time he arrived. He worried on his way down, because if he had to get me out of my wheelchair, where would he put me? Mr. Saksvig just joked, "If I have to put out any fires in your wheelchair, I, at least, want a fireman's hat!"

Now, Sheila, another student, tried to protect me in the lunch room, one day, when she heard someone refer to me as "Hot Wheels". She thought that was disrespectful, and started a fight! But, I thought that reference was endearing.

Some of the students would say to me, "Want to drag Ms. Schaufel?"

I would try to spoil their joke about racing and would reply, "No, thank you, I don't smoke!"

Most of them did not even get the joke, because, in those days, "drag" meant "a puff from a cigarette."

At the beginning of the year in 1976, I received a note from a former student.

Kathy S: *I don't suppose you remember me at all, but let me tell you, I have never forgotten you. You are the best teacher I ever had. How have you been? I'm fine. I'm a senior this year. I'm glad my two younger sisters have the chance to have you for a teacher. They'll be able to understand why I think so much of you as a person, and as a teacher. Beverly says she has you for a teacher now, I'm glad. I hope my seventh grade sister has a chance to have you...* The note made my day!

In two of the eight years I taught, I had two student teachers. Debbie was cute, tiny, and a bundle of energy, and she was great!

The second student teacher was Donnie, who had cerebral palsy, and I knew him from the Orthopedic School. He was very tall and intelligent, but his physical movements were very restricted. He used a motorized wheel chair, but he had limited hand grasp, and finger control. We worked through some of his physical problems by preparing things ahead of time such as transparencies, and having students write on the board more than normal, etc. I learned a lot from him. He did a good job, and was hired by the School District teaching for 12 years in the Kenosha Unified School District, only retiring due to multiple, personal concerns.

About my fourth year of teaching, the School District began requiring continuing education credits to maintain teaching certifications. Six credits were needed every two years if one had a bachelor's degree, and three credits were needed if one had a Master's Degree. I did not know how I was going to fit in the time to take these classes. I was so glad when I had completed my degree at Carthage. I thought I never would have gone back to school again! I liked learning, but... anything different to my schedule took a lot of planning, and now it was mandatory. And, computers were on their way, and functionally, I did not see how I could possibly work them. Even turning them on by myself was impossible. I had to do a lot of typing for various organizations with which I was involved, and I was a pretty good typist as long as it was on an electric typewriter.

I decided to look into a sabbatical leave. I could take time off from the school district, and be paid while I went to school. That would give me enough money for room and board, as well as money to pay for attendant care. So, I signed a sabbatical contract. I would be off for a full year, but had to promise I would return to teach for two more years.

After my sabbatical, I returned to Bullen, and taught for eight years, although it only counted for 7.25 years, since summers never counted. Each year was different. I always swore that if I ever started sounding like some other teachers who were discouraged, or disgruntled, I would quit my job.

On my eighth year, it happened. Many teachers in our school left each year. Two of my students, in one of my smaller math classes of 16, I never saw clean or sober. It was difficult, and very stressful! I even had nightmares that they had me trapped with my students in the classroom, and starting fires!

Then, in March, I had a fall onto the concrete garage floor. My car lift's chains were not hooked correctly. My head had hit near my temple, and my eye was injured, and bloody, on the right side of my face as well as being black and blue. When Pastor Peterson stopped by while I was at the hospital, I told him that I was thinking about changing occupations. He countered with, "What do you think God wants you to do? He has taken care of you well so far!"

When I got out of the hospital, and released to go back to work, I realized that I could not handle the noise of the classroom. The students thought somebody had beaten me considering the bruises, and my eyes, were still looking bad. I surmised that my brain was swollen, because, as it was healing, I think it triggered nerve endings near my brain's old "horror movie memory storage area", and I would hear babies crying, spooky music, hyenas laughing, creaking doors, or hideous laughs. I was glad when those sounds finally disappeared months later!

In May of 1979, I was forced into a difficult decision to turn in my resignation. It was hard, because I loved teaching. While I did not have a job yet, I knew I would get one.

~ 12 ~

Community Involvement

Including teaching, and after the Orthopedic School reunion in 1971, a subgroup of the alumni, along with other people with disabilities from the community, began meeting weekly in the Jane Vernon Elementary School in the Orthopedic Wing to play cards and to go swimming in the accessible pool. Officially, the group was given the name of Kenosha Handicapped Community Center (KHCC), and bylaws were written. It became the first, social group for people with disabilities in Kenosha. For more than a decade, I was there every week on Tuesdays in the evening, between 7-9:00 p.m. Dad helped raise some money from Johnson Motors, where he worked, to help pay for the lifeguard and transportation for those who could not get there except by taxi. City buses were not accessible, and did not run at night.

There was a Tuesday program during the regular school year for the pool. I loved it, because there was a ramp going into it. I would never stay long, though, because I would get so cold during the winter. After I was finished, Susie, or Mom, helped me to dress.

On holidays, we would have special parties such as a Halloween party the week of Halloween, and Santa Claus for Christmas. Mom and Dad came to the Halloween Party, and even Dad got in the spirit by wearing one of Mom's wigs, and one of my dresses for Halloween!

As a member of the KHCC, I was asked to speak at an Orthopedic School PTA meeting to some parents who had young daughters in wheelchairs. They had questions about many things, and these ranged from what should the parents allow their children to try on their own to very specific questions on how do we handle going to the bathroom, and menstruation when their daughters couldn't handle these concerns by themselves. I always thought it would be much easier to have been born a man in these situations. The general questions were simpler as they could all be answered with questions. Was this something you wanted to try at that age? Was there a reason it would be unsafe for this individual to try the activity? Did the person make good decisions? Were the parents overprotective? A person does not know what another is able to do until one tried it, and usually, success was not on the first try. Since each individual was different, I couldn't make any of the decisions for the parents, and only they, and their children, understood their abilities and their limitation(s). If the child thought he/she could do something, and understood the possible consequences, it would never hurt to try. I always wanted to try skydiving when one of my friends, Karen who also had MD, tried it with her boyfriend. The jump went just fine, the parachute opened, and they jumped together. The view as they fell was excellent, however, the landing was a disaster! A gust of wind hit the parachute at a wrong angle, and her boyfriend fell on top of her, breaking both of her legs! But, what counted was that Karen thought the experience was worth it. I didn't want to try it anymore! Come to think of it, I thought even a Ferris wheel would be high enough to make me sick. I would get weak at the hips at any height, and wanted to fall forward. Even my wheelchair with the bathroom was about one inch higher than the chair I had previously—and even adapting to my current chair took quite a while! Pathetic, huh?

The more specific questions of the parents could vary quite a bit, so I spoke to them individually after I finished speaking. Methods of transfer varied and different types of equipment could be used, like the commode in my wheelchair. Catheters might be an option, but often caused infections. Menstruation? Sticky pads for me, but I remember belts! I wondered how cave women took care of this problem! I never moved all day so I did not have a lot of issues. I lucked out with only three days max, and never had to stand or walk with a walker, or crutches during my cycles. Diapers? Use whatever works, and be creative! Some used birth control to not have a period. If there were issues such as the heart, circulation, or hormonal problems due to menopause, then birth control, or hormone therapy, might not be an appropriate course, and could cause more problems than the pills would resolve. Consulting with your doctor on physical concerns would be best.

In 1968, I started attending yearly banquets held by the alumni group from the Easter Seal's camp (WWAAC). The first banquet I went to was in Sheboygan. Susie drove, and my cousin Barbara went with us to help. There was a banquet, program, and dance, but it didn't have good accessibility. I was carried down a flight of stairs, because the elevator was broken? There were over 200 people there with several in wheelchairs. Elevators were always a concern at those banquets. If only one wheelchair could fit in the elevator at a time, and 50 people were in wheelchairs, the worry would be would everyone get to the banquet on time? There was even a Mass the next morning for those who wanted to attend. I think it was at the Sheboygan banquet that I met Arlene who had been in a wheelchair from polio since the age of 16. (At one point, doctors did not know if she was going to live, so they ordered an iron lung to breathe for her). She was 13 years older than I, but she came from Kenosha! We became friends, and we decided to have the 1973 WWAAC convention in Kenosha. It would be a lot of work, but well worth it! The group always planned the locations about three years ahead, so there would be enough time to work out all the details. Arlene also became a very involved member of the Kenosha handicapped group, and took over the major responsibilities when I no longer could attend.

The WWAAC conventions were always fun wherever we had them in the state! One year, it was in Green Bay, Wisconsin. Pat and his wife, Dianne, had arranged to give away a signed football from the Packers as a door prize. I was never really into football, so I looked over the table of prizes. I proclaimed, "The only thing I would not want on this table is the football!" The inevitable happened, and I won it! I donated the football back for the door prizes the next year. Darn! I won it - *again*! I couldn't remember what happened to that football, I must've given it away. Many friends wanted that ball!

Another year, our WWAAC group stayed in the main hotel in Appleton. That year, the Detroit Lions were with us. They would be playing the Packers in Green Bay that Sunday, and we could see into the room where the team players were wrapping their legs/ankles for the game! On Saturday night, we saw at least 30, huge, strong men walking through the lobby. Chadwick was the quarterback at that time. He was cute, but I kept thinking, "Think of what I could do with just a small implant of a fraction of one of their muscles!" Now, I realize that's not what most women would be thinking, but, just for the record, they all had great buns, too!

Later, I met one of the players in the elevator with my friend, Jerry who was a lawyer and blind, and his guide dog, we weren't so impressed. The Lion's player was afraid to get into the elevator with us, asking if Jerry's guide dog would bite. Thus, we knew the Packers were going to win that day. (Chickens!)

Many of the camp staff used to attend conventions, too. Ken Saville, previously a counselor for the Easter Seals Camp, he was, now, the Vice Director of Easter Seals for the state of Wisconsin. He attended many of these meetings helping with personal care, reports to the board, etc. All staff that attended helped as if the group was one close family. (Today, Ken is vice president of Easter Seals Wisconsin).

Mary and I would often stay up all night, and her favorite drink was a Bloody Mary! I think it was her favorite because her name was in the drink! (No one could like tomato juice that much)! Some people would be dancing for hours in their wheelchairs. Others were talking. Many were at the bar. The first time I was editor, I found an anonymous poem about past conventions that went something like this:

> *I will go to the WWAAC convention*
> *and if I do, I promise not to drink*
> *and if I do, I promise not to get drunk*
> *and if I do, I promise not to fall*
> *and if I do, I promise to fall forward on my WWAAC pin*
> *so no one can see I'm a member.*

We would often take a hotel over, and we provided a lot of surprises for the other guests! Everyone would always expect something unusual to happen at every convention.

Joanie could not use her arms, and actually ate with a utensil held by her toes with her foot on the table. I did not see that it was a problem, but I did agree that she should stay away from wearing dresses while eating! I could not believe how agile she was!

Barney could not speak, or straighten out his body, but he always had a huge smile. Yes, you could always tell what he was thinking—girls, girls, girls. At one of the conventions, there was another group having a party by the pool. Barney had just received an electronic talking device on which he could type his thoughts, and the words would be spoken aloud in an electronic voice. Well, he moved his feet pretty well, and would always be pushing his wheelchair backwards with his feet. And, one day, he came too close to the edge of the pool. Someone at the pool party bumped into him, and everything went into the pool. They pulled Barney out first, then his wheelchair. Unfortunately, his talking device did not make it!

I was elected to the WWAAC Board about 9 times for three-year terms. I held every position including treasurer. I spent at least 10 years as editor, or editor helper, and the last 12, or more, as Parliamentarian.

At the 1973 convention in Kenosha, there were 212 attendees. In 2011, there were only about 20. Like a lot of groups, many of the old members passed away. New members were hard to recruit, and there was more accessibility, and activities in the community, so a search for accessible hotels was not needed any longer. Today, we would not be able to find 50 accessible rooms, because a certain percentage of the rooms are designated handicapped accessible. We needed more than the 4 to 10 rooms available, now.

The WWAAC, originally, was formed in 1955, but we finally dissolved the club in 2011. It was very sad to dissolve this group. Even though we gave camp funds every year for something like the electrical wiring, sound systems, picnic tables, clocks, etc., the WWAAC members were able to present a final check of more than $12,000 to the camp director at Wawbeek.

Eddie was also a member of KHCC and WWAAC. He had an idea for another group he wanted to establish—an advocacy group to assist people with disabilities with appropriate legislation, housing, accessibility, etc. He would be president, and asked me to be vice president. He organized a board of about 15 people, requested the assistance of a lawyer named Burton Lepp, and developed a constitution and bylaws. Banging our head against the wall, the name alluded us. But, Arlene and I came up with the name ABLE, Inc.—Abolish Barriers for Lifetime Efficiency. It became a very active group, and I was very busy during this decade with these three groups as well as teaching.

Inevitably, Eddie and I butted heads on some things. He would much rather go out and protest by dragging himself out of his wheelchair, and putting himself in the middle of the street to stop traffic. I, on the other hand, preferred going through a more subdued, traditional, but effective process. His was a good way to demonstrate awareness, but my way was more permanent. I really did not like politics, but I understood politics. Patience was needed as nothing happened overnight! Requests had to be reasonable, specific, personal, and inexpensive at the same time. We were looking for changes when things needed to be replaced!

One of the first things ABLE worked on was ramped corners to make sidewalks accessible. Eddie, Al, Dave, and Frank, a quadriplegic from an industrial accident, did most of the legwork…I mean…"wheelwork". It is perfectly okay to use 'leg' for a person that cannot walk, or 'see' for a person who is blind. It is a language issue, not a sensitivity issue. Semantics might get really complicated if things would change too much, e.g., actually a blind person can see with their ears. Not that their ears heard better, but only because the person paid more attention to their hearing! Imagine dreaming in sound and touch. Anyway, there was a State Congressman in our County named Russell Olson who responded to ramping the corners, or "curb cuts", by thoughtfully saying, "Why should we put in 'curb cuts' for people with disabilities? You never see anybody out in a wheelchair anyway." Gah! We really had a lot of work to do! Years and years of work!

I had presented 9000 Kenosha signatures to Madison on my first day of teaching. Since the first accessibility bill had passed in 1971, "curb cuts" were ABLE's first focus to allow more people with mobility impairments to be involved in the community. Frank went to the city after the "curb cuts" had begun. No input from people with disabilities was sought, so the first ramps were steep and problematic. Before the ramped corners were very far along, Frank decided to take an extra wheelchair for a city official to try the "curb cuts". He had the official sit in the wheelchair to go down the new constructions so a person without a disability would have a first-hand experience on what could happen. The official wheeled down the "curb cut", and fell out of his chair on the road. Thus, Frank showed him, firsthand, what could happen to a person as well as possibly of avoiding lawsuits against the city. Each of the already constructed corner ramps were evaluated as to their usefulness with tape-recorded notes. A more standard plan was developed. The problematic "curb cuts" were re-constructed before continuing with others. Four, or five years later Kenosha was in the forefront, and ahead of the rest of the state. A 5% grade was the maximum slope a person could safely handle. State standards were now set.

Passage of Assembly Bill 1 around 1975-1976 would make it unlawful to discriminate against a person in regard to voting, jury duty, and housing, as well as employment solely on the basis of the person's disability. This all started in Wisconsin and California!

~ 13 ~

1973 - A Busy Year

Work, KHCC, ABLE and WWAAC provided a lot of socializing with both those who did, and did not have, disabilities. I tried to ask my family to do less, and get out more with friends. Eddie could drive with hand controls, so he took me to Madison for something to do with the legislature. In order for me to exit his car, we transferred my car lift to Eddie's car. On the way, Eddie's car started smoking, but with no smell, just below the center of the dashboard. Neither of us knew what was wrong. We stopped the car on the side of the highway to figure out what to do. I told him that he should get out of the car in case it was serious. He refused to leave me alone. He would figure out a way to crawl around the car, and open the door, removing me. While we were discussing this, the smoke disappeared, and we continued on our way without any more incidents.

Eddie was really like a brother to me—and we fought like siblings, too! He always went out with a lot of different girls - he was a ladies' man, and it took him a long time to find someone. In the meantime, Eddie used to come on New Year's Eve, and play Monopoly. Keeping up with his macho image, he would threaten me with "If you ever tell anybody I did this on New Year's Eve, I'll..." Of course, his threats didn't work with me. Then, for a few years, not only Eddie came to play, but so did Al, Dave, and Arlene. Mom made a good punch made of Ginger Ale, 7-up, raspberry sherbet and fresh raspberries along with a little brandy! Yum!

My sister had been dating Bob for over a year, and he asked Susie to marry him on their first date! Mom automatically "suspected" him, so, every time they were out in the car by the back porch a little too long, Mom would flicker the porch light letting Susan know her time was up! Bob always thought she was trying to land an airplane, but it definitely caught their attention right along with the neighbors, too!

I was 26 when I began speaking to my friend, Al, a lot on the telephone. He was 13 years older than I, and a quadriplegic. Getting involved with him seemed safe. Although several people asked me on dates in college, I didn't trust anyone enough to date them. However, one night, called me out to the porch before he left to give me my very first *real* kiss - and he was experienced, good, and he gave me more than one kiss, too! I could hear Mom moving around in the living room saying, "Haven't they been out there long enough?" to my Dad, and that's when he went home!

My friend, Edith, invited me to my first deaf convention in 1973. She my sign language classes, and always had an interpreter with her. I thought it was very interesting that even with so many people in the room, it was very quiet. All that I could hear moving was the wind from the movement of their hands! Some of the couples had children that could hear, and when I

94

spoke to their parents, they would sign for me. Signing should be a utilized as an international language, because it is a single language.

Susie and Bob were married in May of 1973 at St. Mary's Lutheran Church which was a new church and very accessible. I was Susie's Maid of Honor, and even had my hair done for the wedding! The wedding was wonderful, but Dad was nervous taking Susie down the aisle. He calmed his nerves by drinking so he was leaning on her and chewing gum that he believed would get rid of the alcohol smell. Bob's brothers played a trick on him, So that when Bob knelt at the altar with Susie, everyone could see what was written on his left shoe, "Help", and on his right shoe, "Me." The entire congregation saw "Help Me!" on the bottom of his shoes! Mike and Gary stood next to him holding back their laughter, and poor Bob had no idea what was happening!

The wind was blowing about 30 mph on the day of the wedding. I rode in the bridal car touring the city with everyone else and Dad had to take apart my wheelchair, and put it back together again at the reception. There was a large hill, and my Dad pushed the motorized wheelchair while simultaneously controlling the driving lever on my chair. But, the lever stuck, and it took me in circles for quite a while until Dad figured out how to stop it! Once inside the building, I had to redo my own hair, and I really missed my wig! There were many people at the wedding, and Al and I danced. He could always dance gracefully while controlling both of our wheelchairs.

Our whole family began attending St. Mary's Lutheran Church. We never missed a Sunday, and it was good to be an active member of church, again, since the Salvation Army was no longer accessible.

Bob had another brother, James, and both he and his brother were in the Vietnam War. Later in 1973, there was a Memorial Service for Bob's brother, James, who had been declared missing in action. The empty coffin with the draped American flag was an impressive sight. Many years later, the family found out that James was shot, taken as a prisoner of war, and inevitably died due to his severe injuries.

At the end of June, I went to the Muscular Dystrophy camp for the first time. The basic difference between this camp and Easter Seals was that Muscular Dystrophy had a one to one camper/volunteer ratio, but their staff was unpaid. MDA only covered the disabilities under their umbrella. Easter Seals covered all disabilities. MDA rented camping space, so it wasn't always as accessible, and ramps had to be set up on some of the buildings. For a few years, MDA was at a Jewish campground in the Wisconsin Dells. I thought this was particularly interesting as the camp had two kitchens to keep the food Kosher. My understanding was that Kosher meant the kitchens could not mix meat and dairy products. With my future lactose intolerance, I was in trouble on dairy days.

The first activity we had was square dancing on a huge tennis court. All ages of people with MD were present, between the ages of 6 to 30. One of the volunteers, Lloyd, took me as a partner, and did a great job with my manual wheelchair. Almost everyone was in wheelchairs, and we promenaded, and do-si-doed without crashing into them! I also tried canoeing, and Lloyd, and my volunteer, while the canoe was on land, they lifted me into the center of it, and they put a life jacket on me. Next, they shoved the canoe and me into the water! My attendant,

Carol, was at the front of the canoe, and Lloyd, in the back. I will never forget how peaceful it felt with no sound while gliding over the lake except for the occasional sound of water dripping off the paddles. The sun felt so warm on my skin, and the movement was very smooth. I always return to that Moment whenever I want to relax.

Fishing was fun. I had fished before, but only for minnows with a tiny piece of worm. Here, I had to put my own worm on the hook! That was depressing. It was not because I was afraid of the worm, but because the worm tightened himself up so much that I couldn't get the hook in him. The worm was stronger than I was! I could feel the fish nibbling on the worm once we finally had him in the water. I could hook the fish, but not reel him into the boat. It didn't bother me that I couldn't take the fish off the hook. Besides, who wants to take a fish off a hook anyway?

I had the opportunity to sleep on a mattress on the ground one night by the lake. I was worried about spiders, but what the heck. I woke up early asking Carol to set me up. It was just in time to see the sunrise, and watch a mama duck take her eight ducklings for a morning swim. The birds were waking up, and they began to sing. When I went swimming later, I noticed that the lake looked clear and much cleaner from above the water than when I was under it!

I also was able to get to know Lloyd a lot better. He was a very interesting character with a very good heart. He liked to go hiking and fishing in different areas of the country. He traveled a lot and cheaply! He acted kind of tough and rugged, but I spotted him across the last campfire trying to inconspicuously wipe tears from his eyes as everyone sang *You Will Never Walk Alone* - a song that Jerry Lewis sang at the end of the Labor Day Telethon each year. I felt both curious and comfortable with Lloyd.

For the next several years, I alternated going to either Easter Seals camp and the MDA camp, because I was usually in a situation where I could not go to both of them. While I was at one of the camps, my parents would take a well-deserved break, and go on a vacation such as Las Vegas.

In July of 1973, my situation wasn't any different. I still couldn't go to Easter Seals camp, because I was going to Europe. I found a handicap travel group from Florida run by the Fein family. I took my own attendant. There was extra help available from some members of the tour group if needed. I had asked one of my attendants from Easter Seals camp the year before to go with me, but she had taken a job at the last minute. However, Diane volunteered to go with me! Time was getting very short, and I was very lucky that Diane was working at Abbott Laboratories in North Chicago. She could get her passport in three days! Normally, it would take a couple of weeks to get a passport, but Abbott did so much international business with their medication sales and research, she was ready to go in no time! One other friend, Shirley, went with us from Easter Seals camp, and its alumni group. She was in a wheelchair from multiple sclerosis, and couldn't walk, but she could stand, and take care of herself. She often came down to stay with me from Christmas break through New Year's Eve. The three of us were going to share a room, which after a while, we found out wouldn't work. The space in the European rooms was pretty small, especially with two people in wheelchairs trying to get around.

BY THE GRACE OF GOD AND YOU
A Chair Does Not a Person Make

We flew from Milwaukee to New York JFK Airport, then, we transferred to LaGuardia. The travel company had everything worked out so that when we arrived, we were transferred everywhere on time. The airport on the other hand, for some reason, had a seven-hour delay, which meant I was going to have to use the airport bathroom. We took one of the garbage cans that stood quite high, and tried to use that as a stool, since all other chairs were bolted down to the floor. I managed the airport wait, the seven-hour flight to Frankfurt, Germany, as well as the trip to our hotel (12 hours), and all I had in the way of drink was three ice cubes! Now my only problem would be to stay up an additional eight hours, so that I avoided jet lag for the whole trip! But, I was getting tired, now, not to mention thirsty, and I could have chugged half of Lake Michigan!

We stayed in Mainz, so we did not have to worry about the water there, because the city had a newer sewer system than any other city. We took a bus trip to Wiesbaden where Elvis Presley was stationed when he was in the Army. Next, we took a cruise down the Rhine, and saw multiple castles, many German pubs, miles of hills filled with vineyards, and the Lorelei—an extremely dangerous, and fatal rock in which ships often crashed to pass an extremely narrow turning point in the river. The legend shared with us was that a siren called "Lorelei" bewitched the hearts of the sailors, and the sailors would be mesmerized by her voice in song, and it would cause their ships to crash on the rock. They died, and their ships sank.

After we got off the boat, we made our way by bus through the Black Forest to Heidelberg. Many seats were removed from a regular bus so that all the people in wheelchairs would fit. The major problem on the trip was that the bus lift was shipped on the wrong plane, and went to London instead of following us to Germany. So, the extra helpers lifted us in our chairs on and off the bus every time we stopped - and, there were 25 to 30 people with disabilities. Only one had brought a motor to clip on his chair if needed, but most of the time, it was in the baggage compartment. Some of the people in larger wheelchairs had to bring a little device, which was a small crank that would fold their wheelchair tighter against them, so that they could get through some of the narrower doorways.

Heidelberg was a beautiful little city that was overlooked by a huge Castle. Diane and I did a lot of shopping there. I bought a Hummel figurine, and some amethyst rings among other things. The area was pretty flat, but there were no such things as curb cuts on the corners. Getting up and down those curbs was difficult for Diane. It was a little easier to go down the curbs backwards, so I didn't have to worry about falling out of my chair. There was a little German woman using a cane that we apparently, but accidentally, went down the curb in front of her, and getting in her way. She shook her cane at us, vehemently saying something in German that I was sure we were glad we couldn't interpret!

The next stop was in the Alsace-Lorraine area where we saw a perfect example of an old German town with German architecture including flower boxes on the windowsills. We stopped at a Notre Dame Cathedral (there was one in every town) that was unusual, because it had a very easy entrance—only one step on the side. The inside was breathtaking with the gold, paintings, stained-glass windows and statues.

Our group continued to travel towards the Swiss border where we saw the magnificent waterfall of Schaffhausen. It is the largest waterfall in Europe on the Rhine River. The waters cascaded over what looked like a semi-circle of three steps like configurations causing rapids in spots along the way. It wasn't as tall as Niagara Falls, but appeared to cover a bigger area to me.

We went straight from there to Zürich where we heard the Sunday morning church bells for hours! Someone helped us get up that day, because Diane's back was sore. I didn't do much that day except for talking to a Swiss resident who judged Wisconsin cheese as the best in the world! The next day, we passed more financial institutions, than I thought were in all of America. When we got to Lucerne, we went into some watch shops. I bought a ring watch, which I used for years and years. And it became my trademark!

We traveled through the Swiss Alps to Bern, Switzerland, a city that was named for the first animal—a bear—that came into the city. That day, as throughout Germany and Switzerland, we saw many castles that formed cities built within the walls around them. Bern was the first city we had a chance to explore. It was like going back in time 500 years. We crossed a bridge that resembled a river moat around three sides of the city. The outside walls of the city held all of its residents inside, and the city now was bulging at its seams. Accessibility was poor, and I was glad that the person who had set up the tour had already investigated where we could, and could not, go. During this whole trip, I only saw one resident who used a wheelchair. Mr. Fein took us to a restaurant that was on the very top of a hill. We could see everything from there. Our first course? Oxtail soup—yummy! On the trip, so far, we had a lot of veal, which I rarely ate at home. The breads were all very good, but the butter… no taste. I had to salt mine to know it was on my bread. Switzerland was unusual, because it had four languages, but no national language. There were German, Italian, French and Romansh.

Next, we saw multiple mini waterfalls throughout the Swiss Alps. Melting snow probably caused them. One waterfall was more beautiful than the next. I could not bend my head over far enough on the bus to see the top of the mountains from my view on the bus. Turns were very sharp, and multiple crosses where people had died were affixed to the spot where the deaths occurred. We finally made it through to Geneva, Switzerland, where we saw Lake Geneva, fountains, and the United Nations building from the inside.

We moved across the border into Italy. The grass was unkempt, and we could tell right away that we crossed the border, and the area more poor. It would have been 500 miles to Rome, and no places to stop to go to the bathroom for people in wheelchairs. Bathrooms in the whole area were either down a lot of steps, or Roman toilets where you had to squat while you balanced in designated foot spaces on the floor. It was worth going into Italy, even though it wasn't even a day. We stopped at the Gran Paradiso, which had two green mountains (one on each side of a center), two taller and barren mountains (one on each side behind the green mountains). About five feet in front of me, a huge cross that could pump water from the melting glacier that was in the center of a mountain in the distance. We used cups to drink some of the refreshing, cold water from the tap we had not had on most of our trip. We mostly drank eight ounce, $1 classic Cokes, so we would not become sick with diarrhea. We even skipped the tea and coffee, which had water in it.

After returning to the bus, we passed through Switzerland again right by Mount Blanc. Diane reached out of the sunroof of the bus to take a picture of it, and then we were on to France!

BY THE GRACE OF GOD AND YOU
A Chair Does Not a Person Make

We stopped in Lyon, France, for wine tasting at a vineyard. It was Bastille Day on July 14, and we all tried some German wine, which was sour, Spanish wine was sweet, and French wine, which was dry, but very tasty! When we went to our hotel, we could see all of the fireworks going on in the city. Only one of the persons on the tour knew French. After three semesters of French, I, at least, remembered how to ask where the bathroom was, not that I could use it, and if I should turn right, or left, to get back to the hotel!

We decided to celebrate Bastille Day that night. I had escargot for the first time! Wrong choice! I took a really good look at the snails before I ate them. For me, it tasted like a rubbery mushroom in garlic butter. I was supposed to pull out a snail with my fork, and pour the garlic butter from the shell onto my bread. I consumed only one of the nine on my plate. That was all I could handle. That night, after going to bed, I was half-awake, and half-asleep thinking that the pieces of that snail got back together, and was crawling up my esophagus! Yuck! As far as eating goes, the only other unusual thing I found in France was whenever I ordered a hamburger, it had a fried egg on top of it.

Next was the Palace of Versailles, the estate of Marie Antoinette, wife of King Louis XVI. Unfortunately, it was the only day that it rained so hard, we could not even get off the bus! We missed the Hall of Mirrors, ornate rooms, elegant gardens, etc.

On to Paris which was friendlier than I expected, but not that clean. The city still had the outdoor, open toilets—open from about a foot and a half above the ground so you could see a person's feet and more. There was a door, but no top. We walked around the city for a while. We went into a perfume shop where we tried a number of perfumes. The aromas all became so mingled that I couldn't remember which was which!

Our hotel in Paris was right above the Metro line. Every time the Metro passed, I could feel the train's vibration through my wheelchair. No one else could feel it. When I finally made them aware of the vibrations, I ended up having a good night's sleep. No one else could sleep because now the Metro was keeping them awake!

Before we went to sleep that first night in Paris, Shirley was in an adjoining room with the door open and found a little box with three lights on it. She tried pushing the white one. About five minute later, this man just unlocked her door and came into her room. He was all dressed up, and handsome!

We heard him say, "Can I help you, Madam?"

She blushed, and explained, "Sorry, it was a mistake!"

He left before Diane could run in to see what was happening, or to get involved!

Some of the other women on the tour were wondering about the second toilet. One person washed their hair in it, and another used it to soak her feet. It was a bidet, and who would have thought it was for douching?

We toured a lot by bus throughout the city. Some of the people went to the Moulin Rouge that night, but I didn't really want to handle somebody carrying me up a few flights of stairs! Heck! We could get in enough trouble in our hotel room! We did go to and outdoor café for lunch. It was a cozy little setting where Shirley, Diane, and I were sitting at a round table with a big umbrella. We were trying to look sophisticated, so we tried to look as if we knew what we were doing. Just when we finished ordering, the umbrella folded up over all three of our heads!

The waiter came back, and asked, "May I help you?"

None of us could move.

Quietly we all responded at the same time, "Yes, please." We changed tables!

We did have a chance to go to the Louvre, and saw original artwork like the Mona Lisa, which really looked like a postage stamp next to most of the other artwork. Comparing the paintings of different centuries was very interesting. Sometimes the nudity was embarrassing. Winged Victory was there also along with one of Diane's friends from America who just happened to come into the Louvre at the same time we did! Boy, the world is so small!

That same night, and behind Napoleon's tomb, there was a sound and light show describing some of the history of Napoleon and his army. There would be a spotlight on an area so you would hear Napoleon's speech, or a light following the sound of soldiers marching all around us. Impressive!

In each country, I brought back a sample of each denomination of their money. Converting the money was fun for me. I would help other people on the tour convert it. When we had been driving on the autobahn highway in Germany, I learned the metric system as we arrived at our destinations a little faster than I anticipated. Why? Because meters were smaller than yards. I hated converting to Celsius as the first day I heard the temperature, I thought that I would be freezing! But, instead of freezing, the temperature reached 90°. I hated to admit it, but I forgot to convert the second day, too. I wore heavy clothing again! You would think that I would learn!

All Diane wanted was a pinch on the behind before she would get back on the plane to America, or she wouldn't have what she thought would be the full European experience without it! The oldest man on the tour happened to be sitting next to her so he just reached over, and pinched her. Diane was happy, now, so back to America it was! We got on the plane, but this time we didn't have to worry about staying up seven additional hours, we had to worry about not being tired enough to go to bed when we got home.

Once I reached home, and rested for a day, I was notified by Easter Seals that I had been chosen to receive the state Gallantry Award for "courage and determination in adjusting to a disability." I was going Cable, Wisconsin (over 400 miles away) to receive the award on a Friday night at the end of September. I was honored that Easter Seals chose me for the award, but I didn't feel I was doing anything different from anyone else. I was just living my life, and dealing with any obstacles that came my way. I was supposed to teach school that day, and it was about eight hours of travel time. Didn't Mom and Dad really deserve the award more than I did? Dad would have to take off work, too. I didn't think I should go, but Mom and Dad told me that I should go—so I did. I notified the school district, and Dad arranged the time off at his job.

In September, Susie found out she was pregnant with her first child. Right after that, 11 people we knew, and loved, died within a three-month period. Even though we were so happy the baby was coming, all of the funerals took their toll.

Therefore, in October, Mom, Dad, and I made our way to Cable, Wisconsin for the Easter Seals Gallantry Award. The Lodge that we stayed at was beautiful! It had a wooden, cabin-like interior with the magnificent stone fireplace and high ceiling in the lobby. We made it there in time to change to go to the banquet. I felt very uncomfortable when I headed to the front of the room. Mr. Steffenson who was my first, Orthopedic School principal, read my accomplishments. I felt so uncomfortable, and I never even smiled. After it was over, I talked to a lot of people I had never met before who told me that it was nice to hear my story, and told me what it meant to them.

I started to think, "How come I made it this far?"

Maybe, because I never remembered my parents telling me that I couldn't do anything, so I tried everything to find out what I could and couldn't do—just like everyone else! I also had a lot of good role models from the Orthopedic School. Frankie became a music teacher as well as a principal. Les became a writer, and editor at the *Kenosha News*. Larry (even with his lack of muscle control) worked for a while in a group home teaching carpentry! Bonnie worked for an independent living center, and then opened a group home of her own. Maybe it was because I was expected to get a job! I also had no pain, which makes a big difference, and I had good communication skills. I really couldn't do anything by myself. Everything was physically set up for me. Everyone else did the work, and I received the credit? That's not fair! Family and friends support was always needed. What did I do? Huh?

This article appeared in the *Kenosha News* on October 5, 1973 —page 8. If you want to read it, you may. I think I have told you everything in it already.

She Doesn't Use "Handicapped"

Carol Ann Schaufel, a mathematics teacher at Bullen Junior High School, recently received the Gallantry Award at the Easter Seals Society of Wisconsin's annual meeting.

A Carthage College graduate, Miss Schaufel is confined to a wheelchair because of a rare form of Muscular Dystrophy. She has no use of her legs, limited use of her hands, and cannot lift her arms above her head. Her wheelchair is electrified since she is unable to push it herself. Neither can she open the doors or drive a car. At the present time, her Mother, Mrs. Kenneth Schaufel drives Carol to her job. Miss Schaufel attended the Vernon Orthopedic Wing for 10 years. She graduated from Tremper High School in 1965, and received a scholarship from there. She is a member of Gamma Kappa Alpha, Carthage's highest honorary scholastic society.

She graduated from Carthage in 1970 and took a part-time teaching position there until securing her job at Bullen. Both Carthage and Bullen are architecturally laid out so that a handicapped person may use their facilities, as are Lance Junior High School and Tremper High School, the only other local schools where she could consider employment.

Ms. Schaufel is president of the newly formed Orthopedic School Alumni, vice president of the local ABLE (Abolish Barriers for Lifetime Efficiency) group and president of the Kenosha Community Handicapped Center which she started. It is the only social activity club in Kenosha for handicapped individuals.

She is a member of the Wisconsin Wawbeek Associated Activities Club (WWAAC) and attended Easter Seals' Camp Wawbeek every year. She also reads and writes in braille and recently spent three weeks on a tour of Europe for the handicapped.

According to Miss Schaufel the word "handicapped" is a term she doesn't really apply to anyone, including herself. "You're only handicapped if you don't do anything for anyone," she said. The Gallantry award is given each year to a Wisconsin resident who demonstrates courage and determination in adjusting to a personal crippling disability. It is sponsored by the Easter Seals Society of Wisconsin in conjunction with the National Easter Seals Society.

I received congratulation letters conveying the following messages:

Pastor Peterson: *Your accomplishments have meant much not only to others who are handicapped, but to others in our parish and in our community who are aware of your accomplishments. We are proud of you and are thankful to God for the very positive witness that you have made in your chosen profession and in the influence that you have had upon others.*

Carthage College: President Harold Lentz, *We are extremely proud of you here at Carthage college. Your record here as a student, and your excellent work here as a teacher, were most outstanding.*

Bullen, Principal Robert Saksvig: *You are certainly well deserving of this award. Throughout the past three years, you have consistently proven your abilities. I have always been particularly grateful to you for the many contributions you have made to the program at Bullen Junior High. The students you have worked with over the past three years reflect the enthusiasm and abilities that you have brought to the classroom. You can take pride in the significant contributions you have made to your students and to the staff. All of us are extremely proud that we continue to have the opportunity of serving with you as we meet the needs of the young people we work with daily in the city of Kenosha.*

Kenosha Superintendent of Schools, Otto Huettner: *Kenosha Unified School District heartily concurs with the recognition being given to Carol Schaufel. Carol is a lifelong Kenosha resident ... Carol is an unusual young lady who has earned the respect and admiration of her Associates. She is quiet and unassuming and is always pleasant and congenial. She demonstrates a contagious enthusiasm for the teacher-learner process. She has developed teaching methods which promote an excellent learning environment and adapts to overcoming physical limitations imposed by her handicap.*

Reading the above notes, I understood. Many people didn't live their lives. Everyone, disabled or not, could choose to live, or just exist. I chose to live!

In 1973, Kenosha had its first WWAAC convention. On a weekend in the middle of October, we had a banquet, program, and dance for 212 people at the old Holiday Inn by the

BY THE GRACE OF GOD AND YOU
A Chair Does Not a Person Make

Kenosha Harbor. Arlene, I, and a few others worked hard to make everything workable. Accessibility worked pretty well as the doorways were wide enough for wheelchairs. For the bathroom doors which could not accommodate the larger wheelchairs, the management just took the doors off allowing enough space to maneuver in the bathroom. There was one year, at the Madison convention, the hotel did not have enough rooms available, and so I was lucky enough to get a suite. There were so many people that came who didn't have rooms that we split the suite into two parts. Six girls shared the bedroom, six guys shared the living room, and occupied by Steve and the counselor. Five of us were in wheelchairs. Mom and Dad were with me at the convention, too. Mom came to pick me up from the hotel, and saw how messy it was. There were so many cups, popcorn, pizza and pop cans all over the place, that she was embarrassed, and cleaned the whole area before we left!

Kenosha Mayor Wallace Burkee spoke at the 1973 convention, and decided to give Eddie an award for all of his work in getting curb cuts into the city. Of course, Eddie was up to his old tricks. He had an enema bag hanging on his chair that was filled with whiskey and water. He would drink it straight from the tube, or fill his glass of ice by putting the tube in his glass! He did not know he was going to get an award. In addition, none of us even thought to tell him to take his enema bag off the back of his chair. When he was called up to receive his award by the Mayor, his enema bag was in clear sight! He never even used enema bags! Where did he get it anyway?

To Eddie's credit, he did do a lot of work on helping with the legislation and attainment of the curb cuts. What was interesting was that all disabilities were surveyed to see if the curb cuts would be a problem to anyone. Everyone said, "No problem." Once the curb cuts were under construction, a number of people who were blind or visually impaired complained that they could not tell with their canes that they were going into the street. If they had a dog, the dog couldn't tell either. No one anticipated this serious problem. What helps one disability group doesn't always help another. As new curb, or curb cuts, were replaced, it was now agreed that a cement grid would be placed in the top of the curb cut, so people who are visually impaired could identify with their canes that they were crossing into a street.

The Muscular Dystrophy Association began a weekend adult winter camp in the winter of 1973, and I decided to go.

This was the article in the paper:

It was cold and pretty snowy but nevertheless last weekend was a nice one for a winter camping experience at Camp Sydney in Delafield. The campers, as one might expect of people who would be outdoors in Wisconsin on a January weekend, were hardy. There was a difference though, telltale only because they all started out in wheelchairs. They were, all 11 of them, Muscular Dystrophy patients. Watching them out on snowmobiles and horse-drawn sleds, one could hardly work up a smidgen of do-gooder pity. They were having too good a time.... Bundled in a blanket waiting for her ride was M.D. patient Carol Schaufel of Kenosha.

The winter experience was fun, except for two things that did not go exactly as it was portrayed.

1. Being pulled on the back of the snowmobile had some gassy fumes, but was an excellent ride!
2. Everyone else's horse did great pulling their sled, but mine insisted on clopping on a 5-foot tree. My horse went over it, knocking the tree down with its roots out of the ground!

I was definitely struck by the picturesque scene I saw from inside the lodge. There was a cozy warm fireplace next to a full ¾ wall-sized window overlooking the beautiful frozen lake with ice fishermen on it. While I was intrigued with ice fishing, it would be quite some time before I would try it, because I wasn't ready to try that - yet!

~ 14 ~

Traveling with a Busy Schedule

After 1973, my parents took me to Las Vegas for the first time during Easter break. . It was the first time that I flew with my parents, and was lucky enough to get a seat close to the front of the plane, which made the transfer easier. The airport staff placed my wheelchair into the cargo hold of the plane, and I transferred onto a smaller, airport wheelchair that fit between the rows of seats. This made it easier for Mom and Dad to help me into the seat with a two-person lift.

When we got to Las Vegas, the airport staff, again, transferred me into the smaller airport wheelchair, and carried me down a flight of steps that were next to the airplane. Then, I was back into an airport wheelchair to go to the baggage area to retrieve, and transfer, into my wheelchair. We left the airport by cab, with my parents lifting into the cab, and out at the Riviera Hotel. No more transferring until we flew home, but all that transferring was very tiring!

I could not play the slot machines by myself, and as much as I really enjoyed blackjack, I couldn't reach the table. So, the dealer placed my verbal bets taking my head signals - hit was yes, and stay was no. Las Vegas was a bustling city no matter what time of day. All the lights, special themes of the hotels, shows, food, food, and more food were wonderful! There were no low, blackjack tables for people with disabilities at that time. The dealer at the blackjack table thought he was being funny, and tried to make a joke.

"You should get a pillow to sit on," he said, probably, barely seeing my head.

"Actually, I am already sitting on two pillows from the room!" I told him.

The TV show Hollywood squares was being filmed at the hotel where we were staying, and we saw Charlie Weaver, Joan Rivers, and seven other stars at the same time.

Across the street from our hotel, and on another day, we walked to the Circus Circus all the way down the strip to the hotel that used to be called the MGM Grand, until it had a fire in one of the higher floors. Today, it is known as Bally's. We saw the original, and very real, MGM lion who was toothless, and had poor vision, inside a little fence, and anyone could have his/her picture taken with him except me. The photographer was unsure of the lion's reaction to the shiny wheelchair. I was fine with that!

When we were in the Sands Hotel, I sat at a blackjack table with a man who had too much to drink, and he signed several papers for more money. I watched as he lost at least $5000 in a short time. It was very stressful to me, and I left the table. I always gambled responsibly, giving myself a limit on losses, but not on wins. When we left Las Vegas, and were waiting at the airport, I played the slot machines with help winning $100. The plane held a raffle, and if you wanted to play, you put in $1 with the seat number. The seat number that was called, surprisingly, was my seat number! I won the raffle.
It was a fun trip, but at least I came out even!

BY THE GRACE OF GOD AND YOU
A Chair Does Not a Person Make

From 1973 to 1986, went to Las Vegas 16 times! Each time was different. I had a chance to see a Lido show with their spectacular costumes, Wayne Newton, Debbie Reynolds who was cute and funny, Liberace, Glenn Campbell, who was more handsome than I had anticipated in his white jumpsuit, and my favorite, Tony Orlando whose song, *Tie a Yellow Ribbon,* hit the charts. Tony was very weak having just completed a drug program, but he gave his all for the shows by singing and dancing all the way to the back of the room where I was sitting. The girl who was sitting on my right was saying how she was going to get a kiss from him. I thought that would be a fun idea! She missed him, because he passed on our right side of the table. I turned my head to the left, and he kissed my cheek, and then quickly moved to the front of the room. Tony was sweating hard, and he flicked his hair, and some droplets landed on me. When I told this story to my friends, I changed it a little. I exaggerated, "Tony was perspiring, because the kiss made him so hot!" I thought that was very nice of him to kiss me. I knew that he had a sister with cerebral palsy.

We also saw Pearl Bailey standing outside of the hotel, maybe waiting for a limousine. She was very nice, and gave me a kiss, too. Mom and Dad had seen Nipsey Russell, who was a comedian, walking through a parking lot. Mom got so excited all she could say pointing to my Dad while looking at Nipsey, "He likes you!"

In the early morning on one of our trips, Dad decided to get a cup of coffee while Mom and I were getting ready for the day. He told us that he watched a movie that was being filmed in the casino, and he thought it was Clint Eastwood. The person had to stand on something to be taller than his co-star. Since Clint Eastwood was 6'2" tall, we finally realized that it must have been Robert Redford, who is only 5'9".

On another trip, we spotted my friend, and chess mate, Warren, who had cerebral palsy, difficult speech, and was in a wheelchair, and his Mother, Lucille. Dad and Mom were helping him get out of the cab, when I yelled, "Help!" Mom had forgotten to put the brake on my manual wheelchair, and I was rolling toward an eight-inch curb. I had no way of stopping myself from falling off it! Luckily, Lucille saw me first and saved me just in time!

In 1978, I had spent a lot of time with a teacher named Merle. He was single, and I talked him into going to Vegas with us. He liked traveling, but he had never flown before, and was afraid. He didn't want to go alone, so he asked Jeff, a student who had kept in touch with both of us, to come to Las Vegas. Jeff was my student who helped me during the noon hours, and graduated. Merle was excited about the flight, and because of this trip, Jeff and Merle spent many years of flying and cruising. Since Merle had no relatives alive except one older uncle in Arizona, we all became a family. But, our trip had to be cut short. My Grandma "with the kitties" had osteoporosis (as do I, now), and had broken her hip, first, then, she had fallen. Grandma ended up in the hospital, and, of course, no one could help her but Mom. We tried to get a flight back early, but only made it home a day or so ahead of time.

When I visited Las Vegas, I would spend a good 8 to 12 hours per day at the blackjack tables. The rest of the time was spent eating, or sleeping. It was a nice social experience. Sometimes I could even help some of the players who would often ask me questions. Having taught statistics and probability gave me a little advantage—very little, but very helpful. For example, I helped one man win back a couple hundred dollars as the cards were falling just right for him.

About a year later, I was rolling down the street in Milwaukee to get into the Summerfest grounds, when I heard someone yelling behind me. I waited, thinking that I had dropped something. When the man caught up with me, he asked me, "Aren't you the lady that helped me play blackjack in Vegas last year?" I didn't know how he recognized me. I never thought that I would see him again, but he made my day!

In July of 1974, my sister had her first baby. She had a bit of a hard time when the baby was born, because she had a uterine inversion. This is when a uterus turns inside out at birth, and it happens in about one in 30,000 births. Since her doctor was a general practitioner, he called the other doctors in the hospital hoping to find someone to assist him. The only choices were a foot doctor, a psychiatrist, or him to put the uterus inside right! Susie was put under anesthesia due to her pain, so someone else had to make the decision. Her Doctor fixed the problem, and she had no other problems with her other two children. The baby was named Kenneth after my Dad, and his middle name was James after Bob's brother who died in Vietnam. I was his godmother, and his uncle Mike was his godfather. Mike held Kenny during the christening, since I could not do it. Ken screamed during the entire baptism. He hated baths, and wanted no water on his head!

Ken seemed to grow up fast, and was so handsome! By the time he was walking, he was picking up everything on the floor, and putting it in the garbage can. Everything was supposed to have its place! Dad had found one of his own, old toys, a little red metal fire engine that Kenny would ride up and down my ramp for hours at a time. He kept everyone busy!

Fred was ordained as a priest in 1974, too, and my parents and I were present for the ceremony. When we came to congratulate him, he stepped off the riser on which he was standing, and gave the three of us a Lutheran blessing! We also met his parents, and soon after that he was assigned to Texas where he worked with cancer patients in a hospital, and then he continued on to Washington DC, where he was in a parish having Rose Kennedy in the front row every Sunday! He had also performed mass in 1973 at our WWAAC convention.

Before he left for Texas, Fred, Les, and I spent an evening at the Lake Geneva Playboy Club! It was a lot of fun, but I can't remember why we went there, but we didn't drink! I had been to the club once before with Chester, a relative, who was a member of the Playboy Club and Kenosha Yacht Club. We ate in the main dining room, but it was not very accessible. There were two, or three, steps into the building. I must have taken a freight elevator up to the dining room, because I had an opportunity to go through the kitchen, as I had to do in many places. The dining room was beautiful, and I still remembered the rich, purple carpeting that went halfway up the wall!

Right after Kenny was christened, I took another trip to Central America with the Feins. This time, I went with Steve's girlfriend, Barb, who was another Wawbeek counselor. Barb was a very cute, small framed, but a physically, strong blonde. This trip was one hour difference than Kenosha's Central Time Zone. No jet lag on this trip! We landed in the capital of Guatemala, and traveled to some of the neighboring communities. One day, we bartered in the marketplace, and saw some of the country's unique textiles—clothing, hats, or pictures that were in at least seven different layers of colored cloth folded back, and sewn into recognizable designs. I don't know how they did it, but they used a picture the country's national bird, the quetzal, that had a very long, feathery tail. My heart hurt inside to see people on the city streets, having different disabilities, reduced to begging.

We traveled from city to city with each city having their own, brightly colored textile patterns, so you knew where people came from by their clothing design as well as their own industry in each city. For example, making bricks was a likelihood for everyone in one city, another city designed and made silver jewelry, and still another city did all of the weaving for the country. The cities were in mountainous regions which had a number of those beautiful waterfalls created by nature on their mountain paths. Driving between cities, we would see places they called Laundromats, which was an open area with wash tubs near streams, where the people of the region would be washing their clothes. Some of them bleached their clothing by putting their soapy items in the sun to turn whiter. Many of the people walked from place to place with huge baskets held on their heads. There were many back problems as well as many young people with polio, since there were no inoculations. Life expectancy was 40 years. We saw a family of three by their home as we went into another town, and asked to take their picture for two dollars. They were very happy to pose for us! A boy was walking around the city with his goat, selling fresh from the tap goat milk for a quarter a glass, but I passed on it!

We stayed overnight in an area surrounded by three volcanoes. The weather in Guatemala was beautiful—80° almost all of the time! Marimbas played in soft tones like xylophones during the cocktail hour. The Royal Poinciana trees with huge orange flowers also impressed me.

Next, we went to Costa Rica, and stayed a few days near the ocean. Barb and another attendant got me into the swimming pool, and from there I could watch the pelicans scooping up their lunch with their big bills. There were small, dog-sized, shy iguanas running between the coconut trees about 20 yards away. That was close enough for me!

The next day, we took a trip to the top of an inactive volcano, named Irazú. From the top, you could see both the Atlantic and the Pacific Oceans. It was a little cloudy, and we were on top of the clouds! The cooled volcanic ash was very prominent with a lake covering the eruption point at the Irazú Volcano National Park.

The last night there, I tried a fresh lobster, but just couldn't handle it. It contained too much iodine, and frozen were better for me! On our last night in the Costa Rica resort, the fans caused my hair to tickle my face all night. I couldn't brush my hair off my face, so I just kept blowing it off with my breath. In the morning, Barb wanted to take a swim before we packed, so she placed me so that I could see out the window. I still saw little iguanas running around. I was ready to move on to Panama. I had enough of iguanas. I saw Barb walking towards our room when my eyes moved above the curtain. There was a huge spider the size of my fist with multiple hairy legs. Was that what was tickling me last night? Barb appeared, and stood on a chair to kill it with her hand, and a piece of toilet paper! She was brave, and never even flinched!

There were no good roads into Panama, so we flew. We were in such a nice place in Costa Rica that it surprised me to see all of the graffiti on the buildings in the downtown area.

BY THE GRACE OF GOD AND YOU
A Chair Does Not a Person Make

Getting on the airplane was no problem, but the plane trip to Panama was the scariest flight that I ever experienced! The plane was small, and we flew through a bad thunderstorm. I wasn't sure we were going to make it! The ride was so bumpy that our plane dropped altitude a couple of times. I thought that I would be glad when we got back on the ground, but that experience was a little bit of a rocky ride too! The Panama firefighters, who spoke no English, had volunteered to carry us off the plane, and down the flight of stairs to the ground! I was strapped into a small airport chair, but on the way down the flight of steps, the chair tilted, and I had no ability to control my head. I tried to flag one of the firefighter's attention, and I was having difficulty swallowing, but no luck. One of the firefighters finally did hold my head up a little, which helped! The good thing was my wig never fell off!

Well, we made it to Panama, and was it was hot! Barb and I did some shopping, and got back to the hotel just in time to have a siesta. Every day, because of the heat, there were heavy downpours, between noon and 3:00 p.m. The next day, we took a trip to the Panama Canal, and watched a ship go through one of the locks. A picnic in the jungle was next by a very old Banyan tree that had dropped enough roots from its branches to look like it was 400 years old! There were many python snakes in this area that a lot of the children enjoyed playing with in the jungle, but we did not see any! What we did see was a tiny cloud in the distance that hurried everyone onto the bus, and back to the resort before it started raining torrentially. That night was everyone's last night together, so we celebrated with a Coco Loco drink, which is rum and coconut milk that is served in a coconut shell.

I had been having a lot of diarrhea a few days. Poor Barb had to deal with my problem. I discovered, when I returned home, that it was not the water causing my diarrhea, but it was all of the ice cream desserts/milk that we had along the way! I had to take Kaopectate pills like candy all the way home on the airplane, since I could not get to the plane's bathroom!

When I did get home, my doctor put me in the hospital. He thought maybe I had diabetes, but I thought that maybe it was lactose intolerance, which is the inability to handle dairy products like milk, ice cream, so he ordered a diabetic test without all of the needles. If I had to go to the hospital to have blood drawn, I would usually tell them, "If you are not good at this, don't touch me." One of the other doctors in my doctor's office had to take care of me once. He thought I was noncompliant, and scolded me when the nurse told him that I would not let her take my blood, yet she tried three times! When he tried to draw my blood himself, he totally understood the problem! Everyone had a very difficult time taking my blood pressure, too. How could they prove I was alive? I usually avoided doctors. One doctor that saw me stated, "You must almost be dead, or you wouldn't be here!" The doctors ordered liquid glucose, and immediately after I drank it, it gave me diarrhea.

I was lactose intolerant—meaning I could lose weight on a hot fudge sundae! If I had to choose a health problem, this was the best problem I could ever have!

In the meantime, Al was very sick at the Monroe Clinic about an hour to an hour and a half ride away. Before I left for Central America, he was doing some strange things like taping our conversations, and asking my Mom to listen to them. My parents thought I would want to see him, so they took me. When I saw him, I didn't recognize him. His skin looked as if it was stretched over bone. When he came home, I confronted him on his odd behaviors with some questions, and I told him, "If you ever really need a friend call me, but until then, you will not hear from me." Arlene was his friend, before I was her friend. She called Al to see how he was doing. He swore up and down that I put her up to it. I never called, or told Arlene to call, but Al made sure Arlene told me what he thought! Other strange things happened during that period of time. Our address was placed in the newspaper as having a rummage sale. People knocked on our door. We told them, "No, not us." However, the article did help a neighbor. He had a garage full of things that he sold that day—an impromptu rummage sale! I didn't think Al would have done it, though, because an article in the paper would have cost money that he didn't have. I only saw him once more, and years later.

In 1975, the school district began requiring teachers certifications to be maintained every two years. Six credits were needed for any who held a Bachelor's Degree, and three for a Master's Degree. I was already busy with teaching full-time, extracurricular activities, ABLE, WWAAC, a social group at the Jane Vernon School, traveling, and more. I did not know how I was going to add this into my schedule.

Les tried to convince me to be a rehabilitation counselor, because, as he pointed out to me, it was what I had already been doing for years, except my job revolved around people with disabilities. The school district was concerned, because about half of the students were using marijuana two to three times per week. I had seen some problems in the hallways, and heard of others reporting to the principal.

I made an appointment to go see Ann Trotter, the head of the Rehabilitation Department at the University of Wisconsin-Milwaukee. She explained that because I taught statistics classes, nine credits would be fulfilled by that experience. I had completed the GRE when I was at Carthage. The only thing that I was lacking was a class in human development/testing. Carthage, by then, had begun a Master's program. I was to take that class in the summer of 1975. I just had to find an attendant for the year ahead in Milwaukee, and complete the required class, before I was accepted. Everything was ready ahead of time, and I reviewed everything with the school district, so that the district would allow me to be on sabbatical for the 1976-1977 school years. My degree would be in educational rehabilitation focusing on alcohol, drugs, and youth. Upon completing my year of school, I signed a contract to come back, and teach for at least two years. I wasn't really considering leaving teaching at the time. I just wanted to make getting the newly required credits easier. I did write a paper on what I had learned in Central America, and submitted it for credit to the school district, which they accepted for at least two, or three, credits. With the above plan, I hoped to complete my courses in a nine-month school year. I would do my internship in the summer of 1977 at DePaul, and graduate by August 1977, so I could return to work in September 1977.

But, first things first! Eddie had a bad pressure sore, and spent over four months in the hospital lying on his stomach. Therefore, I took over many of his duties at ABLE. I went to visit him, remembering how much the bleach in the hospital sheets used to cut up my elbows. I didn't even have to lean on mine like he did because of the strategic location of his pressure sore. The Kenosha Hospital's front entrance was, and still is, ramped uphill to the main floor in a semicircle drive. When Eddie was released from the hospital, he was so happy that he rolled out the front door, down the hill, fell out of his wheelchair, broke his leg, and taken right back into the hospital! I felt bad for him, but did you ever feel bad for someone, and after that shock wears off, something strikes you funny? It was so horrible, but I just start laughing. Well, it was like laughing at a funeral service for no reason. I was embarrassed, but the image of it was too funny. He had the worst luck! Not long after, though, he married a friend of mine from Oshkosh, also named Carol, who he met through WWAAC. After living in Milwaukee for a while and both of them working at a handicapped housing service, they moved to Las Vegas. I continued with ABLE. In Las Vegas, he had a booth at a flea fair, and gathered a gun collection, which included a working gun from the Civil War. As far as Vegas goes, he continued to have bad luck—in the casino!

In the summer of 1975, I completed my human development/testing class at Carthage. It was good to be back at Carthage and in school.

When my class was completed, Mom, Dad, and I, took a handicapped tour with the Feins to Hawaii. This time, Shirley, my friend who went to Europe with me, and Mary, who was on her first trip, went with us! The weather was always about 80°! Macadamia nuts were served on the plane while flying over the Pacific Ocean. We were greeted with leis when we landed, and then, we took a second plane to our first stop in Kauai staying at a beach resort. Every morning, about 6 a.m., a rainbow would touch the beach in front of us. When we ate breakfast, there were no walls. Birds flew through the restaurant, and pools of small fish guided us through the entrance. We rented a car, because we were on our own that day.

While we waited for the car, we saw an 80-year-old Hawaiian man, who came over to me, and out of the blue revealed to me, "You are in a wheelchair due to the sins of your parents!"

I didn't know what to say. Normally, if he had been a child, I would have taken time to explain.

Since I was on vacation, and his beliefs were very ingrained, I just said, "Yes," and left to get into the rental car that just arrived. Mom was very hurt, and felt guilty, because of the man's statement, and it bothered her for a long time.

The island of Kauai was about 60 miles wide. We knew we were going to see the plush part of the island the next day where over 600 inches of rain a year was a normal expectation. We decided to go to the more barren part of the island. We also saw a blowhole, where the waves are forced up through a rock's hole, which shot multiple feet into the air.

The next day, we had a guide, and went to the hotel where Elvis Presley filmed the wedding scene in *Blue Hawaii*. We saw some of the other plush vegetation, and waterfalls, as well as hearing about the old customs and the history of the Hawaiians, and Capt. Cook, who discovered the islands. If a baby had been born "defective or deformed," the parent would leave the baby alone to fend for himself/herself with the rain, with the animals, with nature, and with little, or no, chance of survival. I actually thought this information tied in with the 80-year-old man's comment the day before. Another guide described how they caught squid. He explained, "A person goes out into the water, and lets the squid wrap his tentacles around his hand. With the squid secured, the native bites the squid's eye, which loosens the suction on its tentacles. He then takes it home to eat!" I wasn't sure I bought that story, but I did eat squid/octopus on the previous trip to Costa Rica in a casserole. It tasted like rubbery bacon to me.

That night, we went to the hotel show at the resort. Mary had a particularly good time, because the Hawaiian man sang directly to her! She was melting all over, and her eyes were very dreamy, especially when he gave her his lei! It made the whole trip worthwhile! She was talking with her smile and eyes all night long!

We got on the plane the next morning for Maui, which is an island, shaped a little bit like the number eight. The airport was in the middle of the eight, so it was very windy. We took a ride to our hotel/ resort that even had a golf course! We passed sugar cane fields where we saw them cut and burned. (A fun fact: Do you know how C & H Sugar got its name? The C & H stands for grown in Hawaii, and refined in California!)

We found a nice area where we all sat on the beach, and my first time, and watched the water. Mom and Mary took a little stroll along the beach. Mom was helping Mary balance on the sand since Mary wasn't used to walking on it. Shirley and I were talking to Dad and a couple of other people from the group, when all of a sudden we heard, "Help, help, help!" We turned to look, and both Mary and Mom were lying on the beach yelling for help! We figured out that a wave had knocked them down, and retreated to make it look like they were just lying down yelling for help. Dad yelled, "Stand up!" and went to help them. They were terrified as the pull of the water really scared them. They thought the ocean was going to pull them into it! Not long after that, we noticed the water was getting close to us. We were in an area where the tide was coming in, and we didn't know it. Mom and Dad helped everyone off the beach. I was last, and a wave did come up, and knocked me backwards while I was sitting on the sand. I couldn't believe how warm the water was and how powerful! It washed a ton of sand into my ears as the wave retreated. I don't think I got the sand all out until I got back in Wisconsin.

We also went to a pineapple plantation where we tasted the fresh pineapple—warm and juicy. I have never tasted a pineapple so good! I think I appreciated it more, because I found out it took a pineapple a year and a half to mature.

I believe it was on this island they removed us from the tour bus on top of a deep valley with gusts of wind so strong coming over the place where we stood that I literally could not open my eyes! The Hawaiian story was that when they chose a Princess, they threw a girl into the deep valley below. If the wind blew her back onto the place we were standing, the gods had chosen her as Princess. I imagine that all of the princesses chosen must have been petite.

On to Oahu, and Honolulu was where Dad was stationed in the service. He really wanted Mom to see this area of the national cemetery, the Air Force Base from the cemetery, and Pearl Harbor. Pearl Harbor and the Arizona were particularly meaningful to me! I always got goose bumps at historical places. We cruised a little while along the shore of Waikiki Beach. This beach was very narrow, and its sand always traveled to the other side of the island due to the ocean currents. The sand is replaced on a regular basis, and we had a good view of Diamond Head. We met up with a former Easter Seals camp counselor, Dave, who took us to see one of the local shows. Of course, we saw Don Ho, who sang his song, *Tiny Bubbles*. We went to the zoo that had the only snake on the island, because a mongoose killed all of them, and a Kodak Show demonstrating the different types of South Seas dances such as the hula, and it was slower than the Polynesian which had very fast hip movement. It was called Kodak, so that we could take many pictures!

BY THE GRACE OF GOD AND YOU
A Chair Does Not a Person Make

One of the couples on the trip was engaged, and both were in wheelchairs. The man had been catching a ride on the woman's chair by hanging onto the chair without his safety belt buckled, and he was pulled out of his chair onto the ground. I believe he broke one, or both, of his legs in the fall. The plane flight back was miserable for him, because of the air pressure on his wounds.

It was our last night, so we went to a luau, complete with music, fire dancers, and a roasted pig. Everything was delicious except for the poi, which really did taste like wallpaper paste. How do I know it tasted like wallpaper? Not that I've ever tasted wallpaper paste, but it was the announcer's description. It did taste like paste, and it smelled like it, too!

I went to M.D. camp that summer. I think this was the year that they had the sword swallower! Amazing to watch, yet it made me gag to watch him after I knew how he did it! With the tip of his tongue on the sword, it started rolling up into a ball-like mass in his mouth. When the sword was removed, it was held tight so it could unroll, and clicked the tip of the sword to be stiff again.

The swimming was great that year, too, and I talked Lloyd into tossing me into the pool's deep end instead of putting me down by the side of the pool, and sliding me into the water. He was a little scared, but gave me instructions on keeping my back bent, which was, of course, no problem! That way it wouldn't hurt as I plunged into the water, which, by the way, was an *excellent* entry! He also tried dragging me through the water while he swam, and held onto my hand between his feet. I was to tug on his foot when I needed air. It was fun!

I met Kristi at the pool, and our conversation steered in the direction of school. She told me that she was going back next year to UW Milwaukee. I felt as if God was making my plans for me! Without asking, she wanted to know if I needed an attendant, since she was going to have to apply for jobs to pay for school! I didn't know why I was surprised, but I was. She would be a perfect match, too. Now, I truly was ready for school!

The one notable change at M.D. camp was that at least three people had passed away. It seemed to happen every year. I felt like I was back in grade school. One of the men with Muscular Dystrophy spoke with me telling me that he was very afraid to die. I found out that the volunteer assisting him was a pre-med student. We all had a conversation on the topic. The pre-med student shared that seldom did a person know when he/she was really dying. The camper felt calmed by this information, and he told us that he felt cheated, because he didn't have the strength to commit suicide. He wasn't saying that he would commit suicide, but that for him, it wasn't even an option, and that was why he felt cheated. He also was one of the few campers who did not have a motorized wheelchair. Lloyd brought him to my home, so that he could try my wheelchair, because it was something he just wanted to do. With adjustments, he could at least go in circles, but the chair needed more adjustments. He never felt this much freedom before. He never had the opportunity to get an electric chair, however, because shortly after he passed away. That was what was hard about MD camp. Every year upon returning to camp, it was sad, and hard, because two to four campers weren't there, because they had died. No one could anticipate who would be missing.

M.D. winter camp was challenging too. It was probably -20° with the wind chill. I, finally, decided to try ice fishing! Contrary to popular opinion, it wasn't just to get hot chocolate, although I did love hot chocolate—actually, chocolate anything! The previous year, a few fish had been caught, but were released. The people that had gone fishing claimed that they could see down into the water, and could see the fish near the line *if* they were under a blanket! I had to try it! I wasn't the only one who went ice fishing. First, a person made a hole in the ice with a piece of equipment that looked like a huge drill. Second, they put a couple of holes about 12 to 15 inches in diameter in the ice for others who wanted to try. Lloyd placed me onto a blanket next to one of drilled holes. Lloyd brought me a fishing rod with bait already on the hook, and he put it into the water. He leaned me forward so I could see into the hole, and put a blanket over both of our heads, and then he leaned over on top of me. It *was true*! We could see the fish by eliminating the sunlight! The water was clear, and not very deep. The ice looked about three inches thick, and I was sitting on it? It was both warm and relaxing in my present position. There was no way I was going to be able to hook the fish, because I couldn't move. After about 10 minutes, Lloyd got up. I didn't realize how much pressure he had put on me, because I felt extremely light as if I was going to fly forward, and end up in the water. I waited a while, and still watched the fish underneath the ice. I heard, "We are breaking out the hot chocolate!" I was ready to quit! I loved the experience. It sure beat last year when my horse took my sled over that 5-foot tree!

Then, back in the lodge, we played Sheepshead. Darn! I never could beat Lloyd at cards, but I did begin paying more attention to him!

~ 15 ~

Politics and Master's Degree

I was becoming more involved with politics. On April 8, 1976, my friend from the Orthopedic School, Les Ryshkus, employed by the *Kenosha News*, wrote the article below:

Leader in Helping Handicap *written by LES RYSHKUS:*

Many Wisconsin residents practice one of their most cherished privileges this week, the right to vote. For many of the physically handicapped and disabled, the act of voting can be a difficult, if not an impossible, task. Although the absentee ballot is available to those unable to get to or into the polling places, most people, able and disabled, prefer the privacy of the voting booth. The Wisconsin legislature recently passed Assembly Bill 1. This bill, which Gov. Lucey is expected to sign within the next two weeks, secures the civil rights that so many take for granted. AB 1 would make it unlawful to discriminate against a person in regard to voting, jury duty and housing as well as employment solely on the basis of the person's disability

IT WAS WITH *this legislation in mind that ABLE (Abolish Barriers for Lifetime Efficiency) held an appreciation dinner Friday evening for legislators at both the state and the city level. The dinner was attended by the State Representatives George Molinaro, Russell Olson, Eugene Dorff and guest speaker State Representative James WAHNER of Milwaukee. Many City Councilman and County board members also attended. WAHNER has been a driving force behind much of the recent legislation for the handicapped. In 1971 he introduced the first bill to ramp curbs making them accessible to those in wheelchairs. In 1973, he was chairman of the Gov.'s Task Force on problems of Problems of People with Physical Handicaps from which evolved one of the first comprehensive reports of its kind on the problems of the handicapped. "In 1971 when I introduced the bill to ramp curbs everyone laughed," said WAHNER. "They're not laughing now." 15 states quickly followed Wisconsin and made ramping mandatory for all newly built or remodeled curbs. Commenting on Assembly Bill 1, WAHNER said, "I think this ranks us among the leaders in the country in securing the same rights for handicapped people as those enjoyed by every other minority in this nation." WAHNER concluded with his evaluation of legislation for the handicapped since joining the legislature nearly 6 years ago, "The progress in the past five years has been dramatic. But we still have a long way to go. Abolishing barriers is something we all care about and have to work on. Groups like ABLE bringing legislators in to talk and to listen will help lead us in the right direction."*

THE ABLE DINNER *also included those at the city level responsible for such things as the ramping of curbs downtown, the $.10 bus fare for the elderly and handicapped, and the* *soon to be accessible courthouse. A program was presented by seven members of the community involved professionally in various fields dealing with the handicapped. Such topics as housing, architecture, transportation, employment, insurance and financial assistance were discussed. Many sides to these issues were discussed, some hopeful, some discouraging. Ed Jenkins, Kenosha Transportation Commission director, spoke of a Dial-a-Bus, a specially equipped bus that could be ready to transport the handicapped and disabled by 1977. Linda Legler of the Housing Authority spoke of her problems finding landlords willing to take in a person with a disability. But perhaps Jack Killian, director of the Achievement Center summed it up best when he said, "People are treated as adults only if they are able to lead a productive life." And that is what ABLE was thanking the legislators for: helping them to lead a richer and more productive life.*

Everything came together when the members of ABLE, combined with many letters, many trips to Madison, and many voices, Wisconsin became a leader in accessibility for the disabled in the country.

We went to see my Grandma "with the mink" at a hospital in Chicago. She was shook a lot, especially with her head. I remembered she was taking high blood pressure pills, but she did not take potassium by eating bananas and potatoes one needs with them. She died.

This was the last summer I attended at the MDA camp, because the administrative policy changed for summer campers, and they only accepted people 18 years old and younger. After this change, June started an adult, MD camping group called "With a Little Help" Taken from the Beatles song, because "we all needed a little help from our friends." The group did all of their own fundraising. Carol was my counselor, again. While dressing me, she found a lump in my left breast, and when I went to the camp doctor, he suggested I get it taken care of when I returned home. I waited until I started school in Milwaukee, since a hospital was right across the street from my 22-floor dorm.

Kristi was ready to start school. Mom and Dad took me to Milwaukee with my personal belongings, and I moved into the dorms. There were 22 floors, and I was on the third floor. Waiting for the elevator was pretty long sometimes! I found out which building my classes were in and did some trial runs to see where I was going to need help with doors, or elevators. Of course, the snow would mean I would need someone to walk with me. My classmates were very helpful! I also signed up for two meals a day for the first semester.

I went home, and returned to Milwaukee for the MDA Labor Day Telethon in Milwaukee. It was the first time that I had ever worked the Telethon. The phone seemed heavier, and it was difficult to write on the carbon copy pledges. Even though I did my best, they called me a couple of times, because it wasn't dark enough to read. I also called the handicapped transportation to pick me up after the telethon, and take me to the dorms. The vehicle never arrived. The bus came for some of the other people, but because I was not a resident of the city, the specialized transportation wouldn't take me. I started to panic. Kristi told me that we could ask Lloyd, since he was there, too. He was kind enough to take me, and he stayed to watch two movies with us when we got home—*2001: A Space Odyssey, wh*ich I never really understood, and *Harold and Maude*. Kristi and I started to settle into a routine. We seldom made it to breakfast, however. She took a job at the pizza restaurant downstairs, and had additional hours of work. We had a good group of roommates, and we a good mix of studying and socializing! Of course, dorms would be dorms. There were the 2 a.m. fire alarms, which would ring, because somebody obviously had nothing else to do. Eileen, another roommate, would always sleep through the fire drills. We did promise her that if it were a real fire alarm for a real fire, we would wake her up!

I found out that Easter Seals in Milwaukee had a swim program at the University that I could take for credit. I received special permission to take 13 credits, since 12 credits were the maximum allowed per semester in the Master's program. It was the first time I ever had a gym class. I learned how to roll over in the water, which was a big accomplishment for me. At first, they told me to roll away from the curvature in my back. That didn't work! I tried and, then, tried it the opposite way, which was my heavier side so it floated to the top easier. In order to flip my body over, I put my arm over my head. I couldn't always be this independent. It depended on how many other people were in the water, and the undercurrents, but I felt successful in a sport! I only took the class for the first semester, because the second semester I had to do a field experience.

There was always so much to do on campus. I enjoyed feeling like a number in a large school instead of being "special". The special services department had a couple of events for people with disabilities. They were just organizing, so I went to some of them. The library was fantastic, but I still had problems doing things on my own there. I spent some time in the union—a study and eating area. Most of my classes were in the building next to my dorm. Some of my new classmates walked with me to and from my classes when the classes weren't close to the dorm—especially if there was snow.

One of the first things I did was go to Columbia Hospital to see a doctor about the lump in my breast. The lump was smaller now. The doctor thought that it might be fibrous instead of something serious. He ordered a mammogram, which was not easy for me, because I had to lie on a hard table, on my sides, smashing my breast with clamps. Everything turned out fine! It was really a scary couple of months worrying and wondering before I had the mammogram.

Shortly after I started back to school, I got a phone call from home saying my dog, Penny, had a stroke. Penny could no longer stand. My parents had to put her to sleep. It was a hard time for me.

It seemed to me like everything I went through in life prepared me for the job I was going to be doing in the future, so that I would be able to understand what people were thinking and feeling. At the time, Kristi had an African American male friend who used to walk around the area with us. It was interesting when I noticed that people were not staring at me, but at them! That felt good! Really, I hardly noticed others staring anymore, since I could ignore it. I always look different doing everything, so I would expect people to stare. Since I knew so many people in Milwaukee that were in wheelchairs from all the state meetings and rallies I attended in Madison and Milwaukee, I found myself staring at anyone with a disability just to see if I knew the person!

Classes seemed to be easy, especially the medical aspects of people with disabilities. They could say a disability, and I could name a person who had it, think about them, and what their limitations were as well as how the disability had changed the person over the years.

I almost had my Master's thesis completed before I started the program. Many of my friends had been having problems finding employment. My thesis was - "Causes of Unemployment for People with Disabilities". My idea was that employers were blaming the union for not being able to hire people with disabilities and the union blamed the employers! Out of all the questions that I asked on my survey, these were the only survey questions that turned out to have a statistically significant response.

I enjoyed getting back into the academic atmosphere, and all of the books that I was required to read. I especially enjoyed *Custer Died for Your Sins*. One chapter was about Indian humor, and the history of the treatment of Native Americans in America. *The Education of a WASP* (the White Anglo-Saxon Protestant) was another book that I enjoyed. I felt that this book emphasized how society perpetuated discrimination involving African Americans, and society itself never learned, nor wanted to learn, how to make relationships better.

Being away from home for the first time other than camping, I had to try some things that I hadn't tried before. Mom and Dad always had alcohol in the house, and Dad had had two drinks every night when he came home from work. I had a few drinks at my sister's wedding, but didn't feel anything. Having never been drunk, I decided I had to try it - once.

There was a disco upstairs where I joined Kristi, Lloyd and a few friends. I had several screwdrivers. I had no idea how I would react, but I just withdrew. Lloyd said that I became quieter than normal. Nothing I wanted to do again. I also tried marijuana, since it was everywhere. It was funny. I never really felt anything in my head, but the wheels on my chair felt like they were floating over the ground! I could act crazy enough when I was sober and clean. I never really tried anything again.

I had previously had some bad reactions to medications. I always pitied those who needed drugs to find happiness. I liked wine, occasionally, but more than one glass would give me diarrhea. I never liked the taste of beer! I never really liked drinking other stuff as that meant going more to the bathroom! For other people, it took just a few minutes to go, but for me, it took 15 to 20 minutes, and was a real waste of time! There is no such thing as a 10-minute shower for a person with a severe disability. It takes me longer than that to gain energy to take a shower.

It was the first time Kristi had lived with anyone with a disability. I asked her if I did anything that bothered her. She shared that she had just written a paper on it for one of her classes. I asked if I could read it. She had written that I said "please" and "thank you" for everything! She got to the point where she was just waiting for either of those words. Ever since then, I would sometimes say "please," and sometimes say "thank you" by not trying to say either too often with the same person. I didn't want to get out of the habit though, because if I was working with someone new, I might forget to thank them, and perhaps the person wouldn't feel appreciated. "Please" preceded, and acted as a good reminder of something they forgot! "Thank you" often meant a good feedback for "you did it right. It's done."

There were two, 24-hour dance-a-thons, and I went. The first one was for Muscular Dystrophy. I had not tried to dance for 24 hours previously, but I only was able to complete the first 20 hours, because I just could not move my body anymore! The second one for United Cerebral Palsy (UCP), however, was a little easier. Kristi took my hands, and kept me moving for about 15 minutes, and I did not have to move my wheelchair nor myself. I made it! The school newspaper wrote:

UCP Cabaret Dance-…… Carol managed to stay on the dance floor for 10 hours straight, give or take a few spare minutes or so. The result of her efforts? $103.50 of sponsor pledged monies. Over $1000 had been raised during the marathon.

I also worked on the UCP Telethon. I thought James Darren looked very hot in his white suit, and disappointed in an actress who cried over the adults and kids with cerebral palsy. You did not have to raise money by using pity. I knew some of the people, and they were intelligent and strong! I took a list of 31 points that I wanted to make with the UCP Board of Directors. The person in charge of fundraising believed funds could not be raised without pity, but the Board of Directors disagreed. My 31 points included suggestions on how to make the CP telethon more positive. For instance, letting people tell their own story as well as the problems on a daily basis, or show how some of the technology works to assist the individual. I watched the show the next year, since I was no longer in Milwaukee. They did a good job.

About the same time, people were starting to be concerned about the Jerry Lewis Telethon for Muscular Dystrophy. I always felt that was more difficult as so many of the diagnoses were terminal. Many advocates criticized the term "Jerry's kids." Even though many of the people he assisted were adults, I always believed that to a parent, a kid was a kid no matter what the age. This show could have been more informational, and medically based.

Besides this type of advocacy, I also had an opportunity to go to some of the political fundraisers. I heard Mayor Meier from Milwaukee speak as well. Unfortunately, I was tired—unusual for me—and his monotone voice put me asleep - twice - during his speech! I was so embarrassed, and I'm sure I made a "good" impression! Later that summer, I was at a fundraiser for Rep. Wahner.

I was having a good time, and had two drinks, when someone tapped me on the shoulder.

"Hi, I am …..."

But, because of the noise, I could not hear him.

"What?" I asked.

"I'm Gov. Schreiber," he repeated.

"Who?"

At least Gov. Schreiber knew I was embarrassed, because my cheeks were probably red from the drinks!

The most impressive political event I attended that year was to hear the Presidential Democratic candidate, Mo Udall, speak. The room was large, and packed with people. The minute the Secret Service men came in, you could hear a pin drop in that room! It gave me a very scary feeling. Udall followed, and more Secret Service men followed. As people started shaking his hand, and he reached the front of the audience to speak, the mood became more normal.

At the beginning of the second semester, I had to do fieldwork. I was approved to go to the Jewish Vocational Center (JVC) in Milwaukee. The staff was very helpful, and I learned a lot. My supervisor was in a wheelchair, too, and was about ready to retire. She gave me many good pointers on how to work with people with severe learning disabilities. The first client I met gave me a great big hug! My supervisor said, "Now, that is not appropriate behavior. You should shake hands!" The introduction was repeated. Appropriate work behavior, the ability to complete simple tasks, and using social skills were taught to me. I was there only a couple of days a week. The only physical problem was that the telephone had a rotary dial. I could not dial fast enough when I would try to call my supervisor, or someone else in the building, and the operator consistently returned to my call. I usually just went to the person's door, because the operator could not forward inside calls.

My own experiences with different agencies proved that there were many injustices for people with disabilities. In order to receive funding for a person with a disability, many sheltered workshops were forced to say that, due to their fiscal situation, he, or she, was depressed. In other words, there was no funding for the physically disabled, but there was for emotionally, disabled participants. There were also issues like marriage. Should two people with learning disabilities be allowed to marry? Did they know what marriage was? What if they had children? Nursing homes would often give patients birth control pills without the patient's knowledge if they were of childbearing years. Where were the ethical lines? My feelings varied with different situations. Marriage? The individuals would have a right to support each other when needed, and definitely, the right to have feelings for each other, just like anyone else, but they may have less ability to control their feelings. Children? Would they be able to take care of a child, or discipline them on an adult level? Mental capability? How many people with low intellectual abilities came out of an institution pregnant by a staff person? It's sad to say, but it happens! It is horrifying to find that some women who were in comas have become pregnant! Where and how do you draw these lines?

I completed my Master's thesis along with the oral presentation. In order to complete my Master's in one year, I needed to do an internship during the summer. Kristi was not going to be in school during the summer, so I started looking at some place closer to home like the A Center in Racine. It was about 15 miles from where I lived in Kenosha. Mom would have to drive me back and forth. Tracy, a person I had known in passing, asked me if I needed an attendant for the summer. God was at work, again, because it wasn't something I was even considering. My school supervisor told me that there was an opening for a summer intern at DePaul, which is an Alcohol and Drug Rehabilitation Center in Milwaukee. So, I stayed in Milwaukee in the dorms, and Tracy was my attendant. She did a very good job, and took instructions well. However, she was in the nursing program, and wanted to move me differently as schooling recommended. I let her try her way, but I knew certain moves were easier. She learned that it was always better to go with the moves that the individual with a disability had worked out to save time, and energy. For instance, if anybody tried to slide me back by lifting me under my arms, I just got taller, but I didn't move. Pulling me backwards with my slacks was much easier, and far more effective. I slid much easier from the bed if I was on brushed satin sheets.

Mom was glad she didn't have to do all that driving. I had reapplied to DVR who had assisted with the second semester, specialized transportation to and from Jewish Vocational Services (JVS). Specialized transportation at that time was $20 per trip, or $40 a day, which I couldn't afford, because my bill would be $80 a week for 16 weeks totaling $1280. For Summer school, transportation would be the same amount, but it was only eight weeks, four times a week at $40 a day.

I found out a lot about myself that second semester. The students would try different counseling methods out on each other. From our class, I was required to have one of the students as a client, and I would become a client of another student. Because of the experience, I discovered that mentally placing myself inside the other person's body helped me understand them.

If I did not feel the same way, I'd ask myself, "And is this how I would really feel in this situation?" What question should I ask to make the client aware? Then, I would confront the individual, or ask questions to find out how, or why, the person came to that conclusion, or feeling.

Counseling by a classmate was always uncomfortable, and I'm quite sure my clients would be uncomfortable as well. One of the issues that my counselor asked when confronting me:

"It seems like your parents and you have the same friends. Your friends are your parents' friends. If something happened to you, what would happen to your parents?"

That had me thinking about it - a lot. Mom and Dad used to have many different people with whom they played cards, but no one had come over for a while. The only visitors I could think of were my Grandparents. When I would go places with Steve and Les, my parents went along most of the time. I wasn't uncomfortable with it, but maybe I was protecting myself.

I remembered a couple of things. At a close, male friend's wedding, I was going through the reception line, and the groom kissed me. He kissed me again saying, "And that kiss was for all the times I wanted to kiss you, and didn't." This man did not have a disability. Whenever I would get close to a man who had no disability, I would think it wasn't fair for him, and stopped the relationship once I started feeling any emotional attachment. Most of my male friends had disabilities. I knew the relationships wouldn't work. I remembered telling Mom, "The only reason that I would ever get married would be to stay out of a nursing home." Even though I had female friends too, and liked to know what was happening, I never really liked, or spread, gossip.

There were many times when I was counseling that I would say something to help another person. And, that was when I realized, "Gee, I should be doing that too!" For example, a person needed to lose weight, so he/she brings his/her own lunch. However, if someone asked the person to go out and eat, it would be okay to accept, and I would recommend that the person have soup, or a salad. Now, if I would find myself in the same situation, I would not be ordering that soup or salad. I would order a hamburger, and a chocolate dessert! How many times have you suggested something like this to a friend, or your kids, and not taken your own suggestion when the time was right?

A Chair Does Not a Person Make

DePaul had a very good reputation in its area of expertise. I would remove an individual during group sessions for individual sessions. I needed to record their sessions, so that my supervisor, or instructor, could evaluate my work.

About the third day that I was involved with group sessions, my eyes began to water, because of the cigarette smoke. The counselor responsible for the group gave me some ideas on how to be more assertive by sharing my needs. It seemed like all 16 of the people were smoking at once, and I told them it was causing me to feel ill. The group agreed that only two people would smoke at a time. People made sure that they did not to miss their turn to light up! Their consideration did help me immensely.

Groups, in general, were always scary to me. I never liked parties. When I had to speak in a classroom, I ran the answer through my mind, first, but by the time I was finished, the topic had passed. I spoke in more often in-group sessions, and started counseling in individual sessions. I needed to learn to participate!

One man, who appeared to be tough, indicated that he really wanted to experience a close relationship. As he shared his story, I said, "It seems to me that as soon as you get close to someone, you start drinking so that you push the person away." He both wanted to be close to someone, and yet, did not want to be close at the same time. He could never "win", or be happy. That was very helpful to him, and a number of other people in the group. It was also helpful to me, as I was doing it to myself, but in a different way for different reasons. I wanted to be close to someone, but had already decided it wouldn't be fair. Who could love me? So, I stopped relationships before they began.

Another revelation came to me in the sessions when one of the individuals gave me a compliment for identifying something that none of them had seen. I just moved away from the compliment, and continued talking. The person declared, "Do you know how hard it was for me to give a compliment—that is not something I do—and how much it hurts that you just didn't accept it—you zero it away?" I learned something that day. Now, and forever, if someone gave me a compliment, I just said, "Thank you," but didn't try to explain it away. That was hard!

There was an older woman whose children placed her in the 28-day alcohol program, but she did not know why she was there. The group's counselor forced her to answer simply by asking her a question.

"Do you drink alcohol?"

"Yes, I just have a little bit in soda every day," she answered.

The counselor continued.

"And how many of those do you have a day?"

"8 or maybe 16 per day," she responded. Her denial truly ran very deep.

When I left the group at DePaul, I thanked each of the members of the group, and told them what they taught me. However, I couldn't tell the older woman exactly what she taught me, because I believed she would not understand due to her denial, because it was so deeply ingrained. Or, would it have helped her? I struggled with the question. Later in my counseling career, I could tell a person important things in a soft way, so the person could "chew on the verbal poison", and know that I wasn't judging, or sentencing them, but adding an antidote for them to ponder.

"Yes, that was me, but now I am... I can... and I will ..." and hopefully, within themselves, they could choose who they wanted to be.

My supervisor tried to make me more assertive, and talked to me about the strength of my voice saying, "Sometimes you speak like a little mouse hiding in the corner of the room. You have a lot to say, but some of it can't be heard." She definitely wanted me to speak up more often, but louder too, and I struggled with that, too. Was this softness an excuse? In the classroom, my voice was loud in front of groups, particularly when I had a purpose, or role, to fulfill. I knew that I would rather listen and learn, especially in the groups. Physically, I felt that I spoke softer, because it was just out of a normal breath. Intellectually, I knew that deeper breaths would help project my voice. Trying to change this was hard!

While I was at UWM, a number of the MDA camp volunteers lived in Milwaukee, so I was able to see several of them throughout the year. Jim, from MDA, stopped in to see me several times to make sure everything was going okay. One day he came wearing a suit. It was out of the ordinary for him to wear a suit, so suggested that we go for a walk to get the truth. He had made a decision to change his life, so he changed his clothing, too, and was going to ask LuAnn to marry him! I was happy for him! I was so glad he shared this with me.

Well, it was time to go back to Kenosha. Guida, Jim, Joan, Kristi, Lloyd, Tracy, classmates, teachers, supervisors, etc. had all made my year at UW-Milwaukee very special. It was time to go back to teaching math. All the new things that I learned, I felt would make my job easier.

I became more confident that I could live alone, and be independent as long as I had a reliable attendant. I did have to learn how to ask for help from strangers, and unknown to me, I had developed "puppy eyes" to ensure the assistance. One person said, "I know that you feel good when you can help someone. A person will tell you if they cannot help when you ask. People, in general, don't mind being asked for help. Most feel good helping others. Most people have more difficulty asking for help than giving it. They don't want to bother people, or they think the person doesn't have the time. You never know unless you ask." I began feeling better about asking for more help, but I really tried not to ask for help that I didn't need. Some people definitely asked for help too much, so people really wanted to avoid them. Some, like Eddie, who had disabilities, didn't want help at all. This gave people with disabilities, who really needed help, a bad name. Asking for assistance was a tricky business.

It was good being back at home with my family, again with all of the familiar faces, familiar surroundings, and on the other side of the learning process. I did not go to my graduation for my Master's degree. I was happy just to wait for it to come in the mail. I went to Eddie and Carol's wedding instead of my graduation. Then, I went back to teaching in the fall of 1977. I still had a two-year contract to fulfill!

~ 16 ~

Winter of 1978-1979

It seemed funny going home when my dog, Penny, was not there. Then, Mom became sick, and she broke her rib, because of a very bad cough. Susie had her hands full with little Kenny, and we had no one to assist me. Our next-door neighbor, Jimmie, came over, and saved the day! For a week, she came over every morning to dress me, and helped me get ready for work, returning every evening to help me as well. We were always thankful for all of our good neighbors!

When Mom was much better, I heard her scream. A mouse was in the utility room. Running into the kitchen, she quickly locked the door - as if that mouse was going to care if the door was locked!

When fall came, I woke up in the middle of the night, because I thought I heard somebody walking in the leaves outside my window. Jerking awake, I felt a little vibration next to my head. I felt something scamper down between my feet.

"Oh, no! I bet it is a little mouse. How am I going to tell Mom?" I asked myself.

I called her as if I needed her to come and turn me, but I asked her to stop at the doorway.

I said, "Don't get scared, but I think there is a mouse on my foot.

She half-asleep.

"Oh, you must be dreaming."

She turned on the light, and saw the mouse run. She screamed, and ran out of the room to jump in bed with Dad - waking him. They came into my room, and quickly transferred me to the living room couch with a two-man lift. Mom said that her feet never even touched the floor! Then, Dad set a trap, and went back to bed. About 45 minutes later, the trap finally "clicked".

Mom said a little prayer, "Thank you God," and went to sleep.

These incidents reminded me of what happened to my friend Joyce when we attended camp. She had Muscular Dystrophy, as well, and less physical strength than I had. Her wheelchair had a place to hold her head. When she was too weak to drive a regular, electric wheelchair, she tried to drive a sip and puff chair, but she still did not have enough breath to start the wheelchair. (She came from a farm where the major business was milking cows, and she was unafraid of anything). We were on a campout at night, and the counselors at Easter Seals camp tucked her into her sleeping bag. As soon as they did, she felt something moving inside her sleeping bag. She knew that it was a mouse, but she wasn't afraid even when it bit her finger!

Joyce was an excellent artist, and she drew the most beautiful, detailed pictures on a small 3" x 2" card. She sent me a card that was decorated with a Christmas tree, sketched in black pen, and had a little kitten coming out of a box with a ribbon around it. She also volunteered in a kindergarten classroom where she kept the little kids busy!

124

We would write to each other, and she set up a little Scrabble game, by mail, with a Scrabble board and letters that she put in a little bag. We would paste these on the small board, and it might take us four months to play a game, since we mailed it back and forth. Joyce was younger than I was, and she died very young. There was a point in her life when she had to choose between being able to talk and being able to eat, because her food kept getting in her windpipe. Her doctor placed her on a breathing machine at night, which was supposed to call someone if she was in some kind of distress. One night, the machine malfunctioned, and she died. I miss her. If I were in her position of choosing between talking and eating, it would be difficult for me! What would you choose?

I always needed to turning at night, and, most the time, I would wake up, and call for assistance. Mom used to hate it when she would come in my room, and find out that I was talking in my sleep. I said a lot of things, but I mostly remembered the time that she asked, "Are you awake." I responded, "I am awake! And, get those snakes off the ceiling." (Good thing there were no snakes, because Mom was afraid of snakes too)!

Many people have choked on their food. I saw my brother-in-law, Bob, save someone's life with the Heimlich method when we were at a restaurant. First, he asked if the woman could breathe, and if she was choking. There was no sound coming from the stranger's mouth, so he put his arms around the woman telling her what he was going to do, then he pressed his fists up under the center of her ribs, and out popped a pea!

I even had a problem when I choked on some lettuce at home. Mom was panicking, and Dad didn't know what to do. I remember thinking, "They're not going to be of any help, so I better think of something!" I realized that there was just a tiny bit of air going into my lungs. If I breathed in too fast, it would drive the lettuce deeper into my throat, and I would choke. Breathing slowly, I hoped I had enough air behind the lettuce to cough it up, because I wouldn't have a chance to do it twice. Good thing I could hold my breath for three minutes! Guess God wasn't done with me, yet, since it worked! I, also, had that exact same thought when the lever on my wheelchair was stuck in forward. I was able to turn my wheelchair just in time to stop from rolling down a flight of stairs!

The school year of 1977 went fine. I was asked to be on the local Easter Seals Service Unit, but I couldn't attend the meetings since I was back teaching and meetings were at noon with no meetings throughout the summer. The Unit wouldn't take no for an answer and indicated they only wanted me to answer questions about camp for local residents that might be interested in going. I knew I could do that.

ABLE was looking at providing some attendant care services in the community. Society's Assets had started providing that service in Racine, but had not reached out to Kenosha. Jerry, a fellow student on my floor in the dorms at UW-Milwaukee, indicated that he would like to help writing a grant to get this started. Later, the two cities' services could be combined if needed. Jerry had a disability called epidermolysis bullosa—a skin disease that caused blistering and the scarring looked like his skin was taking over his hands and feet, fusing his fingers and toes. His skin was very flaky. He had trouble swallowing. Loss of hair and other problems also happened with this disability. Although this disability was rare, I knew two other people who had it. He was interested in meeting them, because he knew no one else who had the disease. He traveled to my house, as he could still drive. We co-authored a $70,000 CETA grant, which was accepted. ABLE hired a director to get the service started.

Finally, in November 1978, my friend Arlene married a man named Bob whom she had met at the WWAAC meetings. He was a relative of one of the other members who always attended the conventions. The relative, Donnie, lived in LaCrosse and had a cleft palate as well as a visual impairment. Bob grew up in Milwaukee and took over his Father's independent grocery store business. Bob was very shy. One day he came all the way from Milwaukee just to leave a birthday card at Arlene's door. (Arlene was very outgoing and friendly. She worked as a clerk from her wheelchair at Great Lakes Naval Base for over two decades. She drove back and forth daily using hand controls, steering with one hand and using the gas and brake with the other. She had an assigned parking place near the door so she could get to work in bad weather.) She called Bob up and he came back down to Kenosha. He continued making his trips down here every weekend for three months until Arlene articulated, "This isn't going to work, coming here only on weekends. We should get married!" They did!

School in the fall of 1977 went well, but the winter of 1977-78 was flakey. We had snowstorm after snowstorm, and even Dad had trouble getting back and forth to work. Every morning, the gas line on Dad's car would be frozen. He went outside at 5:00 a.m. to defrost it with a blowtorch, and came back with no eyebrows! (Just an FYI…This is *NOT* a recommended method to resolve a frozen gas line)! There was a week that I was very sick. We were in the middle of a blizzard leaving a total of 28 inches of snow on top of multiple inches of snow already on the ground. I called into work for a substitute teacher very early in the morning. I was coughing and blowing my nose all night, anyway, and couldn't sleep! In the morning, I looked out my window thinking, "Ah, look at those little sparrows on my windowsill." I soon realized the birds were not on my windowsill. They were actually standing on the snow about a foot away from my window! There was a barrel in the backyard to burn our garbage, and it was, at least, four feet high with only about an inch of it peeking above the snow. When I went back to work a few days later, the snow banks were plowed about a foot above the cars, so I felt like I was traveling through tunnels all the way to work. It was very dangerous to get through all of the intersections. Luckily, we had good neighbors who plowed our driveway clear. Now, we just had to deal with all of the snow on the ramp, back the station wagon up to the front door, transfer into the vehicle with the car top lift, and get out of the car at the school right by the door that held my second electric wheelchair.

After the winter, I wrote the following article for my church's inspirational thoughts booklet:

"And we know that all things work together for good to them that love God, to them who are called according to His purpose." Romans 8:28

But, I'm depressed today and say, "What?" A snowstorm that paralyzes the city is good? A family tragedy is good? Frustration in a work situation is good? How can that be? Have I lost sight of so much?

Let me take time to reflect; see the situation for what it is and how God is working in my life and others. For example, in the snowstorms of this winter I felt life slow down for a few days to help everyone gain perspective and work out problems. I saw the making of new, needed friends who helped shovel people out of their homes. Did you become a "friend" to someone in need and feel good about it? Though you were angry at the snow, did you make peace with yourself and others? Instead of blowing your horn to get a car out of your way at the intersection, did you get out of your car and help the driver who was stuck? Should you have gotten out of the car? Should this only happen during snowstorms?

In the example of a family tragedy, I've seen families pull together who have been apart for a long time to lessen the hurt. I have also seen long hidden tears or expressions of love fearful of being revealed because of society's rules. I saw a man cry. He needed to be human. Did you ever see someone grow in strength and have a better understanding of the meaning of life after a tragedy?

And in a frustrating work situation, I tend to worry about things that don't matter and forget, or run out of time, for the things that do. Sure, I have problems with a few people, but I forget what happiness and strength my presence brings to some. Are you trying too hard to change things you can't? Do you make a difference? Everyone does, you know. Really take time to see how much of a difference you can make.

All things do not "seem" to clearly "work together for good to them that love God," too. Is it just because we want different outcomes? God sees the whole instead of the part. He sees that often expressions of anger and hate reflect that a person loves and cares. He knows that in facing death we live. In forcing us to help others in time of need, He realizes we help ourselves in the process.

My prayer for you, and myself, is simply this: Dear Lord, though I hurt from today, I trust in your love that you will not give me more than I can bear. Help me not to say "why me," but instead say, "thank you for choosing me." Give me not an easy life, but the strength to face and live it. Help me "make a difference" for someone today, but let that difference be your will, not mine for when I follow your will, happiness and peace come. In my heart I know all things work for good, but I forget that often. Help me remember, especially when I hurt from the day. In Christ's name we pray. Amen.

At the time, I also became more involved in the church by helping to organize a local Chapter of the *Aid Association for Lutherans* (AAL)—the name of the group had changed to include another group called *Lutheran Brotherhood. Thrivent* was the new name, and is currently voting on a change, again, to include additional Christian groups. Both groups were insurance companies who provided service to the community. Fundraisers were encouraged for people in need for those who lost their home in a fire, and the insurance would match the funds raised for the event. In order to get a gold star rating for our church group, we had to have a certain amount of fundraisers and activities each year. My favorite breakfast was at Easter time, when Mom, Susie, little Kenny, and I would dye about 20 dozen eggs for our church breakfast. Afterwards, we would take any leftover eggs to people in nursing homes. At the same time, one of our members, Greta, was working very hard on starting a soup kitchen for the homeless, a huge undertaking, and it is still in existence today. In addition, I also helped organize several blood drives, but Susie wasn't a big help. She fainted more than once, even though the medics never took her blood! All she needed to see was a needle, and that was it! I remained active in this group until 1984.

At one point, I was President of all these groups - AAL, WWAAC, and ABLE, which had over 1000 members statewide. In my spare time that year, I also became an Amway dealer. I particularly enjoyed helping people choose the colors of their makeup, and had several party demonstrations.

MDA had started a group called *Teens against Dystrophy,* and additionally, MDA hosted certain events, and often gave passes to them. I had an opportunity to go to one of the Milwaukee Admiral Hockey games, which surprised me, because it was very exciting! I didn't get a chance to see any good fights, though, and I was expecting one. What I wasn't expecting was to sit right above the ice with the clear protective shield that, twice, took the brunt of a well-aimed hockey puck during the game! When the puck hit the shield, all of us sitting in that designated handicapped area jumped. It looked like the puck was going to hit us right in the head. Even those that were paying attention jumped, because of the surprising noise!

Mom and Dad took me to a pig roast held in the park for adults, and guess who ended up cooking? No, it was not us. It was Lloyd! I thought he was drinking a little too much that day, so I wrote him a letter telling him that he needed to be careful. On that day, however, I had the opportunity watch him interact with others who were not even in our party! After everyone ate, I saw him talking to two African American youth. There still happened to be a whole watermelon on the table. Lloyd asked the kids if they wanted it. He had no knife to cut it with so Lloyd broke it with his hands by knocking it against a picnic table! Problem solved.

Laurie, who had MD, called me wanting to have a surprise party for Lloyd's birthday, which was on September 15, before he left for several weeks on a hiking trip through the Appalachian Mountains. His celebration would be a real surprise, since they would celebrate at the end of June! I was to be the decoy. I called him and asked him if he wanted to go play pinochle with Laurie and her husband, Joel. He said that he would pick me up, and I agreed to pay for dinner instead of his gas. He said that he would come early, so we would not be late, but we were late anyway!

We went out to a nice restaurant, and had an excellent time. Lloyd had prime rib while I had duck. After looking at his watch, we realized that dinner had taken up two hours! We got to Laurie's about 1 1/2 hours late! Everyone was eating snacks and drinking when we got there, but managed to quiet down enough to yell, "Surprise!" when Lloyd appeared! He sat by me at first, and fed me some snacks. For some reason, I ended up across the room later. All of a sudden, I felt something fall into my V-neck blouse. I looked down to see it was piece of popcorn! I slipped my hands into my blouse to get the popcorn looking around to see from where it came, but no one seemed too suspicious. I looked around again, and Lloyd smiled as he was about to throw another piece! I smiled, thinking he was a very good shot, and ate the piece of popcorn! Why waste a completely good piece of popcorn?

I called Jim to ask if he and LuAnn could take me back home, because I did not want Lloyd to miss any of his party! Lloyd rolled me to Jim's van, lifting both my chair and me into it. I held out my hand, and repeated a happy birthday. He smiled, shook my hand, and kissed me. I did not get home until about 3 a.m. I was 31 years old, and it was the first time Mom was ever upset with me! I didn't even think about calling her to say I'd be late. Sorry!

I went to Easter Seals camp in July that year. A woman camper was telling fortunes with a plain deck of cards, and she taught me how to tell fortunes, too. She told my fortune, but it wasn't bad! I was particularly wondering if I would hear from Lloyd again. We set the cards up for wishes, and she told me that I would hear from Lloyd by September 15. September 15 came - and went. A few days later, however, I got a little letter wrapped up in a toilet paper roll in the mail. Inside were four pieces of homemade stationary made out of flattened birch bark written on both sides. It looked as if the bark came from a river birch tree, because it was pinkish in color. He walked on the Appalachian Trail for a couple of months, and then, most of the time alone. He did not run into many cities, but when he ran out of money, Lloyd either stopped at a farm, or he asked if anyone along the way needed carpentry work.

I pulled the letter out of its tube-like home. I unfolded it, and read it. "I am sitting here by the campfire thinking of you as a woman." I looked at the date of the letter—September 11. The letter could have been here by September 15! I continued to read the letter about what he what he had been doing, when he would be home, and that the temperatures were getting very cold at night. I started thinking about his first sentence, and felt very warm inside. I didn't want to lose that feeling nor run away from it at this point. He said that he would call me when he got home in mid-October. I looked forward to the call. The fortune-telling camper was right!

After Lloyd returned, I received a notification in the mail that *Teens against Dystrophy* was going to go on a Christmas shopping event. When Lloyd called, he told me that he would pick me up for that event. We went to Southridge Mall in Milwaukee. Lloyd was a Big Brother to someone whom I knew about, but I was surprised he brought him along. It turned out to be a lot of fun. I got all my Christmas shopping done, well, at least for my parents. This time it was a surprise, as Mom usually had to wrap her own gifts! Lloyd even took me up the escalator, since my wheelchair's wheels fit snuggly into the steps. I was glad Lloyd was behind me holding the chair so it wouldn't roll backwards. I would never want to try coming down that escalator!

After we finished shopping, we stopped in for something to drink. We were playing around with the napkins, and straws thinking of the different things that the shapes could be if not restricting their use, or their designated size. We had all kinds of suggestions for what we could make. When Little Brother went to the bathroom, I paid for the drinks, because Lloyd was broke, just getting back from his hiking! Three pops didn't cost that much anyway. He reached across me to get my wallet from my purse that was beside me in my wheelchair. He dug the money out of my wallet, and then had trouble stuffing it back in my purse.

Lloyd hit my leg by mistake, and he said, "Sorry."

"No, that was fine! You can do that again!" I told him, and he smiled.

On the way home, Lloyd must have been thinking about something else, because he forgot to drop off his Little Brother. I told him it would be fine to take him to my house, but Lloyd decided to backtrack about 10 miles, and drop him off first. When we arrived at my house, Mom was waiting for him to lift me out of the car. When I got inside, I said thank you, holding out my hand as a way to say goodbye, and he kissed me instead. This surprised me, especially in front of my Mom. I did want to talk to him more, but I had work in the morning, and there was no time.

In early March, I found out that the state was testing for DVR counselor positions. DVR was anticipating opening up an office in Kenosha. There was also an opening in Racine. I wasn't sure if I wanted to change jobs at this time, but if I didn't take the testing and pass, I would not be considered for a position, so I took it. It would be six weeks before I would receive a score.

In mid-March, I fell from my car lift, which I mentioned earlier. My hearing was messed up, so I couldn't handle a lot of noise. As you know, I also had a very difficult class that was causing me a lot of stress. I also heard the weird sounds in my head from my temple area as it was healing. It was as if the area that was swollen was carrying all my old-time movie memories of hyenas laughing, babies crying, weird screams, squeaky doors, etc. I had talked with my pastor who asked me, "Do what you think God wants you to do"!

I agonized over the decision to stay teaching, or apply for a job at the Division of Vocational Rehabilitation (DVR). I received my test scores in May, and passed. I knew I was going to get the Kenosha job! I decided to turn in my resignation, with no guarantee that I would have a job, just trusting in God for my future. I would finish that school year.

At the end of April, my cousin David died in a car accident. His wake was on May 1. He was very special to me, as was Beth, his wife, and his 3 children—Tracy, Cindy and Brian. Dave and Beth were going to come up to the dorms one night while I was at UW-Milwaukee, but then, they couldn't make it, because he was pulled over, and jailed for drunk driving. David was having problems for the last several years with alcohol. I knew he was having problems with family members with messing up weddings, because of his drinking. His wife was carrying the brunt of a lot of emotional and physical abuse, along with feeling guilty, because she didn't want him to come home "that way again." When the accident happened, Brian, who was about five, was in the car with him. Dave had been drinking and driving, and was killed instantly when his car rolled. Thankfully, Brian was okay, but later, he would roll his toy cars repeatedly on the floor asking everyone how anyone could get out of a car that was tumbling over and over. Fifteen years before, when Dave was helping my Dad with some electrical problems, and for some reason, we were talking alone. He told me, "I don't want you to worry. If something should happen to your Mom and Dad, I will take care of you." There was no problem with my parents at the time, but it was comforting to know someone was so concerned with me. His death was a surprise, and a tragedy, as well as a loss to me, and to other family members. I also learned much from the feelings Beth shared. This tragic experience helped me counsel clients/families with alcoholism, and assured them their feelings of anger, frustration, and guilt were typical, and "normal" in similar situations.

Susie did not go to David's funeral, because her second baby was due. The baby was not born until May 10. Bob and she decided to name the baby after my cousin, but first wanted to make sure it was okay with Uncle Al and Aunt Wilma. The gesture was taken as a complement, so David was named. Little David always loved anything electronic. From the time he could crawl around, and move his fingers, he was always getting into trouble. The second he could reach my parents clock, my parents woke up at midnight, and every night,

BY THE GRACE OF GOD AND YOU
A Chair Does Not a Person Make

David was continually turning on the alarm! Not only was my cousin's electronic interest tied to David, but he also liked crashing his tricycle into the garage. Susie's neighbor, Ron, used to fix my van when needed. Ron would tell us how he would watch little David point his finger at the garage from about half the distance down the driveway. Then, little David would put his head down, pedal as fast as he could, and hit the garage! David would fly in one direction, and his tricycle would fly in the other. He would get up, brush himself off, and do it all over again! Interesting!

Little Kenny was also beginning to get into things. One day, when Susie had to go to the store, our Mom was taking care of baby David. Susie came back, and noticed that there were different colored crayon marks all over her bottom cupboards. She called Little Kenny into the kitchen, and demanded "What's this?" pointing at the crayon marks. Five-year-old Kenny touched it with his finger, examined it, and said, "Huh, it don't look like paint!"

The ninth grade dance in June was very special. Mom and Dad came for the first time, and I asked Lloyd if he wanted to come, too. It was a good thing he came, because my wheelchair ran out of power. I had been moving around so much doing decorations during the day, organizing the kids, getting everything ready for the dance, and checking on the band for the night—no power was left, because we forgot to plug in my chair after work! I really felt disabled, again, since I was unable to move my own wheelchair. The students enjoyed watching Lloyd dance with my wheelchair and me. He mingled really well, and really loved kids. (He really wasn't as tolerant with adults that said or did dumb things)!

When we returned to my house, I had to show Lloyd something in my room.
I asked, "Do you want to stay and talk a while?"
He closed the door of my room, got down on his knees in front of me, and kissed me.
"I always thought that you would reject me!"
I couldn't catch my breath. A thousand thoughts were going through my head at once:

- Why would I reject him?
- Why would he want me?
- I have to get him off his knees. He has to be uncomfortable!
- He's such a good person—a real gentleman!
- I'm not enjoying this, and I should be!
- He needs more than I do.

After I began functioning, again, there was nothing romantic in the way I spoke.
"Maybe you should sit on the stool," I fumbled.
The side of my wheelchair was in the way, so he sat on the loveseat. Lloyd asked if I wanted to sit next to him while another thousand thoughts ran through my head:

- What if I can't hold my head up?
- What if I'm uncomfortable sitting?
- I am so short!
- He understands my disability, but could he deal with it?

131

I flashed back to the time when I was about eight years old, and the girls in the cab Ed was driving were talking about whom we were going to marry. There were a bunch of different responses.

- "I want someone who is rich."
- "I want to marry for love."
- "I want someone with a nice car."
- "Oh, someone with smiling eyes."

Not me, I had to be practical.

"I want to marry someone who could lift me!" I told them.

"I used to be a boxer. I can lift you. Would I qualify?" Ed responded.

Why was I so afraid to get involved? I was such a dork!

The telephone rang, thank goodness! Lloyd reached the phone, and handed it to me. It was the Mother of one of the students, Sheila, who had protected me from the "hot wheels" comment in the cafeteria. The Mother was worried because it was 11:30 p.m., and her daughter was not home, yet. I found out that her Mother, Dottie, was one of my schoolmates at the Orthopedic School. I had seen Sheila at the dance, and she was doing fine. I thought for sure she would be home soon, and hung up the phone.

"No, I think I'll stay in my wheelchair," I, finally, responded to Lloyd's question.

Sliding to the edge of the loveseat, he kissed me, when the phone rang - again! It was Sheila, and she wanted me to know that she had gone out for pizza, and that she was home. I thanked her for calling, and hung up the phone, again. Lloyd stayed until about 3:30 a.m.

Mom got up, and put me to bed.

The next morning, she asked, "Why would a guy like Lloyd want to sit, and neck with a girl like you?"

What did that mean? Was it a comment about me—that I shouldn't have those feelings? Was it a comment about Lloyd—who appeared rough on the exterior with some of his language, but he was very sensitive inside? To me, he looked like Lloyd Bridges with a rounder face. He was one of maybe 11 kids. When he was a kid, a toaster accident burned his skin around the bottom of his chin/jaw area, so I didn't think he could ever have a full beard. He had a six-year relationship that was over, before I met him. He would work hard, and then spent his money on what he'd like to do—fishing, hiking… Women loved him.

A few days later, I asked Mom, "Don't you think a man could think of me in that way?"

She just said, "No, it wasn't about you! Lloyd just doesn't appear to be that type." What type was that? That answer really didn't explain anything.

How did I feel? Surprised, flattered, and confused. I had made myself a promise when I was younger that I would never get close to anyone enough to hurt them, because I was supposed to die at 15. Although I wasn't thinking about that consciously anymore, I knew it affected my relationships. Why did God put Lloyd in my life? Maybe it was just because I was supposed to move forward. I needed to allow myself to feel, and be who I was going to be. Mothers will be Mothers for the rest of your life if you have a disability, or not!

I saw Lloyd again, and he took me to Jim and LuAnn's wedding. Joan, a volunteer I had at the winter camp, sat at our table. She made a comment that Lloyd told her that we had watched the sunrise "that night." I was surprised he would've shared anything. I just smiled as he smiled at me. I had also seen Laurie at an MDA event. She just mentioned that, for Lloyd's surprise party, he had really thought we were going to play cards, and asked her if we could stay over if it got too late. He had said that he would take care of me. Surprised again! I never believed that he was interested in me, but I knew he would be a good friend. I didn't feel like I was going to die young anymore, but I didn't think we were near "serious" at that point. I just didn't think it would be fair to tie anyone down with my limitations. At the time, I didn't see what I could give to anyone in a male/female relationship. I needed so much care—could I be an equal "giver" instead of just a "taker?"

At winter camp that year, I had to find out what Lloyd had meant by "I thought you would reject me." This year, he was sporting a handlebar mustache that was long and waxed! I felt it. It could've been used as an unconcealed weapon! I asked him if we could talk for minute, so we took a stroll through the snow. He sat down on a bench. I asked him, straight out, if he remembered what he said to me the last time we were together, and what he meant with his mysterious statement.

"I thought you would reject me because you were a teacher and I was a janitor," he quietly replied.

I thought I would hold him back from doing things he would want to do. But, he thought I was above him for being a janitor! My heart felt ripped from my chest. The Princess syndrome! I really did keep people at a distance. Many people felt that they were my best friends, but they never really knew me. I only saw him a few times after that. Once was at June's birthday party, and once at a hotel where Dan had a party and we got into my first, and only, Jacuzzi. His Dad had developed Alzheimer's, and had some other physical limitations, and Lloyd became the primary caregiver. He had little time to do anything.

The adult winter camps became part of June's adult MDA gatherings. She called her group - *"With a Little Help..."* Health insurance now was required of the volunteers in case of injury, and Lloyd didn't have insurance.

~ 17 ~

A DVR Counselor

At the end of June, I received this touching letter from my principal:

June 28, 1979

Dear Carol,

As I sit here in my office writing this letter to you, it is hard for me to believe that you will not be returning to BULLEN Junior High School in the fall. It will be hard to replace you and certainly you will be missed.

During your tenure at Bullen you provided service to the school above and beyond your normal duties. Your involvement with the students and staff and your efforts in the area of many student activities reflected on your energy and drive. I personally have always appreciated your efforts and I want to say special thanks for making my job easier.

This year's ninth grade dance was excellent, but with your leadership, I knew it would be. Thank you again, Carol, for the many years of fine service and excellent teaching you provided to the students at BULLEN Junior High School.

My best wishes to you as you pursue a new career. I think you know there will be a place for you at BULLEN Junior High. Keep in touch and have a good summer.

Sincerely,
Robert Saksvig

I also started gathering up some of the job references that I had requested to be sent to the UW-Milwaukee Placement Office to start looking for jobs. Here are two of the recommendations:

From Rep. James Wahner:

I am writing to strongly recommend Carol Schaufel for a position through the University of Wisconsin-Milwaukee. I have known Carol for five years both socially and professionally and she is a bright and resourceful lady. She is also an extremely reliable and thoughtful person who is both a good student and teacher, and has enormous patience. Carol has good judgment and has the tact and diplomacy to get things done and still make friends.

BY THE GRACE OF GOD AND YOU
A Chair Does Not a Person Make

I am most specifically familiar with the leadership role that she played in organizing and directing the work of ABLE (Abolish Barriers for Lifetime Efficiency), an advocacy group developed to work on the problems of people with physical and developmental disabilities. She was a self-starter who initiated many efforts to improve the life of people with disabilities.

From Joseph Mangi (principal):

I have known Carol Schaufel since 1975 when I came to Bullen as assistant principal.

Ms. Schaufel has done an excellent job teaching algebra and general math at the ninth grade level. She has a good report with all levels of students, high, average or low. Her classes are well-planned, well organized, and well taught. For several years, she has had three teaching preparations (3 lesson plans for 5 daily classes), *which is one more than the norm.*

Ms. Schaufel has sponsored many extracurricular activities including the ninth grade end of the year dance and a deaf-sign language club. She gets along with the faculty and administration and gives much of her time to the school and school related activities. She is a happy and thoughtful person and is always willing to pitch in when needed.

It had been two years since I had been at UW-Milwaukee. I really believed that I was going to get the Kenosha DVR counselor position. It looked like God was leading me in that direction. I could not take anymore of God's rough stuff, though, but I decided to look for other positions anyway.

I didn't think Dad had too much confidence in me to find a job quickly, though. He decided to retire from his job at Johnson Motors, and thinking that we could travel, scheduled a vacation in Las Vegas for August! I was proud of him. Not only did Dad retire, he also quit smoking "cold turkey" after smoking two packs a day, which made Mom and me very happy. We stopped getting sick frequently from smelling the smoke fumes in the house! Unfortunately, Dad already had the beginnings of emphysema.

My doctor even got into the act by saying, "Since you aren't teaching anymore, and yelling at kids, I think you should take up something like the harmonica! It would be good for your lungs."

So, I began to play the harmonica, and I learned to play many songs, but always had trouble with flats and sharps in the music. I could not curl my tongue to get those half notes right! Very few songs are in the key of C.

I kept an eye on some of the state job openings. I did check out a job at Gateway in the Adult Learning Center for people with disabilities, but it had too much travel between too many buildings all over the city.

There was no accessible transportation available like door-to-door service, or lift-equipped city buses that were available until years later. I still had an open case at DVR which was needed in order to complete my Master's Degree. My counselor's name was Troy. Troy had spoken to his supervisor about me, and let him know that I had passed my state test for

DVR counselor. There was no specific date on when the Kenosha office would be soliciting counselors from the public. The state's procedure was to check on anyone interested in internal transfers first.

I was just about to begin looking for employment, when I received a call from the Racine DVR office concerning a counselor position. It was already the end of June, so I asked Mr. Barbie if the Kenosha office would still be needing counselors. He said that in about three weeks, the Kenosha supervisor would be calling for appointments on those positions. I declined the interview offer, deciding to wait for the Kenosha call. At the end of July, I was pleased to receive a call for an interview in September. The rest of the summer was less stressful, and we did get to go to Las Vegas!

It was September, and I was nervous sitting in the waiting room of the newly constructed and freshly painted DVR office. Manuel, a newly appointed supervisor, greeted me. He took me into his office for an interview. I didn't feel I was prepared very well. I did know that the salary was going to be $3000 less than I was making in my teaching position—even with my Master's Degree. Budget questions were tough. I had no clue what I would be doing in five years! Manuel focused on the computer in front of him, and he spoke fast with his Puerto Rican accent. He told me to call him a week from Friday about 4:00 p.m. if I had not heard a decision on who would be hired by that time.

I called Troy to see how he thought I did on the interview. He told me not to worry. He said. "You did fine." Well, Friday at 4:00 came with no call. I debated if I should call Manuel or not, but I couldn't handle the pressure, so I called at 4:15! Manuel answered. My heart flipped.

"This is Carol Schaufel. I had not heard from you, so I was wondering if you had filled the counselor position,"

"Oh, Carol," he continued, "I'm sorry I did not get a chance to call. You have the position! Your start date will be October 22."

"Thank you God! I knew you had been working on it!" I humbly and excitedly prayed.

How did I get to this point? First, there was Les working in the field who encouraged me to go get my degree. Who would have guessed that Les would become a Doctor in Rehab, and I'd speak to his classes when he was teaching at UW-Milwaukee. I had applied for school with faith that I would be able to go for my Master's degree. Out of the blue, Kristi volunteered to be my attendant for the school year, and Tracy, for the summer. I took the state testing at the right time to be considered. The Kenosha DVR office wasn't even being considered two years before when I completed my degree. What did I do except pass a few courses! And, the fall! The painful fall that forced the occupation change! Miraculous! The Bible says, "Let those that have ears hear." For me it was, "If you don't want to get beat up anymore, pay attention! Do what you are supposed to do!"

October 22 came quickly. About a week before I started work, I picked up the job's policy manual, and summarized the basic rules and case codes onto two pages of standard size sheets of paper, which I put on my bulletin board. This way, for the most part, I did not have to lift the heavy manual to do my work. It was a quick reference to what I had to remember.

Despite my plans, my first day of work did not go well. I had a very bad cold and cough. I was getting 90 cases to review of which two-thirds of the files weighed more than I could lift! I was dealing with a regular desk and a push button telephone. I had difficulty lifting the receiver! My second and third day, I had permission to work from home, because it was much easier to move my files around while sitting on my bed and it gave me a chance to get well!

The second week was much better. My supervisor explained to me how to handle my caseload by status. He gave me a clear idea of the purpose of the state agency I was under—the Department of Vocational Rehabilitation. The basic goal was simple: assist people with disabilities to gain and maintain employment. Doing the job was more difficult. Each person had specific needs and abilities with the different disabilities' limitations as well as a unique personality. It was sometimes hard to tell if a specific characteristic you were observing was part of the disability or part of the personality, i.e., being overly serious. Did the individual just want to focus on a goal, or was there some underlying depression, which would affect that person on the job making success difficult. On the other hand, the person might be overly confident about doing a job, when a denial of realistic limitations might prevent success. A lack of confidence in one's self, because others have always told them "you can't do that", is the more likely case. Thus, knowing for sure what the person could, or could not accomplish, was something that had to be understood. Some people have pessimistic personalities. Others give up too easily, and never know what they can do, but I wanted everyone to have the chance to try! (Later in my career, the name was changed to "Division of Vocational Rehabilitation" depending how we fell under other agencies on our state chart.)

First, I checked the working files to see if individuals were satisfied with their jobs, what the person still needed for the plan they had written, and if they had been employed for more than 60 days. By the end of the second week, I had closed the files of 15 people - equaling a counselor closing half of the "closed files" for half a year's work! Next, I looked at the cases that were coded as "looking for work." I found an additional five, newly employed individuals, and others were close to their 60-day success mark in their employment. Out of the 65 cases that were left, I needed to decide how many individuals were really interested in working, who needed a new plan, or who were afraid to have their case closed, because they thought that they would lose Social Security. Other cases included loss of contact, as well as many other reasons.

By the end of the second month, I was having nightmares. Questions ran through my mind, and I was pulling out my hair! For instance:

- I forgot to change a certain person's status.
- How can I tell if this is a realistic goal for this person?
- Who am I to tell a person what they can and cannot do?
- How do I break down the job to see what a person needs?
- How do they show me what they can handle?

My job as a teacher was mentally stressful. Keeping track of 30 different students per hour in five different classes per day was mentally challenging, but DVR was far more physical. How was I going to manage all of those files? Another concern was travel. I went to many training sessions statewide, and would go to Madison in the near future. My parents could assist with driving and attendant care, but if I couldn't take my motorized wheelchair, how was I going to it? Could I appear competent or professional without independently moving my chair?

I couldn't use a desk, and I had shelf space that was wheelchair height all around the room. A Lazy Susan was available on the corner which was easy to turn with my hand, as well as it held an electric stapler. Files for each client were place into sectioned spaces with doors for privacy, and wooden box divided into16 squares held all the forms needed from intake through case closure. Manuel also hired an accessibility expert to make these plans and ideas become reality. In a couple of months, my office was finished, and I found that moving around the office and reaching for something, was so much easier! The floor space, a pushbutton telephone with a speaker that could be activated by a rocker switch, etc., made just everything easier to access! A woman, who worked in the front office, was redecorating her office, so I bought those things that she no longer wanted, and they made my office homey. I always thought that having a space that was similar to home was very important in relaxing my clients!

On the other hand, Troy wanted me to try driving. My parents and I were already considering buying a van to transport me in my motorized wheelchair! Now that I was getting a van, I was very glad I was short. It would save a lot of money, since I did not need a "high top" on the van, and that would have been at least an extra $4000 plus! Since travel on the job was required, the DVR would purchase the specialized equipment that I needed.

My parents took me to Sr. Kenny's in Minneapolis/St. Paul, Minnesota to try out different small steering wheels and steering systems. The Sr. Kenny's representative suggested that I go to Grand Rapids, Michigan to see if zero power steering would work for me. The flight from Milwaukee to Grand Rapids was less than two hours long, and I went alone. I do not think I would have the courage to try a flight alone, now! People from the rehabilitation center picked me up at the airport, and stayed in their facility overnight. The nurse's aide awoke me the next morning to get me ready just in time for the driving evaluator to test my abilities. I tried the zero power steering equipment, and to my surprise, it seemed like it just might work! My training was scheduled for a few months later. When summer came, a friend of mine, also a ninth grade special education teacher named Roberta had a friend who lived in Grand Rapids, so she accompanied me. Roberta had a hearing impairment, and wore her hearing aids at night in order to hear me call her so that she could turn me.

To drive my van, I had to complete my driving permit. This time, however, the zero power steering did not work, so, we visited Roberta's friend, and then drove back home. Surprisingly, I wasn't disappointed. Driving would have been nice, and while it didn't feel safe, I was glad that I had the opportunity to try! There were many other driving accommodations, and I was able to see how other people, who had different strengths, met their driving needs.

Other available attachments were turn signals that worked with the person's head movements, six-inch wheels that one could almost hold on your lap, and if one had no grasping power, there were spinner knobs on which one could rest their hand, and drive. I even had a friend of mine, Art, who had no use of his arms from polio, and he drove by using a steering wheel on the floor with his feet!

Dad did buy the van, and we worked out a payment plan. DVR equipped it with a lift and lockdowns. Dad took me back and forth to work, now. The next problem was car insurance if the van was going to be under my name. Every insurance company wanted the name of every driver. That wasn't feasible, since my Dad drove 90% of the time, so his name and driving record was placed on the insurance. It was 1980, and I could have my motorized wheelchair wherever I went! This was a *huge* increase in my independence.

By the time I completed my one-year probationary period at the DVR, both of the motorized wheelchairs had burned-out mechanism, and no longer functioned. They were both about 10 years old, and technology advances made old parts impossible to get. My job's insurance paid for 80% of the next wheelchair, but now instead of the $900, the cost was $6000. About eight years after this, I requested another wheelchair, but the insurance company announced, "We will not pay for a motorized wheelchair because it is a luxury and not a necessity!" The commode seats were not allowed on some of the motorized wheelchairs, because of the lack of space between the seat and the battery, and the concern of spilling the urine, which was highly unlikely! Heck, even getting out of a swimming pool doused the batteries much worse! Eventually, policies were changed, and motorized wheelchairs were accepted by insurance companies, but only every five to eight years, and then, it was one wheelchair, either motorized or manual. Many of the repairs were now included as well, but by far the hardest hit by the costs of wheelchairs was medical assistance.

Besides, working at DVR full-time, I was still involved in all of the other organizations previously mentioned. I also had permission to go to Easter Seals Service Unit meetings once a month, now that I wasn't teaching classes during the noon hour. The third week of the month, I had a meeting in the evenings every night except for Friday. Everything I did seemed to be disability related except for the Aid Association for Lutherans (AAL).

In 1980, I was also asked to be on the Muscular Dystrophy Association's task force, which offered assistance with appropriate verbiage and etiquette for telethon talent. We monitored segments for the comfort and dignity of the hosts and guests. We attended fundraisers, and spoke on issues, as well as upheld policy decisions. On one occasion, I had an opportunity to speak to MDA camp volunteers, prior to the volunteers' camp experience, about disability sensitivity issues and discussing their concerns. The best guidance I could give was if each were to put himself, or herself, into the individual's place, then they would know many answers to their own questions:

- If I (the counselor) were in that position, would I want somebody to assume that I needed help and simply let them do it, or would I want them to let me do what I could myself and to ask me what I needed first?
- Would I want them to ask me how to do something like transferring me into my wheelchair, or would I want a transfer to be done according to a book? Because of the curvature in my spine, my center of gravity was off to my left side! If I was lifted under my arms, which didn't work in my case, I just got taller and didn't move
- If I wouldn't like my method of help, the person I'm helping probably wouldn't like

it either no matter if it were a child or an adult.

At some point in 1980, my Grandpa "with the mink" had been coming over to play cards more often, but I noticed that he hadn't been as sharp at cards as he used to be. One morning, he was found lying on the bathroom floor, wrapped in the bathroom rug. He had fallen, was very cold, and was unable to reach the phone, or call someone. Doris, Mom's stepsister, called him every morning. This morning, he didn't answer. She ran across the street, and called the rescue squad. Grandpa was taken to the hospital, and diagnosed with congestive heart failure. Mom, Dad, and I went to the hospital as soon as we were notified. He actually seemed to be functioning quite well when we saw him. At the hospital, he smiled at me, and seemed very peaceful and calm. A few hours later, the hospital called for us to return, but we couldn't go, and he passed away. At the funeral parlor, Harley, Mom's brother-in-law, told Mom and me about Grandpa's will. I wasn't thinking about a will.

"Grandpa left Roger and Susie $10,000 each, and left you $5000," then, he added, "That's because he loved them more!"

I would never have given the first comment a second thought if he had not made the second one, and that comment hurt!

He apologized, "No, I was just kidding!"

I did receive $5000, but for whatever the reason, it didn't matter. I would much rather have people alive than dead. I am sure it was because both Roger and Susie were married, and had more family costs.

Later, my Grandpa and Grandma "with the kitties" were in a car accident. A very young driver backed out of his long driveway on highway H in the County without looking, and rammed into my Grandparents' car. Grandpa's spinal cord was severed, but not completely. He became an incomplete quad. He could walk with a walker, but had little use of his hands. Being on the farm, he was always very tough. I recalled one time that he had a huge 12-inch gash in his leg from some farm equipment. He just wrapped it up tight, and let it heal by itself! Amazing, if not borderline crazy! But, now, he was placed in a Milwaukee hospital, and they repositioned him approximately every two hours. He never complained, and yet now begged to be moved. The nurse snipped that it wasn't time, but my Mom changed his position anyway, and he was fine. Sometimes, it's not about the bigger picture of preventing pressure sores, but of just being human. Even though he wasn't a quadriplegic, he could feel. I knew what a difference it made even if somebody moved me just a quarter of an inch, so in order to sit up, I wouldn't have to use all my muscles, and it made huge difference! (My friend Dave who was a paraplegic had surgery once with no anesthetic. He couldn't tell if the surgeon was using a knife or a finger, but his body responded to the shock. I've seen someone go up to a person who can't feel, and pinch them hard causing a bruise. I am at a loss as to why they would do this. Just to see they couldn't feel?

My Grandmother "with the kitties" was okay after the accident, but my Mother had a lot of additional work. They had a beautiful German shepherd who had to be fed. When Mom got there, the dog came in the house, and knew no one was there. He never came back again, but it appeared as if the man on the corner had given him a home. Grandma still had an outdoor water pump, which she used a lot, but inside, they had running water. There was only an outhouse, so Mom hired someone to construct an indoor bathroom where their pantry used to be. Grandpa came home for a while, but eventually, Grandma and Grandpa shared a room in a nursing home. Grandma was always jealous of my Grandpa. A nurse would take him away to give him a shower, and Grandma would think he was having an affair! Grandma had hardening of the arteries, so at times she could be mean. She needed the oxygen!

Nationally, the Decade of the Disabled was just beginning as more people with disabilities wanted equal access to be a more productive part of the community. Disabled groups were formed. Frank and I were named as co-chairs to the 1981 "International Year of Disabled" Kenosha Committee by the city's mayor. This was a great committee to be on, because it was very specific to the time of January 1981 through October 1981. In addition, it had a purpose of awareness and advocacy for people with disabilities. This was the beginning of big changes to come in this "Decade of the Disabled."

Frank and I were lucky that Kenosha was pretty much ahead of their time. When the handicapped parking law first came out, Frank and the lawyer from ABLE, Burton Lepp, rewrote the law as, legally, a parking lot could not be designated as "private", since all the places served the public. Supposedly, "private" parking lots were originally exempt from the law. The State accepted the change, and different local individuals monitored malls and other handicap parking spaces in the area. At first, the police said, "We can't go onto private parking lots and give tickets," but with the change in the law, there was much more respect given to the need and correct use for those handicapped parking spaces.

Another project was setting up a panel for high school students to hear from disabled professionals who were working and advocating in the community. Some of our speakers were: Edith Simons (deaf and legally blind, professional advocate); Hazel Johnson (completely blind, DVR counselor); Tim Hanson (controlled seizures, social work); Frank Marrelli (quadriplegic supervisor at the Kenosha Youth Foundation); Carol Schaufel (neuromuscular disability, counselor/teacher); George McCarthy (seizures, Society's Assets); Angie Lehman (blind from diabetes, community speaker); Larry Wroblewski (polio, Director of ABLE); and Bobbie Petrausky (spinal cord injured paraplegic).

All of the speakers gave important information to the students, as well as to the community. A person with controlled seizures shared that he was getting married, and his fiancée's parents stopped the wedding from occurring when they found out about his disability. The reason? No good Catholic would marry a person who….

During the next decade, Edith worked hard to get accessible telephone service for people who were deaf. Because of her efforts, TTYs (Text Telephone), or TDDs (Telecommunication Device for the Deaf, or people with speech or hearing impairments) were made available to people, so they could now type back and forth to each other. The individual could also dial the Telecommunication Relay Service (TRS) so they could type to an operator who would read the message, and make a telephone call for them - even something as simple as ordering a pizza to be delivered. It was a huge accomplishment! It is paid for in a different way. Do you know all those little amounts on everyone's telephone bills, and you have no idea what they are? Now you know! The money goes into a fund, and pays for specialized equipment and services like this! If you are in need of any specialized services, a person can call an independent living center in your area to see how to access the assistance.

To begin, it was easiest to focus on accessibility. The real issues with any disability were employment, and changing people's attitudes. People were always assuming what a person could and couldn't do. For example, servers would always ask the person with whom I was dining, "And, what does she want to eat?" or when I was shopping alone in my motorized wheelchair, clerks would always steer me to the less expensive clothing—assuming I couldn't afford it. Some of these things were very subtle. Remember, everyone's feelings are always similar. We all deal with different things. I always have to think, "Are they responding to me or to my wheelchair?" People could see my wheelchair. Individuals with disabilities that cannot be seen deal with other issues like pain. For example, a strong looking man with a back problem limiting him to lift 10 pounds, hated to refuse a woman that needed help carrying something! But …carry it, or explain the truth can be very hard to do. A person who is unable to read would rather be called a troublemaker than admit he/she could not read! If a person was hard of hearing, he might assume what you meant rather than say, "What?" so many times, and might give a weird answer followed by a weird look! In order to deal with the employment and attitude issues, I coordinated a banquet to pull together satisfied employers with employees who had disabilities. It was a start.

Both Frank and I received certificates of appreciation from Mayor John Bilotti that year, for our "*individual talent, ability and concerned dedication contributed for the Benefit of Citizens of This Community.*" We were lucky to be involved with a new library as plans were reviewed before the building was erected so even the employment areas were made accessible.

Just before 1982 began, I received a surprise phone call from the *Kenosha News*. The person on the other end of the line told me that I had been chosen as the first "Person of the Year." (The award was previously "Kenosha Woman of the Year"). I was still not good at receiving awards, but this one was fun! A reporter came to my house for an interview with the whole family. Susie was pregnant with Mindy, so it didn't look like Mindy was in the paper, but she was! Mom, Dad, Susie, Bob, Kenny, and David were there as well. I was chosen for the award, because of all the work I had done with, and for, people with disabilities as well as just having completed being co-chair of the International Year of People with Disabilities local committee. The News had a picture of me on a horse with the camp director balancing me. They also had a picture of me racing in the "Firecracker 500" Fourth of July Race the year before. (The picture looked like I was really going fast with my hair blowing back in the wind. I was last—but I finished)! The article covered my history as well as included a portrait that had been commissioned, and paid for by the Kenosha News from Kenosha Artist, George Pollard. (Portrait is displayed on front cover). Other portraits were of President Kennedy, Pope John Paul II, and many others. Mr. Pollard was an international artist who was born in Waldo, Wisconsin, and settled in Kenosha to raise his family of three sons and a daughter—all who are artists. He became famous after joining the Marines. His superiors discovered his talent, and recommended that he do a portrait of Eleanor Roosevelt and Gen. Douglas MacArthur. He was assigned to become a combat artist, and his fame grew from there. He died in 2008 at the age of 88.

The day the 1981 Person of the Year article was in the newspaper, I received 32 calls and many congratulation letters in the mail for a few weeks. I heard from the legislators I had worked with, received some telegrams from my Dad's friends, read congratulation notes from some of my students, and plucked many fond memories from old friends. I didn't have to be in front of a group to receive the award, only in front of Pollard's camera for two minutes, so that he could take a picture to do the portrait. About three years later, I found out who put in my nomination for the recognition. It was Burton Lepp. He was the lawyer of the groups in which I was involved.

The only real responsibility I had for receiving the "Person of the Year" award was to lead one of the seven sections in the Kenosha Fourth of July parade! Luckily, they drew my name first, so I led the first section right behind the Sheriff's posse! They had a Jeep already for me to ride in, but I preferred to use my wheelchair, because whenever I sat in a car seat, I was lucky if anybody could even see my eyes. The jeep followed, and the day was beautiful! There were a lot of people along the approximately two-mile route. I heard people call out my name, but couldn't find many of the callers in the crowd. My only concern that day was that I not run over any of the posse's horse apples that clowns were picking up in front of me in a little wagon! I missed 98% of the remains!

Of course, with the good, there is usually bad. I went into the newly renovated *Kenosha News* building, and could barely get in and out of the elevator with help! While meeting a reporter there, I met Howard Brown, the infamous owner of the newspaper, who spoke to me. "It is an honor to meet a Kenosha living legend!" That comment made me feel good, but very old! Could you be a legend before you were dead?

After completing my business at the *News*, I told Frank about their elevator. He went to check it out. He could get into the elevator, but could not get out. He checked on the state code requirements for elevators, and there were none. There was another restaurant in town, which had put in an elevator out in front of their restaurant for people in wheelchairs. It was not usable! Frank got into contact with an elevator company in Milwaukee. They hired him as a consultant and a state lobbyist for a few months to resolve this growing problem. There were monthly meetings with a number of different elevator companies for about five months in a row. Everyone sat down at the same table to resolve the issue of what a minimum size should be for an elevator. In about 1983 or 1984, the first legislation was passed for elevator's minimum size, and basic codes were initiated.

Frank and I were both involved in the Easter Seals Service Unit. Frank was also with the Wisconsin Rehabilitation Association when another project came into being with ABLE. A Kenosha City Access Directory was being put together. Wisconsin Easter Seals had produced a survey of Wisconsin's minimum codes and preferred guidance policies to evaluate accessibility of hotels, restaurants, recreational facilities, government meeting places, and other places that people used for more than an hour. All of us did our share of measuring to make sure things weren't too high to reach, too narrow to go through, had accessible signage posted (including braille), provided handicapped parking spaces, had parking spaces that were wide enough for the use with an accessible van, had clear walkways with no curbs or steps, had nothing protruding from the wall that a person who was blind might get hurt on (as their canes focused on the floor), had usable water fountains, had reachable telephones with a volume control, and a place to set a TTY on for people who were deaf. Also, to make sure that there were wide enough turnaround spaces in the bathrooms for wheelchairs, provided light weight pull on doors, had no protruding pipes under sinks where a person could get burnt, and had no ramps with more than a 5° grade. We recorded just everything that had a minimum requirement.

We also noted preferred situations like lever door handles for people with no grasping power, or motion activated faucets for bathroom sinks. I did not count how many accessibility checks we had to do. I am sure there were at least 10 to 15 people certified in Kenosha to complete the many buildings we had to evaluate. We went out in pairs for accessibility checks, since we would run into all sorts of issues. An error was found with a newly constructed women's bathroom, and one could not close the door on the stall, because someone reversed the length and width requirements on the blueprints. It wasn't the restaurant owners fault! What inspector approved it? Another time, the bathroom was perfect, but behind the door was an unmovable heater so the door could not be opened to allow a wheelchair to enter. On another, the bathroom was perfect, but there was not enough turning space to enter from outside. I was stuck once in a men's washroom. There was a 17-inch stall door. I knew some people who couldn't even walk in it! Someone had to climb over my head with another person in front to get me out of that restroom area. I couldn't even get close enough just to see into the stall, it was so narrow!

After the surveys were done, the Access Directory was completed, and distributed. The directory was funded by Outboard Marine at $700, and the Kenosha Tavern League paid $500. Kenosha always seemed to have more taverns per population than a lot of other cities. At that time, there were 176 taverns in Kenosha! Yes, many people with disabilities like to go to taverns, too.

With the new laws, I was very disappointed with some of the decisions that were made without the use of common sense. For instance, an owner with an apartment on the second floor with no elevator had to make a bathroom accessible. Another incident that I thought made no sense was a person was refused a flight fare of $60 to go to a Madison, Wisconsin, doctor but was given a $240 ambulance ride, because flying was a luxury, not a necessity! Maybe I just thought that was crazy, because I was a math teacher.

In April of 1982, my sister's baby was born! A beautiful blond, blue-eyed girl named Melinda Sue. Susie deserved some credit for the birth, so that was how Mindy got her middle name. Mindy was sick a lot as a baby, and looked like she was going to die around her first Christmas, but she pulled through with flying colors. Even though she was sick, she would smile. By the time she was four, she was tough and opinionated! I would walk around the neighborhood with her, and she would ride on my chair. Occasionally, she would run along beside me. After a few blocks, she would then plead, "Just wait one minute." while she sat on the curb to take a break. When asked if she wanted the Cabbage Patch twins for Christmas, she said, "No, thank you. One doll is enough to take care of!" In general, Mindy knew how to stay out of trouble. Her Mom gave her a whole bunch of kisses, and then saw that Mindy was wiping off her cheek.

With a sad look, Susie inquired, "Are you rubbing off my kisses?"

Mindy thought quickly and uttered, "No, Mom! I am rubbing them in!"

All of Susie's kids played with a child-size fire engine Dad had at our house. They would put the toy up on top of my ramp on the front porch, and let go. It flew all the way down the ramp, and across the driveway. Thus, to Susie's children, our parents were always known as Grandma and Grandpa "with the fire engine" where Bob's parents were known as Grandma and Grandpa "upstairs downstairs" as they had a two-story house! Neither Susie, nor I, remembered what happened to that fire engine. Dad always gave things away without asking how the loss of an item affected the other members of the family! He tried to make people happy! He used to say, "I'd rather help you now with whatever you need to see you enjoy things instead of leaving all my money for you after I'm dead!"

Susie's kids always gave me hugs. She taught them that I could not go to them, or reach them! One time there was a little twist and turn to that story! For some reason I told Kenny, "Oh yeah, I'm going to punch you in the nose!" Kenny came over to me, and put his nose into my hand! He was helping me punch him in the nose!

I always liked chasing the kids all around the house. They would run from the kitchen to the living room to the bedroom, and jump on my bed if I hadn't caught up with them. It was like they were swimming in the ocean while they were on the floor. I was the shark trying to catch my dinner! I seldom caught them. They would scream the whole time we were playing!

~ 18 ~

Work & Community

By 1982, I was comfortable with my job, and no more nightmares! I was ready for some of the questions that the clients asked me. Some of them felt sorry for me, because I was in a wheelchair.

"But I am working and you are not. What is it you are thinking about doing?" was my response.

I would refocus on their disability, abilities, and interests. I always remembered how I felt the first time on the other side of the desk. I didn't really want to hear what I couldn't do. I wanted to hear more about the job, and if I felt that I could do it or not. What would the problems be, and did I need special accommodations to help me do what I needed to do?

The hardest situations were when a person was in denial. I particularly recalled a situation with an individual who had alcohol on his breath. He didn't think alcohol was affecting his life, but admitted that there was the usual family, financial, marital, and legal issues. I explained to him that I couldn't help him until he helped himself. He needed to get and stay sober, decide his life goals, and apply for financial aid. Three years later, a person came into the office and asked to speak with me on a busy day. I did not remember the name, but I saw him anyway. He said, "You probably don't remember me, but I just wanted to thank you." He continued, "I saw you about three years ago." I still had no clue who he was and asked, "Did I open your case?" He smiled, "No, but I took what you said seriously. I stopped drinking! I applied for financial aid, received a degree, and I was working for a while. I just wanted to thank you for that." I was touched! How many individuals' lives do we touch and never know? Those lives live within us and affect our thoughts and decisions. He made my day!

A couple of years after I started at DVR, the blind specialist retired. I was asked to become the specialist. In our city, we probably had 10 to 20 people in our caseloads of about 100 to 125 people with visual impairments at any one time. I took the position along with my regular caseload, and discovered the training was very helpful. Besides additional medical information on conditions of the eyes, I tried glasses that simulated different types of vision problems. Retinitis Pigmentosa, a type of tunnel vision, was one of these. It was as if I was looking through a long tube of Christmas paper in order to find a clock on the wall. Another was Diabetic Retinopathy, which is a progressive loss of vision from diabetes. Spots of vision are lost trying to see in the darkness caused by bleeding, or laser surgeries through the holes of vision that are left. People with Macular Degeneration have no central vision for clear detail, and those who are considered legally blind with 20/200 vision meaning the person could can see at only 20 feet that which a normal vision persons could see at 200 feet. Looking through frozen glass, one could see everything including colors, but cannot see detail. In addition, there are many more types of vision problems. I was familiar with braille, but was never proficient at it. Orientation and mobility was not familiar to me, but was used in order to be safe knowing where you are within the community.

Rod was a DVR evaluator who started his career in Vietnam with visually impaired individuals when they were injured in the field. I learned so much from him as well as each individual client about vision aids that would be helpful depending upon the individual and the specific cause of blindness. Knowing what direction one was walking (North, South, East or West), along with using a cane, guide dogs, and learning what one could and couldn't do, were learned right along with safety issues, and other things. There were independent living aids available such as bacon crispers that cooked bacon on both sides at once, black and white sided cutting boards providing color contrast, talking scales, talking watches, large print playing cards, and sunglasses of all colors of the rainbow. Rod said that the closer to the beginning of the rainbow your sunglass color was, the more glare it shut out. There were just so many additional things including some very heavy, spacey looking opera glasses that made it easier to watch television and see blackboards too! Even transparencies similar to what I used on my overhead projector helped many people. For most people, it seemed that a yellow transparency over black print made the words easier to read. At an agency for the deaf-blind, equipment was available for them to watch television! On television, a captioning device allowing spoken words to be changed into text was attached to something that turned all of the captioning into braille. This allowed people who are deaf and blind to read the paper with their fingers as it was printed! It was very exciting for those who needed it!

Some deaf clients said that being deaf was worse than being blind, and some blind clients said that being blind was worse than being deaf.

My thought on the matter was this.

"It doesn't matter. We don't have a choice of what our disability was going to be. We work with what we get, and go from there!"

Another client told me, "I just wish I could see well enough to drive again!"

"I always wished I could go to the bathroom by myself!" I countered.

"You win!" he told me, after weighing the thought in his head awhile.

Sometimes, the clients wanted to work in any job they could despite their constant pain, limited abilities, anger issues, lack of acceptance of their own disability, attitude, lack of support, fear, or other excuses. For the most part, depending upon how motivated and realistic the person was, I believed that most people could work if they were realistic about the requirements of an employer. For instance, one with a hearing aid could hear the boss in his office, but in a staff meeting the different noises from, e.g., iridescent lights, open window, side conversations and the speaker's voice all fight at a similar level of sound, making comprehension difficult. There were times I would laugh, or cry, with some of my clients. Some of the stories were so sad, and many times, I was the first person a 30-year-old woman or man told about being molested as a small child. Some had talked to their parents about it, but they didn't believe it. Sometimes, the sex of the supervisor affected their work history by the memories. Other times, body odors would trigger a lack of focus. Marriages were destroyed, because of an onset of a disability. For the blind, going through a buffet line caused fear.

Sometimes, a parent or a spouse wouldn't believe the client was legally blind, because their peripheral vision could pick out a white speck on their jeans, but not the salt shaker in front of them.

Jerry was a friend of mine who was a blind, public defender. He once told me to "Never tell a person they can't do something. If they're blind, and want to be a truck driver, just ask how are you going to get a drivers' license?"

The news announced, recently, a self-driving car will be on the market soon. Sensors on the cars prevent accidents, and have GPS as well. This would be a huge boost for the disabled, and just another way we can be independent! I sure want one!

People who blame their problems on others never seemed to go very far. If a person and I were discussing something, and they continually said, "Yes, but...," I knew they weren't really listening, and only trying to justify, or think of an excuse for why they couldn't do something instead of creating a way they could. Somewhere along the line, everyone had to start being responsible for themselves. Sometimes, the disability dictated what was possible or not. It was not good for a person who was hard of hearing to go into a noisy factory where he could further damage his hearing unless good hearing protection was available. Individuals had to learn to explain their disability in a way that made sense to the employer.

What types of jobs were available to people with disabilities? Jobs were just anything, and everything from service to professional. For some people, a part-time, low stress job would be cleaning offices twice a week for three hours a night; for others, a full-time nursing job was appropriate. Whatever the person wanted to do, they had to qualify for and do the tasks that were expected from the employer, with or without accommodations. Yes, if the person wasn't doing essential parts of their jobs, it was appropriate to fire them.

Unfortunately, some people could not afford to work and lose their medical coverage, which could amount to $5000 a month for attendant care, or even for three medications if they didn't have Medicare or medical assistance. Medicare did not pay for attendant care, but medical assistance did. Even insurances would pay for nursing care, but never attendant care. If they were on Social Security Disability, the maximum they were able to earn in a month was $500, which was not a living wage. More recently, you could earn $1010 a month. I have seldom seen any Social Security that has hit $2000 a month. Most of them are $900-$1500. If a person lost their disability benefits along with their medical, the person was already starting out in the hole. Company insurances didn't cover pre-existing disabilities either. After 12 months of work, a person was thought to no longer needed their SSDI benefit or the medical coverage, and if on SSI, a $1 for every $2 earned just automatically was taken off your SSI check. As soon as you reached the maximum amount for SSI (about $600 a month at that time), you lost everything without the benefit of earning while you had a 12-month trial work period. This was why many people had no reason to stop benefits. There have been changes since.

Some people succeeded in reaching their job goal, while others did not for many different reasons—lack of opportunity, natural supports, right equipment, appropriate transportation, controlled symptoms, and self-confidence. There were just as many reasons for why people wanted to work. Some people were very capable, so they just needed some help getting to follow through with their goals. Some people just wanted to get out of the house, have something to talk about, feel productive, get a life, and to be able to pay for their medications. If it was for full-time work or part-time work, I always told them that they were making progress, because their mistakes were further apart! Mistakes would never totally go away. We learn from our mistakes more than from our successes. Heaven only knows I was not perfect, either. It was part of being human. It was part of being an adult. We must be responsible for our actions/decisions and ourselves.

Funny things would happen, sometimes. I wasn't in the office, one day, and a client came into the office. JoAnne, my program assistant, noticed that the bag he was carrying was moving, and asked what was in it. He told her it was his pet python, and he did not want to leave it in the car, because it was too hot outside. Another day, my appointment arrived, and then asked, "Is this the same Carol that used to teach at Bullen?" JoAnne told him, yes, and he gulped. He left with "I will be right back." She watched him go across the street to the bar on the corner. He came back in about 10 minutes ready to meet with me! We never know how we affect people!

Being involved with DVR, there were a number of other agencies and schools where I assisted clients with services they needed at the University of Wisconsin Parkside (UW Kenosha and UW Racine combined to make a four year degree Campus), Gateway Technical College, Department on Aging and Disability, mental health agencies, crisis, and others. A number of my clients needed to build their physical endurance as well as a work history.

There was one local agency, similar to Goodwill, located in Kenosha called the Kenosha Achievement Center. I spent a lot of time there my first year—at least one or two afternoons per month. The goal was to acquire enough skills in the area of food service, janitorial, or clerical for the client to be able to gain and maintain employment in the community. The staff was very proficient and caring. They were all part of the client's team.

The first day I went to the Kenosha Achievement Center for a meeting with their staff and our clients, I was nervous, because I needed some help myself. I met with Lynda and Birgit. Birgit was just about ready to start a new job in another facility. We stopped at the food counter. I ordered a hot dog and chips. I liked to add ketchup and mustard. The three of us sat down at a table. I was wearing my favorite light blue sweater. (I bet you think you know what is going to happen next! You're wrong!) Birgit put the ketchup on for me, but when she squeezed the mustard bottle, it squirted all over my sweater. We couldn't get it off, and I smelled like mustard during all five of my meetings. No one would sit by me!

The Kenosha Achievement Center staff also asked for a couple of the other DVR counselors who wanted to be on the Center's softball team called the KAC Monarchs. I loved baseball, and knew how to score very well, and I was good at keeping track of each individual player. I was the official scorekeeper, but my Dad came to help, because I was still in my manual wheelchair at the time, and before I had a van. Therefore, at the beginning and the end of the first season, it was difficult, because I could not write when my hands were cold. At the end of the first season, they gave me a basket and several colored pens, because, having been to the bar only twice before, they told me that it was hard to distinguish whose statistics were whose. The next year I was to keep score using color-codes, so that it wouldn't be so difficult to read in the bar's lighting! The basket? If the team had a player short, they wanted me to cover in the outfield running with my wheelchair, and catching the other team's ball in the basket! Thank goodness they were never short a player! I was never very athletic, especially bumping over grass!

The staff was fun at DVR also. I recalled one statewide conference that fell on Halloween. One of the other counselors, Rhonda, who was a former nurse, took me to the meeting and helped me. It was a three-day conference. We scheduled a Halloween Party in the evening after the second day's sessions. Rhonda asked what I was going to wear. I just took a garbage bag along. Every time we ate, I kept a few things like used tea bags, a banana peel, potato skin, a candy wrapper, an orange rind, ketchup and mustard packs, a food container (like a pie plate), and a newspaper. When it was time for the Halloween party, we cut holes in the garbage bag for my head and arms. We stuffed my neck with the newspaper, and sewed the potato skin, candy wrapper, and orange rind to the newspaper too. I had the used tea bags hanging from my earrings, and the ketchup and mustard smeared on my face. The pie plate I had bobby pinned to my hair with a banana peel hanging over its edge. I won a prize for the most disgusting costume. I not only looked like a garbage bag, I smelled like one! The judges assumed, "I either had a very good self-image, or none at all!"

In 1982, our church sponsored a Crop Walk, and I participated in the first of two, 10-mile Crop Walks for hunger with Jeff. My motorized wheelchair wouldn't climb a couple of the hills, so Jeff, occasionally, pushed me on the first walk. My hand also was tired, so he also drove my chair part of the way. The second-year, it was raining. We both wore raincoats, and agreed to take my manual wheelchair. About halfway through the walk, the sun appeared, and Jeff became very warm. He took off his raincoat, and made it the rest of the way! I guess I probably should have taken my electric chair, however, we did not know if the rain would damage it! I was surprised to find out that Jeff went to the Orthopedic School for a short time when he was a child due to a hip disease that lead to replacement at very young age.

Soon after the Crop Walk, the women's group asked me to speak. I always thought it easier to speak in front of a group of people that you didn't know well! My supervisor asked me to speak about DVR services to a large group of doctors, interns, and social workers at the Medical College of Wisconsin. It went pretty well, except I think I went over my time limit by 10 minutes.

Around this time, and off and on for three years, I also spoke to Gateway classes concerning some psychological aspects of people with disabilities, my own experience, and services available in the community. Most of the students were in a nursing or social service program.

A *Kenosha News* article *(*date unknown) by Kay Jones covered a story of some experience talking with the young children from Head Start:

"I want one just like yours," called out a Head Start preschooler to quadriplegic Carol Schaufel. "Wheelchairs might be fun for a little while to just try," she answered the youngster. "But not if you have to stay in them for a long time."

Ms. Schaufel, who has been disabled since birth, and Edward Chromik, who lost the use of his legs and hands in an automobile accident three years ago, spoke to Head Start students

Friday as a part of program to help children understand about people with disabilities. It is one of a number of similar programs in the public schools organized by members of the Kenosha Committee of Disabled Persons.

Carol and Ed didn't mind the child's question and, in fact, they encouraged the youngsters to ask questions of disabled people whenever they see them. "You shouldn't be afraid of people with handicaps. You shouldn't be afraid to ask some questions." Ms. Schaufel told the youngsters. Ed emphasized the idea with the parents who also attended the session. "Don't discourage kids from going up to a person with a disability. Don't be embarrassed by your child's questions. The more the general public knows about us, the better it's going to be for us with disabilities," he said.

Carol and Ed believe it is important for people to feel comfortable around those with disabilities because, with greater accessibility, more disabled people are getting out to public places more often.

Ed and Carol answered the children's questions. They let the youngsters push the wheelchairs and gave some of them rides in their laps. Many people have disabilities, Ed explained. "A lot of people need glasses. That's a kind of disability because without them you can't see." He pointed out that children are handicapped too, because they're so small. "Because you are small, you can't reach the cereal box and have to ask for help. Well, we have to ask for help sometimes too. We can't go up steps and we can't reach a lot of things either," he said. But, he said, just because there are some things we can't do, it doesn't mean there aren't a lot of things we can do.

Ed pointed out that he is able to get around because he can drive a van with arm controls. Carol was a teacher at Bullen Junior High School for eight years. She now is a Vocational Rehabilitation counselor. "Even though I can't dress myself," Carol explained, "I can hold a job."

The children were encouraged to try to imagine some other kinds of handicaps, too. They were asked to close their eyes and try to imagine what it would be like to keep them closed for a week. . . . The children also were asked to try to imagine what it would be like not to be able to hear, to see people talking but not be able to hear them.

Shortly after this presentation, I remembered talking to Ed, and we both noticed a change in the way kids asked us questions. They used to say, "What happened to you?" I'd say that my legs didn't work like theirs. Now they were asking, "Have you seen a doctor?"

So many things had to be worked on in terms of accessibility even with doctors. I went to have a mammogram for the second time at about the age of 40. The technician asked me, "How come you did not bring someone with you?" I walked from my office downtown to the hospital by myself to make it on time for my appointment! I just said, "I didn't know I needed to bring someone!" Nationally, females in wheelchairs were having difficulty getting appropriate medical care, because doctor's offices seldom had anyone that could help you get on the table for a full examination, especially pap smears.

Unfortunately, I was seeing a doctor again—a neurologist. He stuck some needles in my neck, and asked me what I did at work. I used to lift my files with my mouth. I did everything with my mouth like move my arms in place to eat, lift my files, opened bottles, etc. The doctor demanded, "No more lifting with your neck!" The nerves in my neck were vibrating, and damaged. I talked it over with my supervisor, Willie, and we set up a volunteer system that was being encouraged by the state at that time. Volunteers could not take over any other staff member's responsibility per the union contract, but they could be my arms. At this time, I met Judy, a former nurse. She was not diagnosed with Multiple Sclerosis for eight years, because they told her the problem was all in her head, and she was just depressed. For a couple of times a week, she was a volunteer for eight years for a few hours. There were a number of others who followed her, too, all providing a service, getting a recent work reference and giving different insight to clients with similar diagnoses. Confidentiality was essential, and part of an agreement that they signed. Eventually, volunteers were eliminated from the agency, since they were not paid, and an agreement was made with what used to be known as social services or welfare (W2) individuals looking for work experiences who were paid for work. Besides these people working with me, I often had field experience students or interns. Occasionally, I would train new counselors. All of the individuals who volunteered, or worked with me in the agency were much appreciated, and I learned a lot from them. Thank you! They each had their own talents and abilities, and were special in their own individual ways. I hoped their experience was as valuable for them.

In the summer of 1982, there was one more setback. I tried something that I never did without someone behind me. I went down the ramp at my house alone, without a safety belt. My hand pressed forward due to gravity's pull. I could not control my chair. I hit the side of the ramp, fell on the corner, and plastered my face onto the cement. My Dad came running, and held my eye tightly as it was bleeding profusely. He yelled for my Mom to call the ambulance. She was in a state of panic, so she asked a woman she did not know who was walking down the street to make the emergency phone call. None of the neighbors remembered seeing the woman. The woman was a mystery, never to be seen again. (Probably a guardian angel). The ambulance arrived, and the paramedics put something around both of my eyes. I thought, "This must be how a blind person feels." I felt isolated. The ambulance came. I thought the paramedics asked some dumb questions. "Where do you hurt?" They could see that as I was bleeding!

"What happened?" Dad had just told them.

"What is your name?" The other questions I was just too tired to answer, but I didn't really know the answer to that last question, and wondered, "This must be how a person who has had a stroke feels!" At the hospital, I asked my Mom what my name was. I thought she said, "Karen." That did not sound right, but I didn't let it bother me. I realized they expected me to be at work the next day. I recited my program assistant's, JoAnne's, home telephone number, but I still didn't know my name. I refused to worry about it. I knew I would recall it later. I wasn't hurt bad, but I looked beaten up - again. One of my clients told me later that he wondered who hit me, and who would do that to a person in a wheelchair!

In 1983, Governor Earl appointed me to a three-year term for the Governor's Committee for People with Disabilities. It was an excellent place to meet people, better understand the legislative process, and have an opportunity to affect change! Ellen Daley, who had a spinal cord injury, was the director, and eventually was on the President's Committee for People with Disabilities. Edith was on the committee with me, and taught me some of the ropes. It was here that I met Ann, a midget with no thumbs, who became a very important part of my life! I was fortunate to have known such role models. (In truth, I could say I was a "roll" model also, but that was something very different)!

In May of 1983, I was put on a panel in charge of screening applicants for the Kenosha Social Service Department director position. There were 53 applicants for the job. Thus, three of us reduced the group to 12 people. We finally recommended that four candidates be interviewed, and had an opportunity to watch that final process.

In 1984, I was appointed to the Kenosha County Specialized Transportation Commission for the Elderly/Handicapped by the County Executive. We analyzed the progress of City, County, and Escort (door-to-door) transportation programs. I presided over some of the County hearings. The commission recommended changes to resolve issues of Public concern.

All the things that I was involved in were very interesting. I felt I could contribute to all of these activities; however, I was starting to wear myself too thin. I started to pull out of the groups that were in the evenings and not directly connected to my job. Arlene and Bob took over the social group on Tuesday nights. ABLE had a very competent, feisty new president named Barb. I knew she would do fine!

I tried to do a few more things that were recreational like going to Six Flags which was about 20 miles from my house. MDA also had tickets to a NASCAR race in Elkhart Lake, Wisconsin. Mom, Dad, and Kenny, now 10 years-old, went with me. Kenny was very excited, because he met David Hasselhoff who was going to start the race. *Knight Rider* was his favorite television show, and here was his hero! David came over to me, and gave me a kiss saying, "Where have you been all my life!" He asked Kenny if he wanted a picture taken with him. David just took Ken's camera, and put one of his arms around Kenny's shoulders, and his other arm straight holding out the camera. David took the picture himself! He was at least 6'4". As he walked away toward the hill, he towered over everyone else. David was easy to spot wherever he was! Mario Andretti and Al Unser were racing that day among others. David got up to the microphone while we were standing by the fence line, and announced, "Lady and gentlemen, start your engines!" Yes, there was only one woman! The sound was as loud as a jet taking off! The sound and the vibrations went right through me, which was probably helped by the metal in my wheelchair. It was thrilling! The course was full of twists and turns so you could see the cars at different points from our position. Eventually, we saw them coming in front of us again. Unfortunately, it started to rain. After two laps, we started toward the van. The race was cancelled, because of the thin tires on the cars. Any water on the Speedway was very dangerous for the drivers. I knew hydroplaning was possible on a very little amount of rain, but it was pouring!

I also dated a person, 13 years my junior, a few times. He was very mature for his age and intellectually challenging. He held a very responsible position at the age of 24. Distance was an issue as he was a couple hundred miles away. Good memories though.

~ 19 ~

Independent Living

I discovered from a friend that one of the members of WWAAC was having some problems. She had very little movement, but active in the community, and using very special equipment. Her Mother was getting older, and told her, "I can't take care of you anymore. I want to enjoy part of my life. You will have to figure something out."

Maybe this was a wake-up call for me!

"What would I do if that happened to me?"

I had helped a couple of other individuals with independent living services. I was 38, and not worried about myself, I thought it was time for me. Mom was 60 years old, and Dad was 64. My parents deserved some time together, even though they never complained about taking care of me.

I started preparing about six months ahead of time by investigating the cost of attendant care. A former schoolmate, who was about seven years younger than I was, lived in Racine. She wanted to move to Kenosha, because her brother had married the girl who lived across the street from my parents. She was eligible for attendant care, and we thought that we could share costs sharing the rent for an apartment as well as sharing an attendant. Gateway Technical College had a few training programs for nurses, so I put my name and phone number on the bulletin board to see if an attendant was available for August. Our names were on the waiting list for a newer apartment building just two blocks from my parents' house. We both passed the credit checks waiting to see what would happen.

I let Mom know what was happening, but she was hesitant.

"I think you should wait until Grandma dies, because she will be so worried!"

I knew Mom would be the one who was really the one who was worried, but I told her what happened when my friend's Mother had told her to leave.

"I would never do anything like that—leave you hanging."

I really thought I would be better off to make plans, now, to see what would, and wouldn't, work. "You can help me figure out whatever doesn't work," I added.

Everything worked just like clockwork, and fell into place at exactly the same time. I remember thinking that "God must really want me to do this because He put everything into place so fast, and I never even asked Him." I only prayed to say hi, to say thank God, or to let Him know if anyone else needed help. Kathy and I got a phone call that there was an apartment opening. Another phone call came a few hours later from a person named Rhonda. She needed a place to live in Kenosha for her Gateway's nursing program. The only thing that I had not thought of was how to give the attendant time off from her duties. Kathy had cerebral palsy, and was already self-sufficient.

BY THE GRACE OF GOD AND YOU
A Chair Does Not a Person Make

At first, I went home every weekend, which made my parents happy, helped them to come to terms with everything. I also think that she missed seeing many of my friends. Mom went through a period of depression, and became physically weaker after that point. She blamed me for it, at first, but eventually realized that the move had been a smart one. At some point, I think dependency switched. As a child, I was totally dependent on my parents. When I began to live on my own, my parents did not know what to do. It as if my Mom lost a job, a child, and a purpose all at the same time. I still talked to her every night on the telephone.

Both Merle and Jeff came over to our apartment. Merle had a new kitten, and brought "Buttons" with him, occasionally. He kept me updated on what was happening at Bullen. We both liked Trivial Pursuit, and had fun playing it. He was the one that was smart; I had the funny fill-in answers!

Our apartment had a flat entrance. The city bus went right through the parking lot, and recently, had become accessible. The back stairs of the bus, became a lift, and the bus driver came back to operate manually. I took the bus back and forth to work every day, and used my van mainly on weekends. One snowy day the second winter, eight different people touched my life helping me get me to work. One of these was a caregiver who got me up and ready. A 15-year old boy, in an upstairs apartment, pushed me through the snow to the bus stop. Others helped as well. The bus driver, the attendant who called my secretary, letting her know I was on my way, and a couple of probation officers who pushed me from the bus through the snow. In addition, last, a stranger who opened the door at my office building. This independent living stuff was not independent, and a lot of times, it wasn't fun! Sometimes, you just have to find the humor in it. The snow was at least 8 inches deep that day! It covered half of my wheels, got my motor wet, and paralyzed my chair for about 20 minutes. While waiting for it to thaw, the snow from the wheels left four little puddles of water. It looked as if there were four puppies who left their famous, notorious marks in my office!

Kathy brought her used furniture for our apartment. I only had enough furniture for my bedroom. It was a two-bedroom apartment, so Kathy and I shared one, while our attendant, Rhonda, occupied the other. Rhonda was from Burlington (about 35 miles away), and finished her degree in one year. I didn't really want to think about changing attendants all the time. We put in an electric door opener, which really helped Kathy out as well as me! We had two garage door openers, and they were attached to both of our wheelchairs. I could push the buttons for the door to open, so I could get in and out. It made us very independent, especially in the summer when we could get out and walk around. Kathy could cook some delicious chicken! But as far as cooking goes?

"She could reach the eggs! I cracked them."

"I could put the key in the door, and she could turn it!"

She had difficulty with her finger dexterity. I had trouble with strength! Once the electric door opener was installed, we needed no keys, since the opener unlocked and relocked the door!

There was one new client on my caseload that I really felt would do a good job. She had little to no work experience, but both she and her Mother thought it was something she would like to try. I discussed this with the supervisor. Brenda was changed to a different counselor. Kathy liked her too. Brenda was just thinking about learning to drive!

Once in a while, Kathy would come to work with me, and set up my files in the morning. When Brenda learned to drive, she took both of us up to the Wisconsin Dells for a training session with the Easter Seals' summer staff. All three of us were very positive people, and got along well.

But, later, Kathy decided to move. Her stepsister had a baby, and wanted her to move back to Racine to help her care for it. One of her other friends also asked her to do the same thing, because Debbie really missed her!

I refigured my budget, and decided that could pay Brenda $100 a week plus room and board. I think the stress of so much change triggered her bipolar disability, which she talked about openly. One of the symptoms of her disability was spending money rapidly. Her Mother noticed this when Brenda spent her savings of $1000 in one day! Kathy was no longer there during the day for her to talk to, and Brenda loved to talk. Brenda was very sweet, caring, and was loved by my parents. She had several medication changes, and these were difficult for both of us.

At the same time, my Dad thought I should consider buying a house, since the market was very good. He took care of my money. He was much better at it than I was! If I were to buy a $50,000 house, at least I would have something for my rent money! I had saved $30,000 for a down payment, and Dad would loan me the rest after about 3 months. With a commercial loan, even with a small interest rate, the house would cost $150,000, if I borrowed from a bank, and paid as a 30-year loan. He saved me a lot of money! We looked for a house for about six months, and although we screened about 80 houses, I only looked at four. The first one was much too small. The second house was owned by the brother of the star on *Hill Street Blues*, Dan Travanti, but it had a white carpet, which was not good for wheelchairs. The third house was excellent, but my wheelchair would not fit through one of the hallways. It even had a fireplace! The fourth house was three blocks away from the last house I had looked at, and bingo! It was the one! It would have to be ramped up three steps, was a corner house, and it had a big yard. Inside, it had a lot of open space. The living room was at least 23 feet long, and 12 feet wide with many windows and lots of light! It had three bedrooms, and a big kitchen with an island! It was the house of a veterinarian, so there was also a fence on the property for a dog if we wanted. And, it was only $55,000!

I was approved for a loan, even without Dad cosigning! This is a very difficult for a person with a disability! Regular house payments would have been almost too expensive, because of attendant costs. I only paid half of what attendants received in Madison, but their costs were paid by medical assistance for which I was not eligible. The attendant could get a full time day job also.

So, a friend built the ramp on the front steps. Dad put an asphalt ramp on the front doorstep. Jeff's Dad had put in the automatic door opener! I had furniture now, since Kathy moved. The only extra thing I did was buy touch lamps for easier access. I had two *Home Interior* parties to decorate my walls!

Brenda had a new boyfriend that was excellent for her. He was the son was the son of a teacher at Bullen, who became the vice principal. Small world. But, Brenda decided to move in with me for a while causing her a lot of stress, again, and she just couldn't pack up anything. About eight of my friends helped with the move taking things straight off the wall, or out of the closet, and put them in the cars. By the end of the day, Dan had even trimmed my bushes! Rhonda and her husband, who particularly worked hard, stayed to make everything workable before they left!

Lawn care and snow were the biggest problems that I had as a homeowner. Having my lawn cut, or snow shoveled on regular basis was difficult. Everyone else's lawn was perfect, but mine always looked like the park. If the park kitty corner from me had dandelions, my yard was yellow with them also! If the park was dry, my yard was brown. If it was full of leaves in the fall, mine was, too. Kenny, or others, helped when they could.

Brenda had taken a part-time job in a nursing home. I knew that she was stressed, because she had some problems sleeping. I heard her up in her room one night. Perhaps she was sleepwalking while she was taking down her curtains one day. She came into my room, and turned on the light.

"I cannot find your gait belt to walk you. What should I do?"

I didn't really want to go for a walk, and wasn't totally awake to respond.

"Just go back to bed."

She did, and the next morning, she was sleeping so hard, I could not wake her up until 10:00 a.m. I missed part of the workday.

At the same time, I got a voice-activated system that turned my television on and off, and changed the channels. It also activated a light switch, as well as answer, or dial, my telephone. The system only worked in my bedroom area, and of course, the system didn't always work perfectly. I had 10 people on speed dial. Occasionally, it would hear the word "Mom", and dial my Mom at 2:00 a.m.! I would tell my Mom it was just a mistake, she laid a pillow on top of the telephone just so she couldn't hear it in the middle of the night! I guess I talked in my sleep more than I thought!

I asked Brenda if it would be helpful for me to get a second attendant to split the work, the time, and the check. She thought that would be a good idea, so I sought another person from the community. The girl who applied was very pretty, and had just lost a lot of weight. As time went on, it was obvious that she was bulimic. Her demeanor was up and down, due to her situation. One morning, I had an extremely bad stomachache on her shift. She was very crabby in the mornings, and told me to wait until Brenda awoke. There was no way that was going to happen. I had enough, and fired her on the spot. I had encouraged her to get help with her problem, because I could hear her vomiting after every meal, and really did not want her to die in my house! She was a good worker, but her problems interfered with her success.

Shortly after the other attendant left, Brenda decided she was going to live with Paul. She had been with me for two years, but I totally understood. They were definitely in love, and he took very good care of her. She gave me enough notice, so that I could find another attendant. I checked with the counselors at DVR first to see if they had any good candidates.

In the meantime, a friend from the past stopped by a few times to see me. I thought things were going along pretty well, when one night he came to see me with no one in the house. We were going to go somewhere, but instead, he kissed me. He unbuckled my wheelchair safety belt, put his arms around me and tears started coming from my eyes. I kept saying, "No. Oh, no." He put me gently on the floor, and had his way with me. It was the first time for me. I didn't fight. I couldn't fight. I blocked him mentally. The doorbell rang, and he stopped. It had to be the paperboy collecting for the week, but the door was never answered. He put me back together, and picked me up just as gently putting me back in my chair. I went through a ton of feelings, but mostly I felt confusion, anger, and betrayal. Did he love me, or was I just there at his disposal? Why would he do this to me? What was I supposed to learn from this?

I remembered, "Everything that happens is part of God's plan. Everything happens for good."

I saw him a few days later. He looked horrible, and asked if I was okay. He must have been on drugs that night, because he was acting as if he cared. Did he look horrible, because he was on drugs, ashamed, scared I'd report him to the police? Why didn't I report him? I never thought of the police. Maybe it was pity! Maybe he was giving himself enough hell! What good would it have done? I'd be okay, no matter what. He was out of my life in my head and in my heart! If there was a man in my future, it wasn't he. I never liked wasting energy on negative thoughts. It wasn't healthy, so I just moved on. Life was too short to dwell on this day.

My attendant cleaned me up thinking that I just had sex. I decided not to share what happened. I just stuffed my feelings and never shared this until now.

I didn't see him much after that, but something very unusual happened which helped put things together for me. I was a regular at a Chinese restaurant, because it was within walking distance of the office. About a week later, this was what my fortune cookie read: "It was not that he didn't love you. It was that he couldn't love."

How powerful of an answer was that to "why", and in an unexpected fortune cookie! What I was afraid of most about relationships was over. I knew this could happen to anyone, but I didn't expect it to happen to me. Bad things happen to everyone, but everything seems to happen for a reason. We need both sunshine and rain to grow and flower. No one should stop living, because something bad happened. I learned from it, and went on with my life. I even shared it, when appropriate, to help others. This was like a death to me—a skill I had developed from an early age. Gather any pain, put it in a box, and get rid of it. Dwelling on things I had no control over was deadly. It wasn't my fault, and God moved me along with a fortune cookie!

John, a DVR counselor in Racine, found a client that he thought would be a good match for the job as my attendant. Her name was Teri. She had a lot of energy and a fun personality. She checked to see if she could handle me by getting me in and out of bed. She did great, and I let Brenda know that I found someone. Teri moved in shortly thereafter.

I had a "Dress to get Wet" party with all of the people who loved the pool and being outside from the MDA group. About 15 people came, mainly from Milwaukee. It started out with little squirt guns, and ended up with 5-gallon buckets! We were outside, but the house still was tracked with a lot of mud. June was there, and asked me if I was having any problems with pain. I said, "Yes." She responded, "Gee, I'm glad. I thought that I was the only one!" I felt that it was an unusual conversation when I didn't understand it, since it was out of the blue. Joan was there, and later, Lloyd came for about an hour later, since he found someone to take care of his Father. Of course, Lloyd was the only one that picked on me. I was the one that got the 5-gallon bucket of water right over my head and my wheelchair! My chair started going by itself towards the curb, and I couldn't stop it! Lloyd held it back while someone found a hair dryer in the house to dry my chair out! I was in a place that needed two, 50-foot extension cords to reach me! I survived, and so did my chair.

A short time later, Lloyd called me to tell me his Father had died. We talked a while. He gave me directions to the funeral home, and close to the airport. So, Teri drove me to Milwaukee arriving early, and knew that we weren't going to stay long. The funeral home was accessible through the back door. As a side thought, there was one funeral home in Kenosha that I didn't like to go to, because I always had to ride in the freight elevator, which they used for the coffins. Lloyd spotted me as soon as I came in the door. He said hello to Teri, and leaned over to hug me hard. I heard him sob, and felt tears on my shoulder. I couldn't handle the emotions—was it his pain, or my need to escape his touch? He finally let me go after what seemed to be at least two minutes. That was two minutes longer than I usually allow myself to feel about anything. Biting my tongue did not help! I needed to leave. He took us over to see his Dad who had been a large man. I knew it must have been hard for Lloyd to take care of him. We talked a little bit about it, and then he left. He said that he'd be back in a minute, but the funeral parlor was becoming full, and I knew no one. We left, and went to check out the airport shops, which were unique, but expensive except for a used bookstore. We spent some time there, before we went to eat.

I talked with Lloyd about a week later when he came to visit and we went for a bite to eat. When we got back home, he set me on the bed per Teri's request. She did not know when she was going to be home to help me, but knew it would be before 11:00 p.m. We talked more, and he kissed me saying that he enjoyed it! Wait! I allowed myself to enjoy that—stop it! I hinted about some of the things that were going on with me, but couldn't really share. I didn't want to tell him about the rape or that I went out with someone 13 years younger! I was 41 years old, now, and not a teenager.

"Right now, I wouldn't even recognize a good relationship if it fell right in my lap," I told him.

Lloyd took a breath, and let it out slowly as he pretended to fall in my lap!

"Funny. Cute! But right now, it wouldn't be fair for me to get involved with anyone. I feel pretty messed up. But I like being with you too." I smiled, and then, he left just before Teri got home.

I knew it was always my fault! God don't let me pull away! Lloyd was rugged, nice, caring, gentle, strong, fun loving, and always said what he meant—a real prize and a real hunk! I just didn't think I could make him happy for long, so I made the decision for him. I sent him away. My heart always fought with my head.

My heart yelled, "Stupid, dummy—no guts! How many hints does he have to give, and how many rejections would he be willing to take?"

"He'll always be there for you—you know that! Let him be happier with someone else. You'll never believe he loved you, anyway. Why put yourself through that?" My head whispered, and unfortunately, my head always won!

159

Teri and I did a lot of things together. We even went dancing one night at the Kenosha Holiday Inn. We worked out a routine. I didn't really know anyone there—which was good. Teri said, kiddingly, that she was upset, because someone asked me to dance and not her!

I had a lot of problems that year with the tires on my wheelchair. Seven of them blew out that summer. And, I decided to get solid tires. They were not as smooth of a ride, but were much more reliable. I did a lot of walking—not only for my job to the different agencies downtown, but at home, I enjoyed going to rummage sales. On Saturday mornings, I would look at the newspaper, and map out my route of a three-mile radius. Both my parents and my sister's family lived within that radius, so my wheelchair would roll a lot of miles in the summer. I was about six blocks from the bus stop. Fortunately, I don't remember it raining. The city bus worked in the spring through fall. Jim, the morning bus driver, looked out for me. One day I got stuck when my hand fell off of the controls. I was so glad to see Jim with the bus coming around the block to pick me up! When the snow, came, though, I used specialized, door-to-door transportation. For the four years that I used the bus, I was on a route with mostly junior high kids, which was fun, since that was the grade level I taught!

Teri got a job as a bus driver for the Kenosha Achievement Center. She loved all of their clients, and enjoyed the work very much. It gave her more money, too. She went out with Jeff for a while. She had another boyfriend who would pick me up out of my wheelchair, and carried me down to my basement for the first time. I had never seen it! He set me on his knee for a few minutes so I could look around, and then, brought me back upstairs without even puffing!

For both of us to get to work on time, Teri would take a half hour to get me out of bed and dressed. I would do my makeup while she took a shower. When she was done, she would put on my hair, and we both went out the door! Right! No breakfast!

One day, Teri was emotionally shaken. The director's body was found in the bus garage when she got to work. He committed suicide. How could he have taken his own life when he had given so many people a productive life with his work at the Achievement Center, Easter Seals, and a number of other agencies as well as with the many Kenoshans with disabilities who needed specialized transportation? The stress of changing times, feeling responsible for so many, and the pressures of life became overwhelming may have all contributed. Jim was very gifted, and he affected so many people with his positive attitude. I admired and respected him very much—what could I have done for him that wasn't being done? A chemical imbalance was suspected. How many desperate people are standing next to us, yet we don't know need help? If we did know, would we still ignore it? Caring all the time was emotionally draining. Was that what happened to him? How could we change that?

In 1986, I continued my work with Easter Seals. I even had a regional meeting at my home, so we could discuss some of the problems and issues to give to the Easter Seals House of Delegates. My living room was large enough to set up my Grandmother "with the kitties" dining room table that she had received when she was married. She had given it to me, and it sat 20 people.

That year, I was named the first Easter Seals Adult Ambassador. With the population getting older, Easter Seals wanted the public to know that they were making a difference in the lives of adults as well as children with disabilities. Gov. Earl declared, "The main goal of an adult representative was to help change negative attitudes toward people with disabilities". By coming into contact with an adult with a disability, people will learn how to react, how to see disabled adults as individuals first. And, I wished to share what Easter Seals had done for me.

I also did a commercial that year for Easter Seals, and it was their 60th anniversary. It ran frequently in the Madison area. I went to Madison to help with the telethon and for some reason stopped at a Walgreens to pick up something. There was a little girl about 10 years old whom I had noticed a couple of different times in the aisle where I was. All of a sudden, she came over and touched me on the arm, then ran away. I did not see her again. All I could think of was that she recognized me from the commercial. I felt like a movie star!

That movie star feeling didn't last long, though, because I did not feel I did well on the telethon. I did fine when interviewed by the host who was nicknamed Crazy TV Lenny from the American Furniture and Appliance stores. He was an excellent host, but I had a difficult time reading the donor's names and ad-libbing. Anyway, I received a letter from Pat Fettig who became a very good friend and board member in WWAAC. At this time, Pat was our Easter Seals' Regional Representative:

Another year as well as another record! The 1986 Easter Seals telethon was the most successful ever! Thanks for all of your help as well as your generous telethon contribution. You helped us raise more than $150,000 which will be used to provide direct services to children and adults with physical disabilities. Our hosts mentioned throughout the telethon and we would like to repeat that $.95 of every dollar raised will remain in Wisconsin, and the $.81 of that will be used to provide direct assistance now.

I'm very pleased that you were able to join us in Madison during the actual telethon. A number of people commented that the idea of an adult ambassador for Easter Seals was an excellent one-and-that Carol Schaufel was the ideal choice. We definitely think so!! I did have an opportunity to view your interviews on videotape-excellent.

Carol, you and your parents are special friends of Easter Seals. You have done so much for us and for people with disabilities. One million thanks for everything but especially, your friendship and your caring.

I particularly wanted to share this letter, because Easter Seals still has the best record of any agency in providing the greatest portion of its dollars to direct services. Pat took good care of everyone!

My public defender friend, Jerry, who was blind, was married to Libby, and she was a member of the Lioness Club of Greater Kenosha. She asked me if I would like to join and volunteered to give me a ride to the meetings. Susan, Kathy, and Deb joined later, and also gave me rides after Jerry changed jobs, and moved to New Berlin. Since I was assigned the blind caseload at work, I thought that joining the Lioness was a good idea. The group was originally meeting in different members' houses. Now, they were going to meet at a restaurant, so I could attend. I worked on a number of different projects. I went to bingo at a nursing home. The job I could do best was sitting by the people that could not hear well. I would yell out the called numbers into their ears! I also worked on the style show, and was even a model for it one year! I was on the Board 3 years and President for one. I was an active member from 1986 to 1994.

This group also won one of 10 international recognitions for a project on which I worked. There were two of us who had disabilities visible to the public. Angie (no vision) and I would go to the different third grade classrooms in the school district, and talk to the students about people with disabilities. We visited third grade classes, because their books had a story about a person who was visually impaired. We went separately, and the kids would ask about everything under the sun. I began my talk by looking around to see if any students had disabilities that I could see, like hearing aids (if I could see them), or glasses. I explained that my wheelchair helped my legs just like their glasses helped their eyes. I would explain that I had trouble lifting heavy files, but with my wheelchair, I could move three or four of their desks with the students in them. Of course, I would demonstrate! They wanted to know how fast I could go—6.1 mph. The students wanted to know the cost. That depended on the chair. Mine was about $7000 at that time. Some people had chairs that were $23,000, because different people needed them to lie down, reposition, help them stand, etc. I would bring an accessibility sign, and would ask them what it meant in different settings. In the bathroom, wheelchairs needed a larger space, so hanging onto the grab bars kept people from falling. They could also pull on them in a transfer making it easier for them to use lower hand towels, or dryers. By a telephone, it meant a volume control, and a place to put a TTY. Just because the sign was there, it did not mean that other people couldn't use them, except for parking spaces. For me, I needed the wideness of the parking space to get in and out of my van. Distance wasn't a problem for me, because of my electric wheelchair. Some people with asthma needed those parking places, especially in cold/hot weather when they could not walk long distances without running out of breath. I would always let the students come to see me get in and out of the van, so they could see how I did things. I let them touch the control that ran my chair, so they could see how light the touch was to drive my chair. I would tell them about my job, travel, camping, and hobbies and how I did them! Having a disability wasn't worse; it was just different. I also let the students know that everyone in a wheelchair was different just like everyone in the classroom. Some were happy, and some were sad. Some were good, and some were bad. Some were even in prison. Some were crabby and didn't like to answer questions. I would prefer them to ask questions rather than to stare. They could help their parents with that!

Twice, I found myself in trouble. Once, I was speaking to a gifted class of third graders. I shared, "I was talking to this man who had to put a vibration device next to his throat to move his voice chords." This one little girl said, "Oh, you mean he had his larynx removed?" I had to step up my language in that class! Another time, a student said he had a limp. He uttered something to me that made me think he was being teased about it. Kids could be pretty cruel at times. Somehow, I asked about that when the student started to cry. I hoped that I commented, "We all try to do the best we can with what we have and shouldn't try to be what others think we should be. We shouldn't care what anyone else thinks if we need to do something in a different way." My thing was always, "Wouldn't it be awful if everyone liked the same food, a certain person, the same job? We were all different and need to use those differences which were our blessings!" Truth: I'm sure I didn't say that. I probably just cried with him instead!

There is one thing that always bothered me. When I was fairly young, and to this day, people always said/say,

"It doesn't matter if we're going to have a boy or girl, just so it's healthy!"

In my mind, that would be nice, but I am really glad I was born.

Others say, "If I had that disability, I would kill myself!"

I wondered, "Why?"

People without disabilities have good and bad times too.

Then I had a horrible thought: "What if I was aborted. What if I were aborted just because doctors knew I had a disability?"

A few days after I went to speak to students, I would always get a big envelope in the mail. Sometimes there would be a pile of notes, and other times it would be a pile of pictures. The pictures were so cute because the pictures would have me doing these impossible things like climbing a tree or jumping rope! But in all of the pictures, there was always one thing in common - an extra-large control stick on my wheelchair!

And for some of you who wonder how third-graders write, here are some examples:

Did you go to the dinner with the mayor? Thank you for the nice speech, I liked it a lot. I gotta go to the library. Bye.

How are you and your roommate doing? I'm doing okay. I know you are. We all had a lot of fun when you were here. We wish you would come back someday because we miss you already.

You aren't different because you're in a wheelchair. We still like you anyway. Be nice.

Thanks for coming yesterday. My Mom is disabled partially. She has arthritis so she can't walk very far. She knows a friend who has a heart problem so we're moving to Phoenix, Arizona.

I really enjoyed your coming to our room. I used to think that people in wheelchairs had a handicap but then you showed us all the things you could do. You taught me a lesson.

I enjoyed your talk a lot. I liked the joke about you getting your hair at Kmart. You must feel pretty lucky to meet all those movie stars. You are a very pretty lady. Did you know that you forgot your sign?

I liked listening to you. I've read about handicapped people a lot but never seen one until you came yesterday.

I'm happy you came to our school. You can really make people understand. My sister is

mental, people talk about her, and some feel sorry for her, but she doesn't care. She can't speak really good because she's mental. You made my day a lot better.

Thank you for coming to see us. You should know me. You moved my desk.

For all of my work and community service, I was also selected to be in the *National Distinguished Service Registry* in the Library of Congress from 1987-1991.

<h2>~ 20 ~</h2>

<h2>Changes</h2>

"Where is my purse?" Teri asked. "I always put it right here on the kitchen counter by the back door." We looked around, and noticed that the dining room window's screen was missing. As I went closer to the window, I could see the screen was lying on the ground outside. It had been a hot summer night. All of our fans were on high, and the window was pushed wide open! Someone broke into the house! Nothing else was missing. I remembered that I called Teri's name in the middle of the night, because I thought she was in my room. Maybe it was the intruder. Teri may have only had about 50 cents in her purse, but her Social Security card was gone along with other papers.

After we called the police, they found Teri's purse in a garbage can across the street in the park. Her wallet was missing. They told us that they believed "it was younger kids looking for cash", but it was still scary to us anyway, and felt creepy. Dad nailed the window shut so it could only be opened enough for air, but not wide enough for a human to enter. Teri didn't feel safe at all, so she borrowed a pistol from a friend, sleeping with it under her pillow. I didn't think that was a good idea, and after that first night, Teri returned the gun to its owner.

In 1988, my Grandfather "with the kitties" passed away. Both he and my Grandmother had shared a room in a nursing home for several years. I know Mom always visited, and she did Grandma's laundry for a long time. Grandma lived seven more years in the same nursing home.

<h2>~ Steve ~</h2>

In 1982, I met Steve, and gave him information on applying for Great Lakes Navy Base positions. Eventually, one of these jobs came through for him. He took a job as a recidivism alcohol and drug counselor first. I saw him quite often in different places. He told me he admired me, and would like to help me if he could.

I saw him in 1986. We watched some movies together and got to know each other. By September of 1988, Steve asked me to marry him. Steve was in the process of getting a divorce, and had some legal problems. He had been up front with me about everything.

Teri had told me to find another attendant, because she was going to get married, too. A woman who was my neighbor tried to help me one day when my attendant was in the hospital. She suggested that I find a male attendant. "That would be easier. He would be stronger."

Every time Steve and I went out together, whether it was a restaurant, a Milwaukee museum, or a place in Chicago, I would see someone I knew. A person would talk to me, and he would fade into the background. He was both impressed, because I knew so many people, and discouraged, because it seemed as if we were never alone. With his alcohol background, his reputation was not always good! He felt that I was ruining his bad reputation, but he was dealing with it! I was proud of him, because he stopped drinking and was sober by the age of 30.

Dorothy, my former program assistant, was at my house. We were watching the Olympic ice skating events. She met Steve at that time, and liked him a lot. Dorothy had breast cancer a few years ago, and I had taken off work to go to the hospital with her when she had her surgery. The surgery went well, but she was unable to maintain her job in Probation and Parole at DVR. After a year, or two, her cancer had metastasized (spread) to her back. She was going through a lot of pain and problems again. She loved the Olympics, and we were watching the 'Battle of the Brains' for male ice-skating!

Dorothy had been laughing because she had a dream. There was a spider on the ceiling, and I was there encouraging her.

"You can get that spider! I know you can reach it and kill that spider!"

"You encourage me to keep going on even in my dreams!" Dorothy laughed.

Unfortunately, about 2 years later, Dorothy went into a nursing home. She was really the encourager, because she was always smiling! Her death was very painful—for her physically and me emotionally.

Steve was Tex-Mex and Chiricahua Indian (Apache), and had a sad history. Both of his parents died before he was two years old. A car deliberately ran over his Father, and killed. His Mother died soon after of a broken heart. Steve had a brother and a sister, who were much older than he was, and were not with him very long. An Aunt and Uncle, who had children of their own, took care of Steve.

"I remembered when holidays came along; they would have me eat first, a big plate of scrambled eggs, while they would have turkey, mashed potatoes, dressing, and the works!" Steve once told me.

One thing Steve was given was a broomstick horse! His Aunt asked him to go to the store one day, which Steve was happy to do. The store was a couple of blocks away, but he couldn't find his horse! He cried, "I can't go to the store without my horse! It's too far for me to walk!" Everyone looked for his horse, and finally found it hanging on the back of a doorknob. Steve quickly got on his horse, and galloped to the store!

Steve's Aunt developed an illness, and died. That left him alone with his Uncle who was a heavy drinker. He would give Steve a dollar a day for lunch consisting of a Coke and Fritos. If Steve would say that he was hungry, his Uncle would say, "All you bring to this house is hunger." Steve knew that wasn't true, because he would see his deceased Father's railroad check with his and his Uncle's name on it for about $65/month.

When Christmas came, he had no Christmas tree, so Steve decorated the kitchen chair with lights, ornaments, and anything he could find.

"I don't know why you're doing that because there is no such thing as Santa Claus! There won't be anything under that 'tree' in the morning anyway," his Uncle grumbled.

Steve retorted, "Oh, yes there will!"

However, Santa never came, and he was devastated!

For being alone, Steve did pretty well. In school, the teacher asked the class what their favorite holiday was.

"Christmas!" a first child answered.

"Easter!" a second child said.

By the time the teacher got to Steve, he said there wasn't anything left except Halloween!

"That's not a holiday, you hoodlum!" the teacher responded.

Steve admitted that he did like to go out on Halloween. The bad kids used to go out to tip over the outhouses, but, all he and his friends would do was move the outhouses just a little bit, causing them to step in #2.

By the time Steve was 14 years-old, he was on his own…and surviving anyway he could. He even worked in a convent for a while! He became a boxer in a special service unit of the Navy. He also became an alcoholic, and had some funny stories. One of these was about the time he bought himself a bottle of wine, and put it into his coat pocket. He climbed the rickety staircase to his apartment and fell all the way back down the steps. He saw something red oozing on his pants, and prayed, "Oh, God, please let it be blood", but it was the wine, and he had no money to buy more. Steve had heard the same story from others before, but now it was happening to him. Another time was when he visited and Alcoholics Anonymous group, which sounded like a sissy group, and its name was "The Valentine AA Group". The tough Irish group was truck drivers who told him to stop feeling sorry for himself and get off his "pity pot". Just stop drinking so you can change."

At this point in time, his unemployment had not yet ended, so he asked a friend where applications were being accepted. The friend told him that there were no job openings at company X, but he should try company Y. Of course, he went to company X, and filled out an application for employment.

"You are in luck! Someone just quit! You can start right away!" the man said.

Steve asked, "Aren't you going to check my references?"

"Do you want to work or don't you?"

"I don't know if I want to work for a company that doesn't check references!" Steve exclaimed.

"Get out of here!" the man barked at him.

Steve got a job as a security guard at a factory. Even though he was scared to death knowing that the last security guard was murdered on the job, he took the job anyway. He was all alone in the building, and was not supposed to bring a gun, but he did. He heard a noise in the bathroom, so he crept up to the bathroom door to peek inside. As he put his head around the corner, he saw someone else put his head around the corner. He withdrew with his heart beating fast, and drew his gun. Again, he put his gun around the corner, and saw that the other man had a gun, too! He drew back once more, and took a breath. Steve put his gun around the corner again, and quickly shot a couple of bullets. Steve heard the other guy shoot. The mirror broke. It was his reflection, and his bullets broke the mirror. An article appeared in The Chicago Sun-Times with the headline "Security Guard Has Shoot out with self." He looked for another job the next day.

Steve got married, and had two little boys. At the age of 30, he became sober, and stayed sober. He had custody of the boys from the early ages of four and five. Steve worked at Kopper's in Chicago for a long time, and then took a job in Waukegan. At that time, he met his second wife. He always said that his Indian Grandfather warned, "Don't trust the white man!" He never said anything about women! Both of his wives were of German heritage, just like me.

Steve was now 48 years old, and his sons were 16 and 17. I really didn't believe in living with someone before I got married, but I did not want to get married if the person did not really know what it entailed with me. Teri told him that she didn't think he could handle the #2 and periods. I had to ask him one question to see how he would respond.

"Does it bother you that I have a disability?" I asked him.

Does it bother you that I'm not white?" was his response.

That question surprised me. I never thought of him as being white, Indian, Mexican, or anything else. No, my disability nor his background mattered! I had seen too many marriages break up when one person had a disability. I still did not want him to marry me unless he knew what to expect. Why was I thinking this could work? The answer made me comfortable—a question for a question! He was divorced twice—why would our marriage work? I felt he saw me, and not my disability!

Steve moved in with me along with his youngest son, Gavino and a pit bull that had not yet been named. After Teri moved out, Mom was embarrassed, because of my living arrangements. Every time Mom saw someone that she knew, she would walk on the other side of the street fearing questions would be asked about me. But, Dad took a different approach.

"Steve can give Carol a lot of things that we can't give her. Even if the relationship only lasts 10 years, she will have had that relationship!"

After a year of being together, I asked Steve if he still wanted to get married.

"I am glad I lived with you first or otherwise I think I would've felt cheated. You are a lot of work, but I love you and want to marry you!" he told me truthfully.

Stevie, Steve's other son, came to live with us a few months after Steve moved in my house. He also had a disability, but his was very different. I would wake up singing in the morning.

Stevie would say a couple of things such as, "Another miserable day! Pops, what is wrong with this house? Nobody yells!"

The poor pit bull had no name for several months. So, I asked Gavino a question after he had rejected about 100 names for the pooch.

"What is your favorite food?"

"Popcorn," he told me.

"Well then that is his name!" And, it was a done deal.

The dog was good to me, but she eventually became overprotective when my attendants came around. The dog was not very bright though, because if she would happen to catch her reflection in the television screen, she would bark for hours until someone would drag her away!

In September of 1989, we added a Doberman puppy, and, this time, Gavino had already picked out the name "Midnight". Popcorn was asleep when we introduced her to Midnight. We laid the puppy down on the floor. Midnight went right for what she thought was Popcorn's food dispensers. Popcorn got up fast and started sniffing! To our surprise, she was very gentle with Midnight.

Midnight was trained to be the outside dog. She had her tricks, too! As she got bigger, neighbors would tell us that every day after we would leave for work, she would jump the fence coming home just before we got back from work! Popcorn would always run in a straight line when Gavino would go running with her. On the Other Hand, Midnight would zigzag from one side of the sidewalk to the other even if she was on a leash. Then, she could run like a deer with only about eight strides passing the eight houses on the block!

We did keep the morning attendants, at first, because Steve had to go into work very early, and because I just needed that female touch! Steve was not good at helping me put on my makeup, or making my clothing look professional. The only other place we had problems was with the bathroom. If I had to go #2, even if it was Monday, he would say, "Can't you wait until the weekend when you are at your Mother's?"

The one bad thing was that I had to tell my Mom was that I would never be on time again! Steve was always late!

On a more serious note, my real fear was wondering how I could be an equal partner in my marriage. Steve would have to do most of the work. I worked, took care of the bills, and paperwork, kept everyone organized, and dealt with the stress.

At work, I was appointed to the University of Wisconsin-Milwaukee Rehabilitation Department Advisory Committee. We assisted with program planning, monitored progress, and initiated change. I was on that committee from 1989 to 1994. I also started working with the Kenosha County Long Term Planning Committee. I have been volunteering with the Department on Aging and Disability of Kenosha County in different capacities ever since 1989. These positions were appointed by the Kenosha County board approval. I am presently on the Aging and Disability Resource Center Advisory Committee.

In October of 1989, I also received the WWAAC Achievement Award, which was presented in Eau Claire, Wisconsin. Steve had not taken me to any of these state meetings yet as he had to work.

~ Marriage Ceremony ~

Besides the normal preparations of a wedding, there were a lot of other considerations. Accessibility was number one, for the guests and me. Finding a hall big enough was also an issue. There were still a lot of places that were not accessible. I often said that if I were to get married, I would have to rent County Stadium (the Brewers ballpark)! We started out with a list of 400 for my side. First, we eliminated children. Next, we needed to know who would not be coming from a farther distance. We invited 12 people from Steve's family limiting them, because all of his family was in Texas. Finally, we assumed that at least 10% would not be coming due to previous obligations.

We chose a date in September for the wedding, but scrapped that date, since Steve didn't think he could lose any weight by then. Our next choice was November 4, and Steve did not lose any weight anyway. I think that date discouraged people that were coming from a farther distance, because of Wisconsin snow possibilities! We whittled the list down to 220, now, since the hall only held 200.

There were cultural considerations I wasn't expecting: Steve's relatives from Texas didn't attend, but the few local Hispanic friends that Steve asked to come would respond with 12 people on an invitation for two! A party was a party to them, but space was an issue. Another delicate matter occurred when Steve chose my morning attendant's husband to be in the wedding, and etiquette required that I should have chosen the wife to be in the wedding party, too, and I didn't. She was very jealous of the person he accompanied, because he was 65 years-old and the girl was 21! His wife dragged him away when it came time for the wedding party pictures, and he wasn't in any of them!

Some attitudes were a problem as well.

"Steve must be marrying Carol for her money."

"It is a sin to have sex with a handicapped person."

And, even Mom asked why I was marrying Steve.

"Because I love him," I told her.

"You never said that before. I thought you were getting married to stay out of a nursing home like you once told me," she responded.

After some of those things were out of the way, the wedding plans were a go. Susie was my Maid of Honor. I chose Louise, next. She was my best friend ever since grade school, and she felt that she could handle walking down the aisle as well as going up the three steps. The third person I chose was Patty who had just given her kidney to one of her sisters. She was a volunteer and friend from MDA. Her roommate's sister was a seamstress in Kenosha, and Rita made the dresses. Steve chose Gavino, his youngest son, to be the Best Man. Domingo, 65 years old, and Ramon, who spoke no English and a boxer from Cuba, was also a groomsmen. I told Susie that she was the only one without a disability, or being young or older! Another good friend, Ann, whom I mentioned before from the Governor's Committee for People with Disabilities, sang at the wedding along with her friend who was blind. Ann's niece, who was 16, played the piano, and became a doctor. The pastor who performed the ceremony was a female. Mindy, now 7, was the miniature bride and David, now 11, was the miniature groom. Kenny and Bob were the ushers. We could not always depend on Stevie, so he sat with my Mom and Dad. A couple of months before, Stevie indicated that he would have a church picture taken us as a family, but he didn't.

Since we had a variety of people coming from different cultural backgrounds of Hispanic, African American, white, and more, and with the additional people who were blind, midgets, in wheelchairs, guide dogs, and more, we didn't know how Stevie would respond.

At one point in the wedding preparations, he chuckled.

"This isn't going to be a wedding. It's going to be a circus!"

His sense of social etiquette was just not there, and he didn't know that this statement hurt me.

"I should be the best man not Gavino. I'm the oldest!" He thought this was funny.

Stevie was about 85 pounds and looked like a thin Jerry Lewis, and always had to fight with him to get a haircut!

There were so many things that could go wrong, and did go wrong, before the wedding occurred that it was unbelievable. The caterer was the brother of a student who "pushed me around" in high school. Two weeks before the wedding, he was arrested and put in jail! We were worried that there would be no food! Then, the DJs got a divorce, and we worried more. "No food and no music!" Another major thing for me was that I couldn't find a cake topper where the bride was not standing! I found one bride sitting on the couch, but that made no sense! One of my volunteers also fired ceramics, so Shirley made a cake top for me where the groom was carrying me making more sense! Steve always carried me onto the couch, or lifted me out of bed into my chair. He was strong for his age even though he was seven years older than I was.

Mom gave me a couple of showers so that different people had a chance to come. Susie did a lot of the work. The Lioness Club also gave me a surprise shower. A member named Kathy made me a beautiful money tree with $1, $5, and $10 bills folded into accordion pleated flowers and leaves, and then they were attached to a tree branch! I was touched! I also had a *Lioness in the Spotlight* article written about me. Here were the parts of the article that were not made public:

According to her sister, Sue, "There's never a dull Moment when Carol's around. You never just sit. She can cram more into 10 minutes than anyone I know! When she was little, if she could've gotten around, she would have been the kind of kid who would have unwrapped a box of candy from under the Christmas tree, eaten all of it, then wrapped it up again and put it back under the tree!"

As my 'source' tells me, "We like to take Carol places because she gets us first in line, especially Disney World and Vegas!" Did you know Carol LOVES to play blackjack? It is said that she would play 16 hours a day with only a few "necessary" timeouts! In fact they said she never wins a lot of money, but they doubt that she lost or ever broke even…….. But she has fun.

Do I understand that you were actually kissed by Tony Orlando Carol... This amazing young woman has done so many wonderful things in her life in spite of her handicap and I'm sure there's more to come from her. In fact one of them will take place on November 4—her upcoming wedding. We as lioness are proud to have you as such an active member of our club. You are an inspiration to us all ... especially when it comes to selling Style Show Tickets!

The bridesmaids' dresses were finished two weeks before the wedding, but Rita had not started my bride's dress, yet. She started it on the Monday before the wedding, and brought it to me with perfect fit on Thursday. For the bridesmaids, I chose the color red, since it was Steve's favorite color, and because the Church rug was the same color where our pictures were taken. I had the bridesmaids wear wrist corsages instead of carrying flowers, because I thought that would be easier for Louise. I did have each of them carry a white Bible. I was always cold, so the top of my dress was warm, white velvet with long sleeves and a V-necked delicately net lace neckline. The bottom was a full, simple satin. Rita had even had forethought about resolving a bathroom problem by attaching a separate panel of the terrycloth material in the back of the dress that I could sit on, and flip up easily in case of an emergency. I had thought of that problem too, but my solution was to get up very late, because our wedding was the third one of the day at 3:00 p.m. We had to be out of the church by 5:30 p.m. for the 6:00 p.m. Saturday night services. On my head I wore a headband of irregularly set white flowers from my temple on one side to over my ear on the other with a short veil.

Luckily, the caterer was out of jail, and one of the divorced DJs was going to be at the wedding! What else could happen? Right! My wheelchair broke! I was fortunate enough to get a loaner, but I couldn't drive it very well, and I had to practice a lot. Then, there was no ramp up the three steps at church's altar. On that Friday, KAC came to the rescue, and I could borrow one! That changed the setup, however, and I had to enter from the side instead of in front of the altar. Now, I would be facing the congregation, which might not be a bad thing!

Rehearsal night came. One of the Lioness members, Jeanne, videotaped the rehearsal of the wedding for me. The only concern was that Mindy did not make rehearsal, because she was exposed to the measles, but she never exhibited the symptoms! She and David came early on the wedding day to practice, and did fine. We had our rehearsal dinner at Country Buffet, which was Mom's favorite place to eat!

November 4th came, and it was a beautiful day in the high 40s. I barely had to wear a coat! Mom wanted to make sure Steve got there on time, so she had Bob pick him up! The men wore black tuxedos with white shirts, red Cummerbunds, and bowties. The photographer, Larry, was there early. Larry was one of my former students. He was just starting a photography business. He did an excellent job with reasonable prices! Larry had a picture taken where all of the groomsmen were holding Steve back as if he was trying to run away!

There was a full church, and I was happy to see so many people. Eddie, the cab driver, came. He had been diagnosed with dementia as well as cancer I found out later. He happened to sit by Louise's Father.

Ed told him, "I was told to come here today for some reason, but I'm not sure why?"

Ann and Kate started singing lyrics that I put together with three different songs.

"You are beautiful so beautiful to me, can't you see"---"You make me so very happy, I'm so glad you came into my life" And then, Steve's favorite song, *Never My Love*— "I'll never grow tired of you. Never my love".

The organ music began. Mindy and David walked down the aisle first, followed by Louise and Ramon. Ed turned to Louise's Father exclaiming, "Hey, I know that girl!"

Patty and Domingo were next to walk down the aisle. Louise had reached the altar. Ramon forgot to take her Bible, so she could lift her dress to avoid tripping on the dress as she walked up the stairs. Ramon spoke no English, but Steve saw what was happening, and saved the day as he caught Louise just before she fell! We had a chair ready for her to sit on the altar.

Then, Susie and Gavino followed behind them.

Finally, it was our turn, and Dad told me to slow down, because I was going too fast! When Ed saw me, he told Mr. Cooper, "Hey, I know her too!"

When we got to the altar, Dad gave me away. Steve and I gave my Mom and Dad a rose for all they had done in my life. I turned the corner to go around the altar to roll up the ramp, and there was a video camera right in my way! One of my former volunteers had brought her camera too, and set it up when I wasn't looking. I was able to get around the obstacles, and had a straight shot at the ramp. In the meantime, the ladies were singing the Wedding Song from West side story.

I finally got to the altar area, and came forward to the table. Pastor Cindy had her back toward the congregation. I bumped the table with the unfamiliar chair I was driving. A short service was given, and the song *On Eagles Wings* was sung. Pastor Cindy later told me, "I thought I was going to fall backwards down the steps, or go up in flames from the wedding Candle!"

The marriage ceremony itself went very smooth until Pastor Cindy gave me a lot of vows at one time. I couldn't remember them! I was looking at Steve, giving a questionable side look to Pastor Cindy that pleaded for help. She read the vows slower this time, and gave me a chance to repeat them as we went along. Gavino had the ring, and gave it to his Dad to put on my finger.

I turned myself back towards the table. Now it was time for both of us to light the wedding candle. Susie turned off my wheelchair as a precaution. David worked my hand to light the wedding candle, and Susie lifted my elbow. After the candle was lit, the ladies started singing the Lord's Prayer. David blew out the candle that was now in his hand, and burned himself with the wax making a funny face. One of the people in the back of the room thought he was crying, because he was so happy for me!

I went down the ramp backwards, so I would not fall out of my chair—no safety belt— and repositioned in front of the altar. The camera was back in the way, but I managed. Pastor Cindy pronounced us man and wife. Susie lifted my veil, and Steve kissed me. We exited by going straight to the chapel where we signed the marriage license. I had not thought about how I was going to sign my new name, but I made that decision at the last minute. As I was signing, I hyphenated my name, keeping both names. I thought I would not have to change my professional name, since a lot of people knew me statewide, but I added Steve's last name, Romero. Carol Romero—it rhymed. I loved the sound of it.

We did not have time for a reception line, so we took the pictures. Domingo was gone, but we got everyone else up on the altar. Mindy and David were getting a little rambunctious at this time so the photographer said, "Okay kids, just get it all out of your system." They both made a couple of weird faces, which I chose to be included in my wedding pictures. Pastor Cindy did the same thing when we had our picture taken with her. No, she did not make a face, but she did give us both a set of horns to share between us. Could Pastors do that?

When we finished the pictures, Steve went to put on my safety belt and coat. Lloyd came over, and gave me a kiss. He advised Steve, "Pretty soon, you are going to want to put that belt around her neck instead of her waist!" Steve laughed. By the way, Lloyd gave us a

173

sympathy card instead of a wedding card!

Mom told me that Grandma was so nervous that she could not make it to the wedding at the last minute, so instead of driving around, we went to the nursing home to see her. Grandma was so happy to see us, she cried. I highly recommend that anyone getting married who has a relative in the nursing home go there. It seemed like it made a lot of people happy—not only my Grandmother!

We went to the reception next, and dinner was ready. Gavino gave a little toast to the bride and groom just before we started to eat. I was hungry, and everything tasted so good! As we ate, the food line formed in front of our table, so I got a chance to say hi to everyone, since there was not enough time at the church for a reception line or enough room at the dinner to get between the tables. Linda, with her video camera, went around the room to get thoughts and wishes from all of the different guests. She filmed our first dance, too. Susie had to teach Steve to dance, since he had never danced before. Mindy sat on my lap, and danced. Everyone was dancing, and had a good time. Everyone commented, "The wedding had such a comfortable and friendly atmosphere with so many different people."

I really appreciated that our neighbors, Leon and Betty, sat, and talked a lot with Stevie that evening. Leon commented, "The only thing Stevie and I agreed upon was hurricane Hugo!" Stevie was happy at the wedding. He loved to talk, and he loved Coke! He could have as much Coke as he wanted. Because of Steve being an alcoholic, soda and other beverages were available, but alcohol and beer were available if guests wanted to purchase it by themselves. No one was drunk! Everyone appeared to have a good time without it.

We cut the wedding cake, and Steve was nice to me. He only put one drip of frosting on my nose. It looked like a fuzz ball in the picture. We threw the bouquet and garter, and were still able to get back home before the last boxing match that Steve wanted to see. He remarked, "If I knew that the wedding was going to be so much fun, I would have enjoyed it more!" Huh? What did that mean?

Steve saw Ed about 3 days after the wedding shopping at Supervalu. Ed came out of the store with his groceries, and stopped to talk to Steve. He had worked with him at a security position as his relief in the past.

Ed said to Steve, "Hey, Steve, How are you doing, man? Oh, do you know Carol Schaufel?"

"Yes," Steve replied

Ed continued, "You know she got married don't you?"

Steve played along, "Yes. Were you there?"

"Yes, I was there. Oh, Steve. You wouldn't believe it! You should have seen the man she married! I don't know what rock he crawled out of but he was so ugly!" he laughed.

"Oh yeah?" Steve said surprised.

"Yeah. I have to go. See you," and, he left.

My Mom spoke to his daughter a bit later. She told her that he carried my picture around in his wallet all those years. Just before he died, he saw my picture, but he didn't know who I was, or why the picture was in his wallet.

Eddie died a short time later. I guess the cancer got into his brain.

BY THE GRACE OF GOD AND YOU
A Chair Does Not a Person Make

~ After the Wedding ~

Things were very different the year before, and the year after the wedding. Gavino was going every workday after supper to practice his boxing, and run every day to keep himself in shape. Steve would drive him to Racine, Milwaukee, or Waukegan boxing gyms at different times. We would travel two or three times a year to statewide, and some out of the region matches. I enjoyed the traveling, but I didn't think Gavino did, especially when he had to stay in the motel with Steve and me. Steve snored - loud. I was used to it, but Gavino would sleep on the closet floor with a pillow over his head to avoid the noise. Fortunately, there weren't too many of those trips. I eventually helped out with the boxing and became a boxing clerk. I sat ringside, and was hit occasionally by some of the sweat or blood from the participants, but my basic job was to put the result of the boxing match into the individuals' boxing books. Steve was funny, because he always wanted Gavino to do his best. I don't think he watched any one of the fights, because Steve was afraid that Gavino was going to get hurt.

In a tough match at Afro Fest on the Summerfest grounds in Milwaukee, he had a very exciting match with a tough opponent by the name of Lachance Shepherd. I saw Steve walking back and forth along the Lake Michigan waterfront waiting until the fight was over. Gavino won!

I had fun, though, listening to the different music and trying out the different foods every time I had the chance. One of the ladies at the office asked me if there were a lot of black people at Afro Fest. The next day I had to go back, so I purposely looked as I did not know the answer. Perhaps 85% to 95% of the people were African American, but I didn't know what that had to do with anything.

We had to go to a regional competition in Indianapolis, Indiana. Gavino was really working out hard to get his weight down to his weight class of 125, and became very dehydrated getting to his weight. He had a very tough opponent who was using a lot of energy in the fight. When it was over, Gavino was shaking, and was very cold! The two of us sat for 20 minutes in the 95° heat, and my favorite temperature, and we had something to drink. He finally warmed up, and was feeling better. What crazy things these athletes have to do to their bodies—crash diets to make weight, Ex-Lax to poop it out, and even letting themselves be punched—not me! Amateur fights were a lot safer, because they were required to wear a helmet. There were only three rounds per match. Fights were stopped by the referee when there was a sign of any problem.

On the other hand, Stevie had few friends, and was always very grandiose, thinking that he had a lot of money and saying that his Grandfather was DuPont. He could be very charming, funny, and people liked him, but a person could never tell if he were truthful. Several psychiatrists had tried to diagnose him, but he did not fall into a specific category. He would tell the kids that he came to school by helicopter even though he was less than a mile away. His memory was excellent. He knew every movie, movie star, which stars were still alive, all the major movie lines, etc. Stevie went to see two or three movies each weekend, and made up stories about some of these movies such as "his uncle Tony". There was no Uncle Tony, so we thought about the movie, *The Godfather*. One psychiatrist told me that Steve's brain was

175

compartmentalized. If something happened to him in one instance and something else happened to him at another time, he could not put that information together. He could not learn from his mistakes. Another person who had worked with him for a long time said Steve and I would be lucky if we could keep him out of institutions.

At first, Stevie would do things that caused a crisis about once every month. For example, Steve indicated that when Stevie was younger, he noticed a huge telephone bill with a number that was called multiple times in one month. Steve called the telephone number to see who would answer the phone. It was the Russian Embassy in Washington DC. Fortunately, the person who answered the telephone recognized the incoming telephone number. After a few Moments, the person told him to stop the boy from calling.

"Would you please have the little boy who keeps calling us and giving us counsel on what we should be doing to please stop calling."

Stevie had found the name and telephone number in a book at the library, so he tried it out.

Another time, Stevie was in trouble for calling 911 and being inappropriate as well as yelling at the operator. The operator sent a squad car to arrest him from where he was calling. He had to do community service hours - some with the Kenosha Achievement Center (KAC) which caused some problems there as well. He told one of the sheltered workers that he was a doctor who graduated from Johns Hopkins University at a very young age. He saw another one of his friends there, and just told him that he was just volunteering and not getting paid for his work.

"Are you nuts! No one volunteers to do work without pay," said one of his friends with a disability.   Then, Stevie was supposed to be doing volunteer work at the Kenosha Youth Foundation, before I met him. He was found in a room sleeping on the couch. He was never able to take his responsibilities seriously. Stevie's favorite thing was talking, so eventually, he finished his community service hours working for me at home. I would let him talk as much as he wanted as long as he was doing something in the meantime. We completed his community service hours!

Things started scaring me at home because we would get a call from a strange person.

"Stevie said that we could find a reference at this telephone number as he is looking to rent a room. Is it true that he is related to Rockefellers?" the voice would say.

Once, Stevie came into my room, and had a serious talk. He insisted that he had a lot of money. I started confronting him while Steve and Gavino were at the gym.

"Stevie, you do not have any money! I know that you think you have a lot of money from what you felt was selling guns to the Contra, but you never did this."

He became irate, slapped a glass of hot tea out of my hand which hit the wall 4 feet away.

"I'll prove it to you! I have a lot of money!" he exclaimed, going into his bedroom.

I heard him in his room rustling through his drawers.

"Where are they?"

He came back into my room almost crying standing in front of the bed where I sat.

"I can't find my bank books," he cried.

"Stevie, you do not have a bank book," I told him quietly.

"Explain to me again," he pleaded.

We went over everything I could think of and whatever questions he had, but he still could not put things together. Schizophrenia? Bipolar? Personality disorder? Steve told me that when Stevie was younger, his goal in life was "To be in Leavenworth". Was it from all the movies he was seeing? I asked him to please clean up the tea from the wall so it wouldn't stain. He did, but Gavino still had to paint the wall.

Being responsible, I had checked with my doctor about birth control pills. They were not an option for me, because of my disability. Hormones were not recommended when I went through menopause. I couldn't remember the reasons, but the reasons made sense at the time. It was something about the side effects, poor circulation, and my weaknesses. For menopause though, I was looking forward to having hot flashes, because I was always so cold. I only had three flashes when the time finally came at 58 years old.

Birth control was a more serious problem, though. Fortunately, I was very regular and very in tune with all of my body changes. I knew we shouldn't have sex one day when Steve became romantic, because I felt a slight fever, but we continued anyway. Steve didn't think he could have children anymore. We always had to be creative, and careful since Steve had the job of working both bodies at one time. I knew I was pregnant the next day, because I felt a pain like a spur digging into my right side close to the right of my bladder as soon as I was in my wheelchair. I called the doctor.

"There is no way to tell if anyone is pregnant this early! You wouldn't be feeling anything," he told me, but I knew!

I can't say that I was happy or sad about the possibility of a baby. It just hurt, and I knew I was going to lose the baby. Steve took my urine to the doctor's for confirmation. The doctor called me.

"Congratulations! You're pregnant!"

He told me that he did not have the expertise to handle the situation, so he gave me a couple of names of doctors in Milwaukee. I would talk with both.

First, I told my parents. It hit my Mom hard.

"Oh, no," Mom shrieked, "You are going to have to have an abortion!"

Mom didn't believe in abortions, and neither did I. But in my heart, I knew that I was going to lose the baby. The first doctor indicated it would be hard for me to carry the baby, because I would have to stay in bed all nine months, and that might make me weaker. Because of the curvature in my spine, there wasn't room for the baby to grow, either. Mom was worried.

"No, you can't try to carry the baby. You will die," she said to me.

I knew I couldn't take care of the baby. Heck, I could not even take care of myself or even keep plants alive. Many of my friends in chairs had babies, but they didn't have curvatures, the pain I had, nor the weakness. Steve couldn't handle any more than he already had on his plate with Gavino, Stevie, and all my care. What was I going to do? It had to be my decision, not Mom's. I asked God for an answer to make me do what he wanted me to do. He guided me before. I had a dream. It was a beautiful, sunny day, and I saw a tiny casket float out of the top of my closet door, out of my open window, and watch it float to heaven.

The next day I became extremely weak, and could barely move my chair. I called the doctor, and went for the abortion. I cried as I approved it. Susie had one miscarriage before she had Mindy. She was surprised to see in her record that her baby was aborted. Losing that baby was also called an abortion. It was a natural abortion, but she did not make a decision to abort the baby. I always felt that was what my dream was about. The baby was telling me that she couldn't make it. Yes, I always thought the baby was a girl, too.

Mom and Dad took me to Milwaukee where the abortion took place. The pain was worse in my stomach. I felt like I was suffocating the baby. The pain was there, but it felt different as if the baby was aborting itself. I will never know. The nurses at the hospital gave everyone a last chance to change their minds if they wanted to keep the child. That was very difficult going through again, but I totally understood why and thought that was generally a good idea. I thought about all the people that had babies, and then only abused them. I thought about the people that wanted babies, and couldn't have them. I was taken into surgery, and fell asleep.

I went home the same day, and was very groggy. Mom asked if I wanted her to stay. She thought that Steve would be going to the gym with Gavino that night. I told her that she did not have to stay. I would be fine. I really thought Steve would stay with me that night after dinner, but he didn't—as if nothing was different. I went through it without him. Fortunately, he laid me down on the bed. I slept until Steve and Gavino returned from the gym. There were some things which were never going to change. Men! Steve was much more considerate of me after that night. I still think of how old the child would be, what she would be doing, etc. That never goes away. No one can live life in a bubble. Memories always break our bubbles. We can never see the whole picture. Judging was God's job.

Why would I bring this up to share with you? This loss or giving a child up for adoption was a difficult bereavement. There are many people I knew who had gone through this alone. My relatives will just be finding out! Unless people experienced the pain, they had no idea what I was going through. I heard hurtful statements all the time—never responding to them. During elections, especially, you get all these convoluted ideas on abortion from who? Males, who will never be in that decision making position, and with no female input!

~ 21 ~

Changes x 2

Steve woke up easily, and he was always good about turning me at night. I never had to wait long for him to help me with anything, but then his job changed, and he left for work at 3:30 a.m. An attendant came to get me ready for work at 5:30 a.m.

I took the city bus back and forth to work during nice weather, and the KAC specialized transportation when it was colder. Steve eventually found a local job at the Southeast Wisconsin AIDS Project, and our hours became a little more normal. He was an outreach worker helping individuals be tested for HIV/AIDS and talking about prevention, giving out condoms. When anyone would ask me what my husband did, I would say, "Oh, he goes out looking for prostitutes and drug addicts!" I knew how serious the problem was, and went to a lot of training in this area, when they still thought HIV/AIDS could be spread by mosquitoes. There were the three causes for the spread of HIV/AIDS:

1. Sexual activity between infected gay men and eventually to the heterosexual community.
2. Sharing of dirty needles that were reused with intravenous drug use, at tattoo parlors, or in hospital settings. I knew one woman who contracted AIDS seven years when she was in a hospital in Burma.
3. Cheating spouses brought it home to their unsuspecting partners.

I heard many horror stories where heroin addicted Mothers with HIV were arrested for child abuse in New York the minute their babies were born. At first, there was an assumption that all of the babies carried the HIV/AIDS virus, so the babies never really felt a human touch. After 2 1/2 years, the children had developed their own immune systems and only one third of the babies born actually had the HIV/AIDS virus. I offered to serve clients who had HIV/AIDS that applied at DVR. Many were not eligible for our services, because their limitations were either not severe enough at the time to become eligible, or too severe to be able to work. A few of the people with the disease were angry and just wanted to pass their disease on to someone else, or just decided to continue with their drug use. Many were very easy to work with, because they felt as if they had another chance for a new life and a chance to do it right. By the time the multiple drug medication cocktails were developed to help slow down or control the disease, more was known about T-cell count and virus load. The people that had the most difficulty making progress on these medications seemed to be the drug addicts who were just not used to doing things on a schedule. Medications had to be taken within a short time frame on a regular basis, or the person would become immune to the "drug cocktails" they were taking. There was a limited amount of ways to mix the drugs, and the individual had to make sure that he or she could become immune to all of the options.

In working with the group, my only concern was tuberculosis. If diagnosed, were they on their medication for TB at least 24 hours before they saw me so I wouldn't get it? I also asked if the person had hepatitis, but I was immunized for hepatitis B.

Steve hired Susan for our housekeeper for a couple of hours a month. She had AIDS, could not work a regular job, and was the sister of one of the younger students at the Orthopedic School. Both Susan and Jimmy had a determination to survive and succeed. Susan always wanted to tell her story, because it was different from many of the other stories that had been made public. She came from a good family, but loved the extra money as a teenager selling drugs. A circle began as she used drugs, needed more money to buy drugs, and then led to prostitution, sometimes several times a day, to feed her addiction. She didn't care if she was going to be safe, or beaten in the process. It only mattered that she got the money to buy and use drugs. Many addicts sold their children, or even their little babies for sex for drugs, and she was proud that she never sold her own son for the money to buy drugs! Susan didn't care what happened to her - until she was diagnosed with AIDS. How many people had she infected with HIV/AIDS? Maybe none since she wasn't the "injector," but the beatings? She was brave enough not to care what other people thought about her, and shared her story in the newspaper and in the high schools, sharing her story with your child. Susan got married after her diagnosis, but neither her son, nor her husband, contracted HIV/AIDS. She passed away a few years after the marriage. I missed her inspiration and strength.

Stevie did not graduate from high school. It wasn't that he wasn't smart; he couldn't pass tests, stay focused, and use what he learned. The school system never liked diagnosing a student too young with an emotional disability, because they did not want to stigmatize the individual. Stevie would not even take an aspirin let alone the medication prescribed to help him.

"Nothing is wrong with me," he stated.

Stevie tried to complete his high school diploma at Gateway, but it just didn't work. Someone dared him to moon someone for $10 on campus, where a rape investigation was ongoing. That ended his high school career, and he was banned from that facility.

Just before his eighteenth birthday, I helped Stevie apply for Social Security fighting me all the way. He was very surprised that he got it so easily and so fast.

My nephew, David, was in third grade, and having some problems with writing. He would write everything backwards so it could only be read when held to a mirror - just as Kenny did when he was little. Both had Dyslexia. David was a little character, and one day, his teacher called Susie, and asked if she had written a note for David. Susie told her, "No." He had written a note signed with Susie's name that said, "David cannot stay after school today." David was supposed to stay after school that day for detention, and he had just gotten his bicycle back. He didn't want to be grounded, again, so he wrote the note, and his handwriting gave him away!

Nationally, and in 1990, the Americans with Disabilities Act passed. Wisconsin was ahead of other states in the area of accessibility by making progress, and refitting buses one at a time. The more the buses were used, the less they broke down. Some timelines for accessibility were also set while others took longer, and one of these was the train systems, which did not have to be accessible until 2020. The majority of the accessibility plans that were in the bill were very reasonable for new construction while older buildings were grandfathered in until renovations could be made for accessibility. Bathrooms also had to be redesigned if a person might be inside of the building for more than an hour at a time. The Act gave people with disabilities their rights, and accessibility was the easiest part of that bill. Employment, education, and attitudes, because of myths, were more difficult to address.

Work was as busy as ever. On an average, I touched at least 300 cases per year although the active cases ran anywhere from 70 to 125. I enjoyed staying busy and trying to keep on top of my caseload as much as possible. One year was very sad for me as three of my clients passed away. One was a young woman with diabetes who had a small child. One died after a third bone marrow transplant. The third one took his own life.

I always felt, "Could I have done more? Could I have seen something coming?" Each time someone passed away, a friend, a relative, or a client, I would step back and enjoy each person around me more instead of worrying about just getting the work done. One of the people I worked with at UW Parkside let me know that one of the students that I was working with wrote a paper about me. The topic was to write about a person that had influenced your life. She let me read the paper. The client gave me a copy later. It was interesting to see how he felt, and what he assumed as well as how he saw my struggling movement (I had always been unconscious of it). Greg wrote an essay for class in 1990, and recently approved it so others could read:

10/2/90 ***Carol, a Lasting Impression***

Carol is a person who did not accept defeat. In spite of her physical disability, she manages to not only live life to the fullest, but encourages others to do the same.

I first met Carol back in late '84 or early '85; she was a job counselor at the Department of Vocational Rehabilitation (DVR for short). I was messed up at the time, recovering from a motorcycle accident. Physically and mentally I was feeling pretty down. It was a time in my life where I needed guidance along with a few friends. Carol helped me along the slow road of recovery and helped me appreciate what life can become if one refuses to give up.

Carol is confined to a wheelchair. She has some kind of disease that has paralyzed her from the waist down. Her legs are short and still. Covered by her brown polyester pants, Carol has brown hair and brown, penetrating eyes. Her disease causes her to have painful looking spasms every so often. Her head jerks back, then angles to the right, as her eyes look away from you and into some faraway site during one of these attacks. She puts her hand to her mouth and seems to almost bite her index finger as a reaction, or some kind of forced countermeasure to combat the effects of her muscular spasm. I felt so sorry for her when I first met her.

Her brightly lit office was only a few steps from the check-in window of DVR. When I would call, she would answer on her speakerphone that set on her desk amongst stacks of job applications forms and client's files. "Carol, DVR," she would answer. Her soft voice sounding distant, shuffling papers and the other office sounds seemed to have more authority than her voice.

Carol was easy to talk to. She seemed genuinely concerned. I felt helpless during my first meetings with her. I was drinking every night to drown my sorrows and to ease the pain in my leg. Carol emphasized my staying sober. At the end of almost every session she would inquire, "How's the drinking?" often putting my response in her notes. I often lied to her, telling her I was staying out of the bars. I did not want to disappoint her. Carol's piercing brown eyes seemed to look right through me when I lied. She was hard to fool—probably because she dealt with so many people.

Carol was concerned with my future; I was concerned with catching the ultimate buzz. After quitting one of the jobs she helped me find, I casually mentioned that I was thinking about college. I was afraid of big changes in my life and did not think I had the ability to stick with anything. She encouraged me and said that I could do anything if I set my mind to it. I did not really believe this, but Carol seemed to. Carol took care of the financial arrangements and I started school soon after.

In one of my counseling sessions with her, I revealed to Carol that I was constantly worried about what people thought about me. She told me it did not matter what people thought, if I believed in myself. She illustrated her points, saying that if she listened to peoples comments about her disfigured body and took them seriously, she would be nowhere. She also revealed to me that she did not like people pitying her. I was amazed at Carol's strength of mind.

Carol could make me angry. When I told her about my seemingly endless amount of problems, she would often reply, "You're feeling sorry for yourself." She was usually right, but it still made me angry—angry enough to do something about it. If I was truly sad to the point of tears, Carol would comfort me. She seemed to know when I was looking for excuses and when I was truly down and out. Carol was hard to fool.

Carol always seemed busy with clients. I am sure I could not handle her huge work load with the same amount of gumption. When I entered her office for one of our sessions, sometimes she would ask me to put away a file for her, as I took my file out of the drawer. I hope that her other clients opened up and told her their dreams and desires, for Carol seemed to be genuinely concerned with people accomplishing their goals. In my case, there were times that Carol seemed more concerned with my physical and mental well-being than I was. Visiting Carol was like visiting family and I often thought of her as such.

I secretly felt for Carol at times. She never knew what it was like to walk or run. She is forced to control her limited movements by the joystick on the right arm of her wheelchair. Carol would counter that with a "Don't dwell on what you can't do, but on what you can." Carol's physical condition instead of slowing her down seems to be a catalyst to her insistence on moving ahead. Her motto is to accept what you cannot change and change what you can.

Over the years that I went to DVR, I have met many of Carol's other clients. Their faces show the effect Carol has had on their lives. They seemed to beam with hope, a common condition that occurs after hearing the words, "Carol, DVR," enough times. When I mentioned her name to someone who knows her, that person is no longer a stranger, but a friend. He too has a similar respect and love for this lady. The common thread that ties us together is Carol—a lady that does rehabilitation and a person that does leave a lasting impression on our lives.

~ Meeting New Relatives and Following the Boys ~

"I almost co-starred in the movie with John Wayne!" Steve had told me.

Manpower had a 'cattle call' for 5000 Mexicans to storm the Alamo for the movie, *The Alamo.* Steve was so excited that he wanted to be first in line!

"I was a lot younger at the time," he continued, "and I thought, gee, I bet they are paying at least $1000 for that! Heck, it's John Wayne!"

Steve was first in line—so early, in fact, a policeman asked what he was doing there. Before the policeman got too far in his questioning, more people started to come, so the policeman left. Steve was called into his interview, and was asked only one question.

"What size uniform do you wear?"

"How much will I be paid?" Steve was asked with stars in his eyes.

"$1."

"$1! You've got to be kidding?" Steve was startled, and he left. He never starred with John Wayne.

We heard all kinds of stories as we packed to visit Steve's sister, Flo, in Corpus Christi, Texas. Gavino had gotten his driver's license, and Steve and he took turns driving to Texas. Stevie did a good job, too, once we could get him into the van. At the right time, Mom appeared, and calmed him down. She also calmed me down when I lost my patience, and called him 'poop head.' Stevie wanted to fly to Texas, so he didn't have to ride in the van. We started early, and drove all the way to Austin, Texas, before we stayed at an Embassy Suites Hotel to watch the basketball championship game on TV. Next, we stopped in San Antonio and walked along the River Walk, went to the zoo, and investigated the Alamo. On the way out of town, our van broke down a couple of blocks from the dealership! The van needed a water pump, and fortunately, they were able to fix it immediately. While we waited, we stopped at a great soul food place that served the best barbecued ribs you would ever want to eat!

When we got to Corpus Christi, we called Flo and Olivia, who was his deceased brother's wife. They met us, and led us to Olivia's house where we stayed for about a week. Her porch was easily accessible with a straight shot from the up position on the van lift. The whole family was very friendly and fun loving. We had a good time cooking out and eating food I had never tasted before. Olivia was an excellent cook! We spent some time with Flo, her husband, Ramiro, and her son, Roland. They took us on a shopping trip to Mexico, and because the driving was crazy, Roland gave someone money to make sure the van wasn't vandalized. The peso rate was about 8 to 1 at the time, so we had to calculate how much everything cost. Olivia took me to a flea market in Corpus Christi. I have always loved the designs of Native Americans, so I bought some Native American items to decorate my house and office. One last cookout included bisque and sweetbread meat grilled, and brought all of the relatives together.

BY THE GRACE OF GOD AND YOU
A Chair Does Not a Person Make

We traveled to a lot of boxing matches. The best boxing matches were located between two buildings on a vacant lot in Chicago's Hispanic district. Few of the people spoke English, and the store signs were all in Spanish. I felt like I was in a different country. I picked up several words in the language too—very few of them were swear words, but you know how that goes. It was the first time I had also met Stevie and Gavino's Mother. She was very nice, but quiet. I knew she had our telephone number, and I told her she should call the boys occasionally, and in the first two years Steve and I were together, she never called them at all.

That year I was also chosen as the Wisconsin First MDA Personal Achievement Award recipient. A person was chosen based on outstanding educational, professional, and volunteer accomplishments from each state. The national recipients had some excellent life stories, and I was impressed and inspired by them! Their pictures ran at different times throughout the September telethon, and mine was on at 3 a.m. It would have been good if no one had seen me, because I did one of those dumb things again. Vince Gibbons (Fox 6 News) was the newscaster at the time, and had just had a mild heart attack. I had worked with him earlier, and sent him a get-well card with a note. He had mentioned how difficult it was for me to write. There was a videotaped story on how difficult it was for me to type on my job, but not using a mouthstick yet. All of that was okay, but I had just been by the Kenosha Achievement Center, and all of the participants there knew I was going to be on TV. They did not have much money, and I told one of them that they could give whatever they wished, but they didn't have to give, and could watch the entertainment like everyone else. I usually gave $25 or $30, but for some reason that year, I decided to give only $10 to make them feel better, since it would be announced on the show. I thought I could give more money after the announcement, but I didn't think that was helpful for the general audience. I should have given more, but I felt it made some people feel more comfortable giving whatever they could!

I worked with Peter Barca on a regular basis, he placed people with disabilities in jobs. He ran for U.S. Congress, and I enjoyed going to the fundraisers and election functions. I always took Stevie with me, because he loved the feeling of being involved with something "important", also helping with the Easter Seals Banquets and Lily Day, too. Peter had a degree in special education, and he included Stevie as well. Peter won the election over Mark Newman. I was very proud of my Mom when election surveyors called her. Mom told the Newman supporters.

"No, I know that is not true.....Peter did this for this reason…That was done as a compromise… That was not what happened!"

"Well, I am glad you have so much faith in your candidate! Goodbye," the Newman Supporter told Mom, and finally giving up, ended the call.

I always thought lying and misinterpretations in ads and politics should be illegal. It is a type of bullying and the citizens lose. Just do what the people want not what lobbyists try to control. Common sense in politics would be nice.

At the same time, Stevie went to Kenosha with a friend who stole a car from one of the car lots. The car lot had left keys in the cars making stealing the car easy. They drove it to Illinois with Stevie in the car. Allegedly, the friend saw the police coming, and told Stevie to drive. The friend got out of the car, and Stevie, having no license, ran into a mailbox. The police asked what he was doing.

"I am taking this car to a chop shop!" he told them making it a federal crime, because it covered two states.

The judge understood that Stevie had a disability, so he put him on probation in Illinois. His statements were full of fabrications. An example was that his Mother was dead on one report while on another, he stated that she lived in Spain. She lived in Chicago.

Stevie also used a telephone booth, a phone at McDonald's, and our home phone to call in three bomb threats regarding the Zion nuclear Plant. These places were all within a few blocks of our home. The police knocked on the door, and arrested him. Then, I saw the Boeing's telephone number on our caller ID. Somehow, I felt that was next.

I was wrong. Stevie had sent Boeing a resume, or a sketch of an airplane. I think they were interested in hiring him. I didn't have to deal with that problem. I did have to deal with the next telephone call, though. Stevie had forged a $1500 check he had taken from my checkbook. He used the money as a down payment on a car, and insurance by using Gavino's "remembered driver's license". He also took my credit card number to order an advanced resume that cost over $300 based on mine. He falsely claimed that he was the director of the Wisconsin Easter Seals and California simultaneously. It was time to let him take on the responsibility of what he had done, because we couldn't keep fixing things for him. His Social Security ended, and he spent time in Columbia, Wisconsin where the serial killer, Jeffrey Dahmer, was murdered, and Plymouth that had a prison closer to home. Even in prison, Stevie sent threatening letters to judges, the president, and the Pope. He was upset because he wanted to be in a maximum prison closer to home than a minimum prison farther away. The letters and conviction put him into federal custody, and the judge sentenced him to a federal mental health facility. Since there was no room available in the mental health facility in Minnesota, Stevie called us.

"Pops, you will never guess where I am! I'm in McKean, Pennsylvania."
For 3 years, Stevie had been in state facilities followed by the start of his federal sentencing.

Gavino ended his boxing career in 1993. His record was 39 wins, and 9 losses. This year, he won the American Boxing Federation Regional Championship when we traveled to North Platte, Nebraska. Eric Morel was with us on that trip also, but measles grabbed him, and he returned home without his fight. Eventually, he became a world champion. After the boxing matches, we had the chance to go sightseeing. We visited Buffalo Bill's home where his Wild West Shows took place, and included Annie Oakley and Chief Sitting Bull. We also visited a Wild West Cemetery in Ogallala where some headstones read, "he died with his boots on", or "died by mistake".

The funniest part of the trip occurred when we were packing the van to begin our trip. Gavino was going to be traveling with the team, and Steve told Gavino to put our big telephone bag in the car. He did, and told us to have a good time. We didn't look into the bag. We felt that we might need a telephone, because we were going to be traveling through an ice storm. We made very good time before the ice storm hit at the Illinois/Iowa border. From there, we crawled along, and finally gave up. We were getting nowhere fast entering Iowa City. We opened the telephone bag to call for a room reservation, but instead of the telephone, there were about 500 condoms! Steve had forgotten that he had used that case to carry the condoms for work. Did Gavino know that the telephone was not in the case? Is that why he said to have a good time?

Regardless, though, we found a place to stay overnight, and the next morning, it was still icy, but we could drive a little faster. We saw 55 accidents along the way caused by the icy conditions combined with the snow that had already fallen. And, well, we were accident number 33! Steve hit an icy patch where we spun totally around once, and landed in the center ditch. On the spin, my wheelchair only moved about 1 inch. By the grace of God, there was a tow truck right in front of us! The tow truck driver said that it was about a two, or more, hour wait for another tow, but the driver also volunteered to pull us out for $50, and we were on our way in about 10 minutes.

After that, Steve drove slowly, because he was traumatized. Two little old women tried to pass us on the left. As the vehicle drove next to our van, a woman rolled down the passenger side window. She was so frustrated at our slow pace, she threw a cup of coffee at Steve's window.

Since Gavino had won the regionals, we also traveled to the Olympic training grounds in Colorado Springs, Colorado. Gavino flew with the team, but we drove. Stevie stayed home to take care of the dogs. I was so happy when the Rocky Mountains appeared as we traveled into Denver. When we were in Colorado Springs, the Olympic training ground was right below Pike's Peak. As we walked down a hill, we looked back up at the mountain, and the peak looked even higher! The grounds were incredible, and it was very exciting.

I always seemed to be in the way of one man who was warming up, and security told me to leave. His name was Oscar De La Hoya. Gavino lost the first two rounds of his final match, but won the third. If he had won the last match, he would have faced De La Hoya in the boxing ring! Oscar went to the Olympics from there—then, he became a boxing superstar. The story that I liked best about Oscar was that he always carried a food stamp in his wallet to remind him of where he came from. Humbling! We all need that at times, and no one succeeds without the help of others. Could you imagine having to make your own clothes, grow your own food, build your own car, etc.? Every time I would meet with a client, I would think that this person couldn't read, yet he could fix his own car. Wow! I couldn't do that.

~ 22 ~

Gambling & Support

We took some side trips, before we made our way back home from Colorado Springs. We tried some buffalo burgers in the old section of Colorado Springs. For me, buffalo meat was a lot like beef, but drier because of less fat. We saw the Garden of the Gods with all of the precarious rock formations. We also took a trip up into the Rocky Mountains, where we could sometimes see the peaks of 20 mountains at one time. The scenery was breathtaking! We came across a tiny town called Crippled Creek, and thought perhaps we should be riding into town on horses crossing a train track and passing a depot on the "top" side of town! We were looking down hill at a small street with a few Western designed buildings on each side, and there was even a saloon and a casino. Steve didn't really know how to play slot machines, but he let me play blackjack for a while, and I made $50. He was a little impatient, because he had nothing to do, so we only stayed about 45 minutes.

The following year, we went to see Eddie and Carol who were living in Las Vegas. We stayed at their home part of the time, and then, finished the rest of our time at the Stardust. Eddie picked us up from the airport with his accessible van. We stopped at a casino, and he taught Steve how to play the slot machines. Eddie probably thought that Steve "crawled out of a hole" somewhere, because he did not know how to play them! Steve proceeded to play one slot machine for more than two hours using only $10 - and, he was hooked.

For the next three years, whenever we went to see Stevie, we would make it a fun trip, and stopped at the nearest casino. When Stevie was in Wisconsin, we would go to Ho Chunk in the Wisconsin Dells, Oneida in Green Bay, or Rainbow in Nekoosa once or twice a month. My goal was to win whatever Steve would lose.

There were storms in the area, and while we were in Green Bay, they lost power for a couple of seconds. In Keshena, another bad storm knocked out the electricity for about 15 minutes. Steve fell asleep in the van when it began to hail. He left the van, and entered the Casino. The blackjack dealers held flashlights, and covered their money trays. When I had to use a bathroom that had a small stall, or an individual unisex bathroom, the security guard would warn the women in the ladies' room that a man was coming in to help me. When the room cleared, Steve had enough room to help me. One older woman grumbled, "Gee, you can't even take a dump around here without being rushed!"

For my job, I also had an opportunity to train three, or four times at the Wisconsin Indian reservations, which also had casinos. Thus, we traveled to all 15 casinos that had blackjack. The most important things were the training sessions. During our vacation, Steve and I would sometimes stop to join the powwows to dance, eat corn soup, wild rice, or beaver stew. The first time we stopped to try fresh and warm fried bread that we found surprisingly delicious, and I wanted everyone I knew to try it.

BY THE GRACE OF GOD AND YOU
A Chair Does Not a Person Make

One of the Reservations was 500 miles from our home in Redcliff, Wisconsin. Many of the tribes produced good boxers. It was the first time I sat in an actual 'talking circle.' First, there was a cleansing of everyone's thoughts with tobacco smoke, which sent the prayers to the Great Spirit. While in training, each of us swished a feather sending the smoke towards us to clean our thoughts and heart. Explaining the rules, one feather was passed throughout the large group of 40 or 50 people, and only the person with the feather could speak, and we learned how to listen. No one judged what the person was saying, and it was a safe place. No one could interrupt, or be interrupted, so that their ideas were not lost. In such a large group, there was a limit on speaking of three minutes. If someone abused the three minutes, the person was given a look, a glance at the clock, or other hint. For a smaller group of five or six, 10 minutes might have been given.

That was a very difficult task for me, since I was always multi-tasking. Women who were menstruating were not allowed to sit within the circle, but they sat behind, because they had the power to give life. I was almost at the end of the circle, and anxious about what I would say.

"What should I say? What if I sound stupid? It is going to take forever for the feather to reach me."

As the feather was handed to each, I listened. Everyone had a lot to say, and shared some of the things that I was thinking. It was an amazing way to purge your thoughts, and by the time the feather was handed to me, I was relaxed. I told everyone that I was anxious at first, and listening to everyone speak was relaxing, and I was saddened to be near the end, because the sharing would be over. When the last person spoke, the leader asked if anything "was left unsaid". After we were finished, everyone felt so relaxed, and it was time to leave.

I thought, "What a great way to start a training program, by putting a person right in the culture."

We learned many things over the years at the Reservations. We learned how to make a canoe from scratch from the trees around us. The canoes were submerged in the lake with the summer tools in the late fall. In the spring, the canoes were taken out of the water, and used again. We also learned about building wigwams, which had rounded tops as opposed to teepees, which were pointed.

Tobacco was especially a good gift for the holy men of the tribe. The Menominee would pray over the animals that they killed for food thanking the animal for giving up its life so that people could eat. They never felt that they owned the land like the white man did, and the Native Americans were charged as caretakers of it while they were present. They were allowed to eat that which was on the land, but didn't believe in waste. Every inch of the animal that was killed was used for food, fur for clothing, and even bones for tools.

They explained the difference of the white man's clock, which was in hours and minutes, compared to the Indians' concept of time. Indians told time by the sun, as well as in terms of the four seasons of summer, fall, winter, and spring. They were never in a hurry, but 'relaxed', and stopped to talk to people along the way. All of the wigwam openings faced east to warm their living quarters first thing in the morning, since seldom did cold winds come from that direction. A family of a Mother, Father, and one or two children usually lived with one of the remaining older parents. The elderly were honored with respect, even if the parent was "going back to their own childhood".

There were 11 tribes in Wisconsin, and when the government put tribes on reservations far from their homes, much knowledge was lost. In order to mask their great sorrow, Native Americans developed a great sense of humor. I remember one story about a tribesman who caught a fish so big that even the picture of the fish weighed 10 pounds! However, the sorrow continued when the government took the children from their parents, and forced them into white mens' schools where their language was not allowed. Children were often offended, because the same word in the white man's tongue might have a different meaning. For instance, For instance, "Drink this moo juice" meant "Drink this milk". But, to a Native American child, 'moo' meant "the warm soft squishy stuff you might step in on a nice summer day while running across a field of cows". Their religion had the gods interacting with the people, and they were given human qualities. Storytelling was a big part of their culture in respecting their heritage. It was important that they knew their ancestry, who begat who, for multiple generations back. I thought this was a beautiful way to honor, and respect their elders. Few can trace their ancestors back through three generations.

Because of the white man's firewater (alcohol), and whereas they used small amounts of maple syrup, the white man's processed sugar in their foods caused alcoholism and diabetes. Many would accept the white men's doctoring only if it was combined with the spiritual treatments of their medicine man. Being white, I think the government could have done a much better job protecting the environment if they would have given this responsibility to the Indians instead of just taking their land and putting them in unfamiliar places. They also took care of their elders, and never put them in a nursing home. Family, not things, was more important than profit.

I used that which I learned in training sessions in my office. I decorated it with Indian pictures, dream catchers, quotations, and other things so people might feel comfortable. It made the office feel warm and friendly. Although Kenosha did not have a large Indian population, I did have more people share that portion of their heritage after I put up pictures. Trust was always a problem with the Native Americans, and I could understand why.

Mindy, my niece who was 12, was called the Dolly Parton of the 5th Grade - and not because she could sing! She fell at the end of the school year, breaking her shin in a few places, and put her in a wheelchair all that summer. She wasn't able to put weight on her leg until November. Yes, we were looking more and more alike every day!

When Kenny was 17 years old, he was involved with a young police group called the Explorers, and very active. He found the group very interesting, and he became interested in school again. Kenny was headed for one of the numerous Explorer activities, and 5 teens were in the car driven by his best friend. Unfortunately, there was a tragic collision, and his best friend died from his injuries. While others in the car were hurt, Kenny was seated in the center of the back seat, and he only had scars from broken glass on the back of his head. From what I understood, due to the damage of the car, that it was a miracle anyone lived! Ken graduated from high school the next spring, and began a job in security that July.

Almost exactly two years from the date of the accident, Kenny became ill, and he was hospitalized. Bipolar was diagnosed, and he has had a very difficult time with it through the years. He shared a lot of things with me that helped me understand an inside perspective, and I was grateful. Stabilizing medications was just one issue. With too much medication, he would become "zombie like", while too little would not help, and could cause side effects like gaining a lot of weight, dry mouth, or tics. His arm became bent and inflexible due to one medication. When people feel "functional" on the bipolar medications, there is a tendency to stop taking the meds, and the person reverts. At one point, Kenny had taken his morning medication, but he couldn't sleep. And, didn't sleep - for five days! He was unaware he had not taken his medication. Both Mom and I knew something was wrong, but Kenny didn't. After asking me a simple question, which I answered, he put his hand on my shoulder very hard, looked me in the eye, and asked his question again. It was as if he couldn't hear the answer, was confused, or the answer didn't process.

Later, as Kenny told us:

"When you don't know that there are no medications in your system, how can you be responsible for your own behavior when you can't process information?"

A person with Bipolar Disorder appears depressed, confused, or is misunderstood, and it is hard to make friends while adjusting to medications. Some clients had their own way of knowing when an "episode" was beginning, and they needed a trusted individual to help them through it. Most individuals cannot identify the problem on their own. Symptoms preceding an episode are different with each person. Possibly the person would have a lack of good hygiene, stop cleaning their house, spend their whole savings at one time, be sexually promiscuous, become overly religious, etc. Kenny's episodes were often based on thinking he was protecting others. Maybe it was because of his interest in police work, yet his actions scared people instead. For example, at his apartment, he saw people getting out of an unfamiliar car. He knocked loudly on his neighbors' doors while telling them to "keep your doors locked"! He thought he was helping. The person doesn't always remember an incident, because it was so intense, he does not remember it except for small pieces.

Even the parents and relatives don't understand that the person with Bipolar Disorder may see a situation differently. Others avoid the person altogether, because they can't keep up with rapid thought process. For both the families and the person, there is a long and difficult learning curve, which the individual might not fully understand.

I was always very glad that I just had a physical disability, and could just ask for help when I needed it. With a mental illness, a person seldom realizes that a symptom is occurring without the assistance of another person. I always admired people that took care of their mental disabilities. A psychiatrist was just another doctor that must be seen for general health maintenance. Their medications assisted with good health just like any other doctor's meds. So many people didn't, and still don't, understand.

Alone, Steve and I took our second trip to Texas in 1995. On our way to Memphis, we stopped at Elvis Presley's Graceland home, and toured the inside of the home, the grounds, the airplanes, and Elvis' grave. From there we went to Tunica, Mississippi, which was less than an hour away. Steve remembered where all of the newly constructed casinos were along the way. I remembered the massive amounts of mosquitoes at night at the casino entrances, because the casinos were built on the water. Tunica had been the poorest area of the state when we were there before, and it is the richest today. We traveled from there to Gulfport, Mississippi, where we went to two casinos, and then drove east to Biloxi where we tried all 10! These casinos definitely had the best food we ever ate. Next, we crossed the bayous into Louisiana, and down to Corpus Christi, Texas, where we visited Steve's relatives, again. We visited Steve's brother's grave, since he had not been there, and stopped to see Selena's grave. She was Steve's favorite Hispanic singer, and had been murdered by her fan club president when she was 23 years-old. My understanding was that Selena was a Jehovah witness, and why her gravesite was very simple - a black marble headstone with her first name written in silver on the side of it.

We returned to Kenosha on the Fourth of July weekend, and along the way, we saw fireworks all around us from Memphis to Chicago. Sometimes we could see the fireworks going off in more than one city at a time.

In 1995, "Grandma with the kitties" passed away at 95. It was also the first death from my family for Gavino and Steve, and they carried her coffin. She was my last Grandparent to pass, and it brought back a lot of memories. One Halloween, she picked up a pair of eyeglasses from the table.

Putting them on, she asked, "Whose glasses are these? I can see out of them really well!"

"Grandma those glasses are a part of the Halloween costume. They have no lenses!" I whispered, and we both laughed.

By the time Grandma passed away, she was legally blind from Macular Degeneration (no central vision), and she was almost deaf. Once, when Steve and I went to see her, I had to stay in the car. Steve went in to take her something, and Grandma asked where I was. Steve told her that I was "outside".

"She died? What happened?" she said, startled, but Steve finally made her understand!

There were a lot of summertime fairs at Grandma's nursing home. Mom went to see her at least three times a week. My Grandma was thin, but she loved her sugar, and could eat a whole pack of Oreo cookies in three days. As I was growing up, she always put sugar on my tomatoes and French toast, which made them perfect! I guess it was a German tradition!

Dad began to have strokes. Mom and Dad visited on our regularly, scheduled Christmas Eve morning brunch at our house. Dad was sitting on the couch, and Mom was in the dining room setting the table. Dad's speech became garbled, and there was a loss of muscle strength on one side of his body. I realized what was happening telling everyone he was having a stroke, but I didn't think of calling 911, so Mom called them. The rescue squad arrived in less than three minutes.

Dad had thought something was happening to him, because he had had two minor car accidents in the previous two weeks. He knew he wasn't thinking right and had Mom do the driving. In the beginning, Dad's stroke left him temporarily paralyzed on his right side and caused difficulty swallowing. He stayed at the hospital for several weeks in St. Catherine's rehab section and had to relearn how to do everything. He was very determined, and tried everything they told him. Before his stroke, he was an intense person about getting things done, but after his retirement, he mellowed a bit. Once a person has a stroke, their personality undergoes a change. In many cases, if a person has a negative personality, it becomes worse. We expected his personality to become worse, but instead, he became very easygoing and accepting.

The following April, a newspaper article was written from our local Easter Seals group, and both Mom and Dad were on the Easter Seals Service Unit. The beginning of the article tied into what was happening with my Dad.

Kenosha News April 1, 1995 (a shortened version)

Handicapped Having Trouble Voting—Seeking Polling Place Access

"You and I are one accident away from becoming handicapped," said Richard Guttormsen, principal of Jane Vernon School and chairman of the Local Easter Seals. "It's a shame," he said, "that the handicap has to struggle for their rights"... "Voting rights—the ability of handicapped people to enter a polling place without physical obstacles—are one of the areas in which changes should be made," according to Carol Schaufel, a disabled Vocational Rehabilitation Counselor. "Many people with disabilities vote absentee ballot," said Schaufel. "I prefer to do it in person so people are aware that the handicapped vote too... I would be pleased if voting places were made more accessible so people in wheelchairs, like me, and those with other handicaps could just come in and vote... I hate to be singled out at the polls...I'm singled out enough. If everything were accessible, I wouldn't look so different." Some polling places had flights of steps, some places brought out a paper ballots. Even if you could get into the building, you would need assistance in reaching.

The city clerk had already been working on changing several places within the district... GUTTORMSEN said, "It is a misconception to think that structural changes are always needed. Non-handicapped people don't think in these terms. But with a little thought, all places could be made accessible in some way." – – – Many places were identified to make them accessible with little cost along with another person to witness the voting. Voting machines are not accessible ...

Frank had worked hard on accessibility in voting for people with disabilities simply by identifying the buildings in each ward where they could vote. Fortunately, my polling places always had flat entrances, especially in schools and libraries, but I always needed assistance in the voting booth, because I could not reach the ballot. Frank preferred voting by absentee ballot, but I thought it was important to be seen voting in the community. People with disabilities have voting and buying power. It is very influential when one out of every 10 or 11 people have a disability!

In 1996, I was asked to be on the board for Leisure Independence Network of Kenosha (LINK). It was a 3-year program sought by the Kenosha Achievement Center to assist people with disabilities in transportation, companions, costs, accessibility information, and recreational pursuits. The board oversaw the US Department of Education Federal Recreation Grant. We monitored the Program Director, and checked the budget for program compliance with Federal procedures. It was an exciting program with great flexibility, allowing individuals with disabilities to participate in activities of their choice. Requests varied from shopping to a once-a-week walk along the lake.

Gary, who was a rehab counselor at KAC, and I took a woman, with a learning disability who lived with her Mother to the County Fair in my van. Her Mother requested that her daughter not win any fish at the fair. Of course, being at the fair, she ate, and tried a lot of different things. And, naturally, she threw Ping-Pong balls into fishbowls, and won two fish. She was so excited that it just tickled us to watch her. After all, she was doing the one thing very well. On the way home in the van, however, there was some depression, and she worried about what her Mother would say about the fish and what she would do to her for bringing them home again. I told her not to worry.

"What could be the worst thing that your Mother could do to you for bringing the fish home? Maybe the fish would have to live in the bathtub, because you no longer had a fishbowl. Maybe, if your Mom is really mad, you might have to live in the bathtub with the fish for a few weeks!"

The woman laughed, and came up with her own plan.

"I could always give them away as a gift," she said.

Good idea, why didn't I think of that?

At one of my board meetings, I was very sick and taking cold medications. I lost my vision when clouds in my eyes covered my sight for about 15 minutes. The cloud dissipated slowly into a donut hole, which got larger and clearer until the 'cloud' went away. I was very scared, because it had never happened to me before. It continued three or four times, before I went to the eye doctor. His wife and I were in the Lioness club, and he called the condition 'visual migraines', causing one to lose vision without pain - and, then the Doctor told me that his wife had them as well.

193

~ 23 ~

Technology and Traveling

Madison wanted me to use more technology on my job to assist accessibility with the computer. For a few years, the voice activation program, called DragonDictate was used. I was leery about asking for it, because the original cost of the program for only one computer was $10,000, and other workers needed it as well. Eventually, the cost dropped dramatically, and it was installed on my computer. The whole DVR agency was going paperless, and using my mouthstick to type would be impossible without voice recognition. I could no longer type everything by using my head and neck letter by letter! While others in the state were getting Carpal Tunnel from so much typing, I thought that I was getting Carpal Tunnel of the jaw!

After the program was installed, it took three days to train it with my voice. I enunciated words, numbers, and letters into the computer three times each with one second in between, and therefore, it sounded very choppy.

"I—had—an—additional—disability."

After using the system for at least three years, The *Kenosha News* published the following article on the voice system that I was demonstrating to Gateway Tech computer students:

*March 31, 1996 Miss **Hathaway: Take a Letter** by Barbara Henkel*

High tech office broadens horizons. Miss Hathaway, the fictional, longtime suffering banker's secretary on the old 'Beverly Hillbillies' television show, lives on in a Kenosha business office.

Miss Hathaway is the affectionate name Carol Schaufel-Romero has given her voice-activated computer. Just as Miss Hathaway was known for her efficiency and expediency, the voice recognition system gives Carol more efficiency and speed in her job as a rehabilitation counselor for the Kenosha office of the Wisconsin Department of Vocational Rehabilitation. Schaufel is one of just thousands of people with disabilities who have been able to get, or in her case, maintain a meaningful job through the assistance of modern technology. Schaufel, 49, has a progressive neural-muscular disorder that resulted in her being in a wheelchair since the age of six. That hasn't prevented her from working for DVR for the past 15 years. Before that she was a ninth grade math teacher for seven years at Bullen Junior High School. She has a Master's Degree in mathematics from the University of Wisconsin-Milwaukee, earned after graduating magna cum laude from Carthage College, where she taught statistics for a year.

A quick mind is amply evident in trying to keep up in notetaking during a recent interview. Carol explained how the progressive nature of her disability over time has limited some of her clerical abilities important for keeping track of her caseload. But the state accommodated her by providing assistance to do some of the more physical aspects of her job, such as making photocopies and retrieving manila file folders. Then in 1993 her office was equipped with computers and she was expected to do most of her own typing and file maintenance. Enter DragonDictate, a software computer program, one of several designed to assist the disabled. Schaufel speaks into a microphone, "Voice Counsel, start WordPerfect." In the same, if not less time, then it would have taken to type up a memo, Schaufel has completed the task. That's partly because some shortcuts are built into the system. The computer recognizes some frequently used key words. "You can train it to type a complete sentence based on just one or two keywords," she said.

There are quirks in the system. If someone sneezes in the hallway outside the office door, the computer may pick up that sound. (It typed the word if.) Because she was trained on her computer at the time when a space heater was in use in her office, she now must keep it on because the computer recognizes that background noise. Should her voice change considerably, due to a cold, for example, her voice counsel won't recognize her words. It has the ability to record up to 10 different voices, so in that instance, in a few hours, Schaufel can retrain the computer to recognize her new voice. So far she hasn't come down with a cold, so hasn't had to do that.

Her computer recognizes the word "oops" as meaning what was typed wasn't intended. It defaults automatically to spell check, providing a list of alternatives with similar sounding words that Schaufel uses most often. The spoken command "choose 10" may come out "Houston" or "Tuesday." "It types what it thinks you said. Sometimes we all have to laugh at what it says," Schaufel said. "It gets really funny sometimes."

Schaufel's speed is such that at times the office printer gets backed up. "I can do letters, memos, casenotes and emails."

DragonDictate or a similar program is not necessarily the tool every disabled person needs, Schaufel noted. The Kenosha DVR office serves 708 persons in the Kenosha and Walworth counties. "Very few would need DragonDictate, though some would probably like it," Schaufel said. One woman is using the system to complete her college coursework. Some in Milwaukee use voice activation attached to their computers to turn lights on and off in their home, or to answer their telephone. "It gives them access to their world." DVR tailors a program according to the person's particular needs for the job goal. "There is a lot of different technology out there," Schaufel said. There are tactile keyboards with some keys in braille or with bright colored letters to assist the visually impaired. There are different kinds of mouses with a variety of switches, such as rocker or those that are heat sensitive. A person may be able to sip and puff on a device which can transmit signals to the computer. In another system the user wears a head band with a light that focuses on the keyboard. Keystrokes result from the person focusing one's eyes on the particular key needed. For instance, to assist people with carpal tunnel syndrome, there are keyboards that split apart and one hand lies on each side. On another, a person may insert their hands and use them like paws," she said.

Although Schaufel's neck is her strongest body part, her arthritis of the neck is aggravated if she uses a mouthstick too much. "If I type continuously with it, it is hard on my neck," she said. She points out that her mouthstick is an example of how not all adaptive technology is expensive. Here it is simply a wooden dowel, wrapped with black tape on one end and with a rubber page turner attached to the other with a rubber band.

BY THE GRACE OF GOD AND YOU
A Chair Does Not a Person Make

Carol said when she first became aware of Dragon Dictate seven years ago, the cost was $10,000. Now it's closer to $700, but requires more memory and megabytes than previously. Much of the hundreds of adaptive software available were developed because there was someone with a need, Schaufel said. "A lot of these were developed for people with disabilities, and others use it now as the cost comes down like touch lamps,"

... "There is so much out there right now." Schaufel said. ... "That this is a good time to be disabled." It is also beneficial to employers who have an employee who has become disabled. "The cost of equipment is less expensive than the cost of retraining," Schaufel Romero said. In speaking to groups, the advocate for the founder of ABLE— Abolish Barriers for Lifetime Efficiency—stresses, "What I try to teach is that having a disability is just different: it isn't worse, it's just different. People look at me and wonder how I can do what I want. We're the same, but we have to do things differently."

"Although we (DVR) are looking at how to accommodate for the disability, we're really looking at a person's abilities and work with those. You have to believe in yourself. You're the same person with the same intellect, with or without a disability. If you want a career, you can have one." And newer technology is helping. The goal of DVR, and people like Schaufel, is to assist people with disabilities in maintaining a meaningful life. "For some people, sometimes maintaining their health and energy level is the more important goal," she said. "All of our goals are about establishing a work setting, but that may not be full-time work."

DragonDictate wasn't infallible, though, and after three days, any typing was permanent. One of my clients wanted to be a "phlebotomist", or a person who draws blood, but the computer program "heard", and typed "lobotomist", or a person who takes out part of the brain. I was really happy that the file was never audited!

Training DragonDictate, while speaking in a normal voice, was much easier the second time, and only took about one hour. When an updated program was installed, it was called DragonDictate NaturallySpeaking: Professional. It was more accurate, and training it took only 10 minutes by reading a small article. When I was ready to buy the program for my personal computer, in order to practice, my nephew, David, found an older version of the program on E-Bay for $8. By the time I bought a home computer, DragonDictate total cost was $100.

Another accommodation that I was allowed in my office was a space heater. I was always cold, especially my hands and feet, and I put it underneath my desk. One day, I smelled something hot, and looked down to find my moccasin was smoking! Yikes! I moved the heater to the side of my desk for obvious reasons!

Stevie was moved from the Wisconsin prison to the prison in Pennsylvania in 1997, and Steve and I took a trip to see him. At one point, Steve, Stevie, and I were placed into a separate room with a guard. Guess I looked suspicious. With both state and federal charges against him, the Federal Government took over Stevie's case. The judge recommended that he be sent to a mental health facility, but there was no space available in Minnesota, so they sent him to a non-medical, federal prison about 100 miles south of Niagara Falls.

Visiting the Federal Prison in Pennsylvania was our first trip to a federal prison, and there were a couple of days a week when we could not visit. We saw Stevie the day before we got very sick with colds. The next two days were non-visiting days, so we just spent a lot of time in the motel room. We always tried to see Stevie a couple of days in a row when we were so far away from home.

Visiting a federal institution was not much different than visiting in the state except that I was required to transfer into one of their wheelchairs. This was impossible, because balancing without proper support was very difficult. Without a strap behind my legs, and with ankles that had contractures, I could not keep my feet on the pedals without catching my feet in the wheels. We notified the prisons beforehand that I was in a wheelchair, and then, we filled out papers for the inmate we came to see. At security, a metal detecting wand was waved over me, and my chair made a lot of noise! Not a surprise, of course. At a signal, another guard unlocked a heavy door which automatically relocked with a loud noise behind us. Our hands were stamped, and Steve helped me to raise mine to an electronic device allowing me to pass through the heavy metal doors. The stamp was only visible under the device. Once we were all checked, another heavy door was unlocked, so we could enter into a courtyard through, yet, another door, which locked and relocked behind us. We handed the paper work to another guard inside who assigned us to a table, or area, so we could visit with Stevie. Another guard notified Stevie that we were there, and then, Stevie would be processed, and allowed to come into the visiting area, which took about 10 or 15 minutes.

We were not allowed to bring anything with us except for a clear plastic bag of dollars and change for the vending machines. Stevie wasn't allowed to handle money that he received for prison use. Instead, money was sent to a different address by mail through Western Union or Money Order. We would go to the vending machines to see what kind of food was there, and then, we returned to tell Stevie, and he would decide what he wanted to eat. We would go back to buy the food, and use the microwave, if needed. Stevie was mainly happy just to get a Coke, because that was his favorite drink. He also liked the small pizzas, rib sandwiches, and some different items. Stevie told funny stories, but most of the time we visited about changes being made in Kenosha and answering when he asked us about certain people.

After visiting for three hours, we would retrieve our paperwork, and reverse the process in order to leave the prison, and hoping that the stamp had not been washed off their hands when we used the locked bathroom. A guard returned our ID cards, and we were on our way.

We visited with Stevie one more time, and since Steve had never been there, we decided to go to Niagara Falls. Niagara Falls was one of my favorite places. We drove across the Rainbow Bridge from Niagara, NY, which is close to Buffalo, and into Canada presenting our driver's licenses. We found a motel room in Niagara Falls, Canada going to the casino first, because Steve was more interested in gambling.

The next morning, for whatever reason, Steve decided not to take his Paxil for his anxiety, panic, and depression issues. He decided to throw his pills away, but I told him to put them in my backpack instead. We started our tour of the city of Niagara Falls, and went underneath the Horseshoe Falls which was a place I thought most impressive! This time there weren't any steps, and just an elevator, but raincoats were still needed. With his raincoat on, Steve enjoyed the spray on his face from an outside platform and staircase. We walked through the tunnels, but the rapidly falling water in front of him caused him to panic, and we had to get out of the tunnel as soon as possible. He really felt trapped under the tunnels, and the noise was deafening. I told him to take one of the pills he put in my backpack instead of the garbage. He took them without hesitation, and started feeling much better. Thank you God! What would I have done if they had not worked?

The next day, we drove the car around the city, so that we could see the two falls from different angles. As we went down a hill, Niagara Falls looked extremely large in front of us, and Steve wished that he had taken his medication sooner, so he could have enjoyed the previous day.

As we left Niagara Falls and Canada, Steve realized that he lost his driver's license. We didn't know what to do, or to whom to report the loss, so we just drove all the way home. Our route took us along the Great lakes in New York, and we passed a lot of vineyards. We also passed a beautiful view of the Cleveland Indians' Baseball Park. Chicago was the best place, however, because we were close to home.

Soon after our return, our eight year old Doberman, Midnight, surprised us.

"I think she's pregnant!" Gavino told us.

We never had her spayed, because we always kept an eye on her, and since she was registered, we also thought sometime in the future we might want to breed her. Twice a year, she would wear Stevie's little jockey underwear around the house with a hole cut out for her tail, and the underwear was a perfect fit!

Steve saw a dog around Midnight, and suspected of being the Father about two weeks before we left to see Stevie, but discovered that it was a female. I borrowed a book from the library about pregnancy, and read it from start to finish. As Midnight's due date came closer, she would do everything to leave the house, because she had already started a nest in her doghouse for the puppies. The night she delivered, Steve brought her into the house, and put her in Stevie's bedroom. We could hear Midnight frantically making a nest by ripping up the rug and using some blankets we left. She began her labor. Her labor cries were blood curdling throughout the night, but she was stubborn, and didn't want any help. By 5 a.m., seven puppies were born. Gavino noticed that the dog's stomach still felt like it had some puppies in it. Steve and Gavino took Midnight and the puppies to the veterinarian in the van. Midnight birthed another little puppy on the van floor, but it didn't make it. Another pup was born at the veterinarian's office, but also died. Midnight delivered two boys and five girls

When we entered Midnight's bedroom, there was no odor, and everything was clean. She'd eaten the puppies' placentas, which were supposed to be good for a Mother dog's health. Who taught her to how to take care of all that stuff? Not me! I think Midnight was too old to be a Mother, because she stepped on her puppies all the time. She had her favorite too—a very chubby little male that ate - a lot! There was also the runt of the litter, which Midnight really didn't want to feed. That little puppy had to fight her way between the others to get to a "food faucet", and hide under the others while she grew!

As all of the puppies grew, Midnight's favorite would run, and jump right in the middle of the plate of food spattering it all over for the other puppies to eat and hoarding food of his own. Midnight didn't let her puppies suckle very long. Once they were eating solid foods, she just got angry with them if they wanted to feed.

Merle visited on a regular basis, and the first time he walked into the puppy's bedroom, he was trapped with all the puppies around his feet. Merle was yelling for help so he could get out of the room without a "Great Puppy Escape"! There would always be a puppy or two that would get out with him, and he would have to shove the puppies back through the door.

When my Dad had another stroke, he could barely walk with a walker or a cane. But he really loved dogs, so whenever Dad would come over, we would let the puppies out of the room. They would surround him, and tease him by untying his shoes, which he couldn't reach anymore, and loved playing tug-of-war with his shoe laces!

Midnight would always protect me when the puppies were around, and would discipline them if any of them were playing too rough. Eventually, we sold all the puppies except for one named Gurdy that we were thinking about keeping. She was always getting into lot of trouble, and one day, she managed to get onto the kitchen counter, and she knocked down a jalapeno pepper. We saw it fall on the floor, but just watched as she smelled it, and took a bite. Her mouth was probably on fire, because she started barking at the pepper, running circles around it, and probably expected it to attack her. She was so funny! But, when the pepper didn't move, Gurdy thought she'd try to eat it again. She bit it, again, and repeated her attack until she finally calmed down, before we took it away. But, she was just too big for me to handle. One of my volunteers at work always wanted a Doberman, and so, Gurdy had a new home. Gurdy lived a long life, and was always glad to see us.

In 1997, I met Heather, Gavino's supervisor at a trucking company. Gavino had problems with alcohol and drugs, and had no license or car. Heather would drop him at home after work. She seemed more mature than Gavino, and ready for a relationship. She had a two and a half-year-old little girl by the name of Alicia who already knew exactly what she wanted and how to be her own advocate! Five months after Gavino started going with her, Heather came to me, and told me she was pregnant. While Gavino spent some time in jail for a DWI, Heather stayed with us. She had been living with her Mother who was now in the process of moving due to a divorce, so Alicia became my granddaughter right away!

Whenever Heather left the house, Alicia would cry, climb up on my bed, and lay on me until she went to sleep. When she wanted me to read to her, she would grab a book from Sesame Street, crawl up on my lap, put my arms around her as I couldn't do that by myself, hold the book up, and turn the pages. Once in a while she would tease me by holding the book upside down!

When Alicia was being potty trained, her Mother wanted her to start sleeping in her own bed. In the middle of the night, Alicia would crawl into my bed, and lay on my arm. In the morning my hand would be in a puddle of water. One of Heather's friends, Sarah, would visit with her children once in a while. Alicia would tell a story about Midnight, because Sarah was afraid of dogs, and was worried that Midnight would bite. Alicia would comfort her. "Sarah, don't worry. Midnight has no teeth!" The stories that girl could tell!

Alicia could be very dramatic even at a young age. We would both pretend that we were speaking Spanish like Grandpa. It really looked like both of us knew what we were talking about—no way!

Sarah's boy was a little older than Alicia. He had some cookies he wanted to share with her.

"Alicia, my Grandma made these cookies. Want one?" he asked.

She took offense and said, "My Grandma reads to me, let's me ride on her lap, plays games…and my Grandma can beat your Grandma up!" Alicia!

It was so much fun to have a young child in the house again for Christmas. When my sister's kids were young, they would spend a night the week before Christmas. They would sleep under the tree begging to open just one of their seven gifts each. David didn't care what he got as long as he had the biggest package.

Heather went to the hospital when it was time for her baby to be born, and her labor was hard. Gavino was still on Huber, and he did not know about the birth until the following day. I saw the baby the next day—Evelyce Marie! She seemed so tiny, and Steve was a proud Grandpa! When Gavino finally saw Evelyce, he was very happy, too. Even though he had accepted Alicia as his child, he really wanted a baby of his own. Alicia and Evelyce were both christened on the same day. The girls looked so pretty in their white outfits! It had been a long time since I had been to church, and it felt good to be back, again. Steve was reading the Koran at the time. My faith was always strong—church or not. God guided my life. It made life easy—all I had to do was live it.

When Evelyce was six months old, Evelyce, Alicia, and I were in the *Kenosha News*. MDA was changing TV stations for the telethon, and the *News* gave an update on what was happening with me and my growing family at the same time. For the picture, Alicia had to balance, and stop Evelyce from falling off my lap.

Fall 1998 *Kenosha News*
Can-Do Attitude Goes a Long Way Advocate for Disabled Knows Answers
by Debbie Luebke Metro

Are babies born with wheelchairs? This is just one of the many questions Carol Schaufel fields when she visits third-grade classrooms to help children feel comfortable talking to people with disabilities. Since she has used a wheelchair, because of a neural muscular disease, for 51 years she knows the answers to many of their questions. She also knows how incredibly sweet a child can be.

Her three-year-old granddaughter Alicia likes to ride on the back of her wheelchair and seems to know instinctively when Grandma needs assistance. "She knows when I have trouble with my arms." Schaufel said. "Sometimes she feeds me. When she was about two, she sat in my lap and put my arms around her because she knew I couldn't do that." But Schaufel prefers talking about what she can do, not what she can't.

It's an attitude that's earned her numerous honors throughout her life. Among them are the first personal achievement state award from the Muscular Dystrophy Association in 1992, 1981 Kenosha Person of the Year, listing in the National Distinguished Service Registry in the Library of Congress and the 1973 gallantry award from the Easter Seals Society of Wisconsin. She served on the Gov.'s Committee for People with Disabilities from 1983-86 and was instrumental in starting Abolish Barriers for Lifetime Efficiency (ABLE) and the Leisure Independence Network of Kenosha (LINK). In her job as a DVR vocational rehabilitation counselor for almost 2 decades, she earned the respect of her clients and colleagues.

When she received the 1998 Allan Bullamore Humanitarian Award from the Kenosha Achievement Center recently, her boss, Willie Riley at the DVR commented, "She's been instrumental in assisting persons with disabilities obtain employment and provide the assistance needed to help them obtain a better quality of life." Carol does not waste energy with negative thinking but rather uses her resources to make sure success is achieved. She appears to be driven by the challenge of the task. There seems to be nothing in her life that saps her enthusiasm for living. She gives new dimension to the concept of grace and strength under fire. Carol is a person that one is blessed to know."

She also helps with the small stuff for groups she belongs to. Last spring she sold lilies for Easter Seals at a grocery store. For the Jerry Lewis MDA Labor Day Telethon that begins tonight at 10 o'clock in Milwaukee, working in a game booth at the festival. The telethon runs until 7 p.m. Monday on CBS Channel 58.

Her first realization that something was wrong with her body came when she was about six years old. "I remember looking up at the ceiling and feeling weak. I couldn't raise my arms. My Mom said I walked early, but I always fell and hit my head." She walked until she was four, then she got around on her knees for another two years. By the time she was six, she needed a wheelchair. Children in the neighborhood came to her house to play. She couldn't get into their homes. "I caught colds easily...I still do, and my Mom put a blanket over my legs. I hated that." When she was two she nearly lost her ability to speak when she fell on a park bench and almost severed a portion of her tongue. After she attended the former Orthopedic School, her parents, Ken and Shirley Schaufel, advocated for her to be able to attend Bradford High School. "Administration didn't want to let me go because they were afraid I'd get too tired and the bathrooms weren't accessible. But my parents said, 'Let her try.' They always advocated for me to do things."

She earned a Bachelor's Degree from Carthage College and a Masters from UW-Milwaukee. After teaching ninth grade for eight years in Kenosha, she joined the DVR staff in 1979.

"I always shied away from relationships," she explained. "I had 15 friends die by the time I was 20. I did my job, but I didn't want to get close to people. I'm shy...a bad person to have at parties. I'm a better listener." But she found a good friend in Stephano Romero, who is now an outreach worker for the Southeastern Wisconsin AIDS Project, and they married in 1989. They have two sons and two Grandchildren.

As a girl at a summer Easter Seals camp, she learned to swim, a hobby she still enjoys. She's traveled to 40 states and 10 countries. She also discovered myths and stereotypes about people in wheelchairs were still around. One of her math students was told by her parents that all people in wheelchairs were mentally disabled. In Hawaii she encountered a man who told her, "You're in a wheelchair because of the sins of your parents."

BY THE GRACE OF GOD AND YOU
A Chair Does Not a Person Make

For four years before she got married, she lived on her own. For two years she had a roommate with cerebral palsy. "We did well together. She would reach an egg and I could crack it. I could put the key in the door, and she could turn it." An attendant helps her with necessities like going to the bathroom and taking a shower. Although she has arthritis in her neck, she brushes her teeth by moving her head back and forth. About seven years ago, she discovered she couldn't raise her arms to her face. Most of the time, she can eat on her own.

At her office she has a voice-operated computer, a rocker phone switch and a mouth stick to help her type on the computer keyboard, turn pages and point. "When you're disabled, you have to be creative and organized. But you have no privacy. If you get a letter, someone else has to open it."

The reason she's worked with MDA for many years is because the research they're doing assists people with many different disabilities. She said. "M.D. is not like other disabilities. It's much more final then some," Schaufel-Romero said. "It's important to have the support groups and people out there willing to let people become what they want to become." For her the most rewarding part of her job "is seeing people become themselves. So often they're told not to do something. They just have to think of how they can do things differently. Some of the reasons people want to work is to feel productive and be out with people. I'm just human. But I want to empower people to help them feel as free as possible."

Heather, Alicia, and Evelyce moved into their own apartment with Gavino soon after the article was written, and I really missed them.

At work, my supervisor, Willie, and I did an article on myths about people with disabilities and the workplace. In short, an employer could fire a person with a disability who did not do the job. If they were not on time, missed too many days, or were unable to perform the job duties, the employer treated these employees like everyone else. Not all people that had disabilities were sick more often than others, and those with disabilities should not apply for jobs for which they were not qualified.

Technology could help people with disabilities with their jobs, "*but we found the majority of technology has a very minimal cost. Our agency is willing to work with the employer for that employee for a period of time and determine what is needed for the person to perform the job and the best method to acquire the technology... The agency can assist with the cost. If on the job training is required, DVR can help pay a person's wages for period of time to prove he can work.*" People wanted to work. "*Some want to work just to stay busy. Some, because they needed money. But everyone gets a sense of fulfillment when they work. Generally, when you hire a person with a disability, you're getting a motivated, hard-working person.*" "*Some people with disabilities have been told for so long that they can't do things that—when they find out they can—they are overjoyed!*"

I usually ended up supporting our family's costs.
Steve would always say, "You bring home the bacon, but I bring home some biscuits!"
Heather was helping with the housework and some of the cooking. My morning

attendant would get me up and out of bed. Steve took care of the rest—getting me back and forth from work, getting me to bed and turning me at night, as well as working his own job. He was a good cook too.

Sometimes it was hard to get Steve to do things, though. The time when we had to get rid of our mattress, he just laid the mattress against the side of the garage. I saw it still there a month later.

I wondered, "What would move him to get rid of it?"

I knew he always picked up fast on discrimination of any group. I also knew a great majority of Mexicans who were much neater than Steve, but it sure did the trick!

"When are you going to get rid of this? It's been over a month. I DON'T want this to look like a Mexican house!"

The mattress was gone the next day.

On the other hand, if Steve wanted me to do something when I didn't want to do it, such as going to a meeting or staying in bed on a Sunday, I would get my hand up to my mouth, and drop it on the table as if I was pounding it.

"You are not going to bully me!" He would laugh.

"Do as you are told and there won't be any problem," he told me.

He should have known better. I didn't listen.

In 1999, Steve and I took our second trip to Vegas to visit Carol and Eddie. They picked us up at the airport, but it was a sad trip. Not only was the Columbine shootings on the news, but Carol had a bad area of skin that would not heal. She went to the doctor while we were in Vegas, and it was cancer! Eddie had lost part of his leg and a foot to cancer a couple of years before. It was so good to see them again, but the circumstances were not good. They had taken care of both of his parents before they passed away. Now, Eddie had a hard time dealing with Carol's illness. They finally moved back to Oshkosh, Wisconsin, where Carol's family lived. Eddie stayed by her side until she passed away moving back to Kenosha where he had a few relatives left. I had a chance to see him occasionally. He told me that he never knew how much he loved his wife until it was too late. We could all learn from that.

In the summer of that year, we took another trip to see Stevie who was relocated to Fairton, New Jersey. We decided to take a trip, and took Beny, who was a friend from Guatemala, and happy to travel. Steve began having trouble with his diabetes, and didn't like to drive for long distances. On the way to New Jersey, we stopped in Gettysburg to investigate the city for a day. So many original buildings, all of the graves, bullet holes, and history! We also saw the countryside, an Amish community, Cape May (where Steve had been stationed in the Navy), and, of course, the boardwalk in Atlantic City. The casinos there were nothing like Vegas. There were no individual decors based on the title/theme. Beny and I walked a long way down the boardwalk, and towards the ocean. From there, we could look back under the boardwalk. Sadly, it looked like a few people were living there.

~ 24 ~

Dad's passing

For the last few years of his life, Dad had lots of strokes, and emphysema left him with only 11% function of his lungs. Dad knew he was having some problems when he was placed in hospice in August of 1999. I disagreed with the service telling him that the reason he was there, was he only had six months to a year to live. He was so organized that when he first retired, he already had his affairs in order. Mom and Dad also had their funeral arrangements paid for and planned, which made everything easier.

While Mom and I were playing Scrabble, Dad would go to the bathroom using his walker, but his foot would sometimes take him in a different direction than he planned. Instead, Dad would just follow his foot into the bedroom! I admired him, because nothing seemed to bother him. He would just do what he had to do, and well, que sera sera! It was the first year that I missed the MDA telethon, because we didn't know what Dad's health would be.

When Dad had his first, bad seizure, and we called for assistance from hospice. The woman claimed he was "dying now". I was sitting between the bedroom door and the hallway, and could see him in bed. He came out of his seizure smiling and waving at me as the she spoke.

"I think we should really take him to the hospital. He seems to be doing well. Look!" I told Mom.

Everyone went into the bedroom, and when he had another small seizure, we called the ambulance to take him to the hospital. In the emergency room, he had a very bad, 45-minute seizure. I felt helpless. There was nothing I could do. I could not even reach out to hold his hand. Susie saw a single tear drop from his eye. He knew what was happening. Mom seemed pretty calm, but she could not handle seeing Dad in the ER. She was prepared for it, and yet, she wasn't. Dad was admitted to the hospital, and we spoke to his lung doctor. Dad was not placed on life support per his *Living Will* request—"do not resuscitate". He was made as comfortable as possible, given large doses of morphine, and wasn't fed by mouth, because he could no longer swallow.

Daily, Mom would sit with Dad during the day, and Susie would stay for a little bit in the afternoon. Then, she would take Mom home around 3:30 p.m. I would usually go after work, so someone would be with him. Kenny went daily, as well, and could move him easily. He seemed to have an instinct about how to make him comfortable. Many times, we were all there, and I never saw Dad have another seizure. He seemed very happy. Kenny had just married, and his wife, Linda, helped a lot, too. Dad was very loving, and showed everyone a lot of affection - especially Mom.

One evening when I came into the room, the nurse was feeding Dad. I asked if she had seen the "do not feed sign" above his bed. She wasn't paying attention, and I could hear him gurgling. Someone came into the room, and removed some of the food and water that was trapped in his throat! I always felt someone needed to be there.

One day, I came into Dad's hospital room, and it looked like he was talking to someone very tall. His back was turned away from me, and his face was towards the window.

I heard him say, "I can't go yet, I don't know all the languages!"

I waited a while to see if he was going to say anything else, but he didn't. I came around to the other side of the bed to ask him the normal question.

"Dad, who were you talking to?"

He responded, "Mom."

I was thinking that he was talking about my Mom, but when I talked to her later about it, she thought for sure it was his Mom who had been 6 feet tall. The languages? We guessed the languages of heaven? Mom said that when she was in his room, he was always reaching for something. She asked him what that was.

He said, "I can't reach the doorknob."

"The doorknob to heaven," Mom thought.

The doctor kept Dad in the hospital for nine days. We were glad that he did not have to go to a nursing home. I canceled my WWAAC convention reservation, and we waited. We lived in the hospital—at least it seemed that way. I would call and report to my Uncle Al every day. I was disgusted with one of the nurse's aides one day when she complained, "What is this floor turning into—a geriatric floor, or a nursing home? Everyone is dying!" What a stupid statement! How inappropriate when patients and visitors could hear. Unfortunately, I could smell death coming.

Early the next day, we got a phone call from the hospital that Dad had passed away on September 23. Of course, he died at 3 a.m., the same time he used to get us up and ready to take all of our long trips. He was on his way home.

Pastor Shadduck met with the whole family the day before the wake at Mom's house to discuss the funeral, and celebrate Dad's life. He was there to help us adjust to Dad's death. There were tears and laughter—blessings and closure for all.

The wake was large for a 77 year old, because he had been involved in so many things. Alicia was four now. At the wake, she looked at great Grandma (my Mom), and asked, "Where is the other Grandpa?" Alicia knew something was wrong, since my Dad wasn't moving or talking to her, but she didn't understand. The newspaper said the funeral was at ten a.m., and I didn't realize visitation was before the funeral, so I missed the church visitation, and arrived when the funeral was ready to start. I was just in time for the service. While waiting for the family to walk into the church, I saw the funeral director take Dad's ring, watch, glasses off, and shut the coffin. A fear of loneliness came over me. The church was full, and I held Alicia on my lap. She held the hymnal for me, and we followed the coffin to the front of the church.

I had a difficult time, but I cried alone. Mom appeared strong, but kept a smiling picture of Dad on her kitchen table talking to it when she needed. She would say, "Yeah, you sit there smiling. Look at all the work you left me here to do alone! Bills, thank you notes ..." Mom wanted to write all of the thank you notes herself. She got rid of all of Dad's clothing and things within three months except for one shirt that still had his scent. It comforted her.

Mom showed us a note that Dad left to Susie and me. It told both of us how proud he was of us and that he loved us. He wrote, "Always help each other, and never fight over money!"

Besides Dad's death, I was under a lot of stress personally. A few months before Dad passed away, I realized that I had not received my credit card bill or my bank statements for a few months. I called and requested them discovering that $1000 in cash withdrawals had been made at the Kenosha dog track. I had to figure out how to replace this $1000 for property taxes. Steve had been going to the dog track without my knowledge. His addiction had definitely spread to all types of gambling. We had a big fight, and I stopped anyone from receiving cash with my credit card. The savings account was going down, too. I felt I was losing all control. I definitely was losing trust in him. Steve was terrible with money. He could never keep any in his pocket. I was physically losing strength. I could still feed myself, but people would have to put the food in my hands. Even a tostada was getting too heavy to handle, and I started dropping it.

Right after Dad passed away, I made a conscious decision to use my energy and strength in a different way. I stopped feeding myself. I also could no longer go in and out of the house by myself, because I didn't have the strength to push the electric door opener button. When I lost the ability to feed myself, eating just wasn't as much fun. Most people liked to mix their food, so they mixed mine. I got used to it. I usually just turned my plate as I went when I feed myself, because I couldn't reach over the top of the plate very well. Some people fed me fast; some people fed me slowly. I used to take large bites when I fed myself, because I didn't want to use my energy up on a lot of extra movement. I spread napkins on my chest (like a bib), which did not make me feel very adult, but invariably, people would spill, or miss my mouth. Now, I knew how babies must feel! It still was a better alternative than getting my clothes messed up and looking bad all day. Some people fed me with spoons, but I always used a fork, even for Jell-O! When I would get really frustrated, I'd tease the person who was feeding me. The person would ask me what I wanted to eat first. I say that I ate alphabetical, and it would "blow their mind". The person would ask, "Is this under 'M' for meat or 'C' for chicken?" When a person was used to feeding me, I could just look at what I wanted, and they would know what was next. The truth? Most of the time it really didn't matter what was first.

In 2000, at the end of summer, we got a call from Stevie who declared, "Pops you'll never guess where I am! I've been transferred to Leavenworth prison in Kansas!" He sounded excited as if he had completed a major goal in his life. He wasn't very far from Kansas City, Missouri, so we decided to take a week's vacation, and went to see Stevie the first day that we arrived. The next two days we could not visit, so we visited a museum in Leavenworth that was very interesting and sad, highlighting and honoring the Buffalo soldiers—the Black soldiers who fought up front in Indian and other wars from 1866 and beyond. Then, we checked out the casinos in Kansas City. The next day, we thought we would do some more sightseeing before we could see Stevie again, but Steve was very sick with a cold and cough. I spent that day in the motel room while he slept. I knew that Steve was trying to tell me something that day, but he didn't. He went out to bring some food back to the room. I really didn't want to know what he was going to tell me, so I prepared for whatever was coming. What could it be? Was he going to ask me for a divorce?

The next day, we went back to see Stevie. Leavenworth prison was made out of a massive amount of cement as well as electrical barbed wire fences to deter escapes. They had an open lift for people in wheelchairs. It rose straight to the top of 20 steps that were in front of the building to an entrance near a waiting room for visiting inmates. On the day we arrived, however, the lift was broken. Steve went into the building to ask for assistance, because we might have to leave without another visit. My wheelchair weighed 254 pounds without me and I'm not going to tell you what I weighed! An administrator and a guard came out where Steve entered the building, and I was frisked. Then, they shut down the electrical charge on the gate, opened it, and took me towards a flat entrance into the building. The building area was filled with empty, but barred cement cells. I did not talk much, since I really didn't want them to keep me there! We arrived at an antique elevator that had a narrow door with three steps in front of it. Two more recruited staff carried me up two steps, and squeezed my wheelchair through a narrow elevator doorway. When the elevator button was pushed, it took a while to go up one floor where there were no steps. My escorts left me in the waiting room where I finally saw Steve, again. Did I really just break into Leavenworth prison? Didn't most people try to break out?

After we saw Stevie again, our next stop was Jesse James' family farm in Kearney, Missouri, which had a lot of history. The most memorable were another break-in and a thunder bucket.

The pouring rain had stopped, and the tour guide wasn't really familiar with a portable ramp for visitors in wheelchairs. First, she put it on upside down, and it sunk deeply into the mud.

I asked her, "Is there a back door?"

"Yes!" she said.

We walked around the old farm house where there was only one step. I suggested that she flip the ramp over the opposite way, and I rolled up it onto the back porch. The guide tried to open the back door with no luck. It was hinged at the top, so I suggested that she go inside, and unlock it.

"Good idea!" she said.

After we "broke in" and joined the rest of the tour, we saw Jesse's living area, which was large. There was a hole that went into the ceiling where the slaves slept. I must have been hot up there. In the bedroom, they had a large pot, which they called the "thunder bucket" which was appropriately named! It was used as a commode when people were sick, or couldn't go to the outhouse.

From Kearney, we drove to St. Joseph, Missouri, where Jesse's wife and family lived. It was also where he was shot to death in the back while he was hanging a picture. We didn't have to break in, and a ramp wasn't needed.

Steve felt better, and his cold was going away. He started telling me again that his doctor wanted him to share something with me. Huh? What? He still waited until we got home, and then I put pressure on him to finish telling me. Steve's surprise? Not only did he use up my whole savings of $15,000, but borrowed $18,000 against the van I had purchased a year ago, and he had another $100,000 loan with my signature on paperwork. I screamed and cried! His answer was suicide. That was totally not appropriate. People have to stand up to their decisions and responsibilities. I was angry, because he had made the same promise, twice before, not to gamble. I could understand addiction, yet I would never totally trust him again. At that point, my feelings changed permanently. I was alone and afraid, and Steve helped me find legal counsel. I was angry, but that did not mean I wanted him dead. I went through a bunch of mixed emotions. I finally decided on divorce to separate the money.

My van was going to be repossessed.

"We can hide your vehicle in our garage until things get worked out," a couple of people suggested.

That was crazy! I was not a criminal! I called a top banker where the bank held the van loan. Coincidently, I knew him through MDA, and he straightened it out. I still had to pay $9000 - again - to keep my own van. I had made a mistake, and let Steve sign the van paperwork, so the van was actually under his name. I changed that fast. The $100,000 was dropped, because of a technicality. What a fiasco!

I spoke to Lloyd once every year or two even after I married, and I called him. He told me to get Steve out of the house immediately. I couldn't do that, even though it was everybody's opinion. I felt that I would be fine if I separated the finances. When the divorce was finalized the following year, Steve said to continue just as if we were still married. I didn't think I could do that.

And, then he added, "We would take care of each other."

I could do that and agreed.

"Yes."

I went to his next psychiatric appointment with him, and let the doctor know what my plans were. The doctor was a good man. How did I feel about Steve? I still enjoyed gambling, but never gambled crazy. I would go with friends, but I never wanted him to go gambling with me again. I could never complain about his care of me. It wasn't that he didn't complain, because he always complained, but he was always there when I needed him. We were friends as well as family—that was what I felt.

Lloyd always seemed like family, too. I believe it was around this time that he told me he was having some problems with seizures while he slept and taking medication. Whenever I called him, I would just say, "Hello", and he would recognize my voice immediately. It always surprised me. I would call to just say hi or check on how things were going with everyone. I would plan on talking five minutes or so, but he would talk about a half-hour or more. He always took time to talk to me, never thought I was bothering him, and made me feel strong.

Lloyd told me that June had passed away. I was not sure what year she passed, but her death reminded me of how vulnerable I was. She was ill, and I remembered that June always slept near the edge of her bed. I was told that she fell into some blankets on the floor and smothered. Even though June had a live-in attendant, the aide didn't hear her call.

Recently, and I don't scare easily, I smelled smoke in the middle of the night. The smoke alarm sounded as I called for Steve, but he never answered. I tried to use my telephone to call his cell phone, but my voice recognition was masked by the sound of the smoke alarm. Steve walked into my room. He was cooking bacon, but I was only able to smell the smoke, not the bacon! He was opening the front door for the smoke to escape; he could not hear me call, because of the blaring alarm. I was worried that smoke had overtaken him, and just waiting for the fire to reach me! What to do next time? Always have a cell phone by me? No. Not feasible in the middle of the night, because I can't reach for anything.

Involving work, two other things happened. First, I went to a Social Security hearing to assist one of my clients. The judge indicated, "Let the claimant's record show that the DVR counselor is in a wheelchair." What did that have to do with the client's case? Nothing at all!

Occasionally, after he retired, Merle drove me to wherever I needed to go for DVR in the summers. When we got home, he took me into the house, and set me by the telephone in the living room. I told him he didn't have to lock the front door when he left, because Steve should be home in a half hour. An hour went by he didn't come home. The phone rang, and I thought for sure it was Steve. I reached for it when my driving hand fell off my controls, and I missed the speaker button. I tried to move my other hand, but it also fell down over the left side of my wheelchair. I was stuck; I couldn't move at all. I was happy that I learned patience, or I might have panicked, and that would be no help at all. After a while my arms started to become numb.

I thought, "The worst thing that could happen was if something happened to Steve, and I'd be stuck here alone until morning."

The telephone rang, again.

"I called before, but nobody answered. I called Merle to see if he had brought you home, yet. We are both worried about you. Merle said that he left the front door unlocked, and was going to be coming shortly to see what happened." It was my Mom leaving a message.

Moms were great, weren't they? God Bless Moms! They always knew when you needed help. I was so happy to hear her voice and to see Merle. Steve called just as Merle arrived to let me know he would be home soon. He was interpreting for someone at the jail.

Whenever I was in a precarious situation, or I was just being myself, Steve would compliment me and say, "You are more of a woman than any woman I have known, and you have more balls than any man I know!" He always told me that he was happy to have me in his life even though I was a lot of work!

Steve took me into the Dells when I had to go to another conference. This one was an answer to my prayers. They were considering a new program called the Medical Assistance Purchase Plan (MAPP). I might be eligible for this program since I was now single and had no savings. The program would allow up to $15,000 of savings and a person could buy into medical assistance if a person had been made medically eligible for Social Security. I knew that I would be physically eligible for Social Security, but not be eligible for a financial benefit, which I didn't need because I was working. The program would be looking at salaries 250%, or less at poverty level. I could have been eligible for that and my final premium was $50 a month. My understanding was that retirement funds were not counted. Medical assistance was the only insurance program that paid attendant care, and I was eligible. Steve had diabetes, the beginnings of dementia, and he was 61 years old. He couldn't get me up and out of bed any longer. If an attendant didn't show up, I couldn't get to work. I also found out that there was some assistance for feeding me lunch at work through a special medical assistance program so that people with severe disabilities could continue working. If eligible, I wouldn't have to ask staff for lunch help.

When I got back home from the conference, I started applying for the Social Security Determination on my physical status in January, because it would take about four months at the time, to determine my eligibility.

The divorce was finalized in May of 2001, and my Determination came in June. God was working overtime again. Steve was retirement age, so he retired, and applied for Social Security Disability. It was possible that some problems were from his boxing career.

I encouraged a lot of my clients to apply for the MAPP program, simply because it would be very helpful to them. I recalled talking to the administrator of the program about money that I had saved during my teaching days. My Dad had taken care of this money, so I didn't know its origin. When I first applied, we both thought it would not be a problem. I never thought of bringing it up, again. My other savings were gone, but I did have a burial insurance, and that counted. It looked like we had covered everything.

I now had access to the only medical insurance that covered attendant care. Nursing care was covered to some extent by every insurance company, but I did not need nursing care. Attendant care coverage cost a lot less. The only problem with attendant care for people with chronic issues was that the limitations, the need for service, and the cost would continue for the rest of the person's life. That was why other insurances did not cover attendant care, and also the reason why people quit their jobs to become eligible for medical assistance. It was impossible to cover attendant care, along with normal living costs, without a job that paid very well, and was dependent on the number of hours of care needed.

Through the independent living center, Society's Assets, a nurse evaluated my needs, and determined that approximately 6 hours per day was needed. I needed two hours to get up, two hours after work for personal care, eating and getting back in bed, and about two hours during the night which was about an hour to get comfortable in laying down, personal care, and turning up to four times during the night. Steve was in the home, and covered the last 2 hours of the day. We were divorced now, so he could do that job.

Finding a person to commit to 5:30 a.m. was difficult even with the help of agencies, because not many of the clients on MAPP worked full time. Occasionally, people had to get up very early for medical tests. I was still able to hold needing to go to the bathroom until after work at 5:00 p.m. I only needed an hour for lunch during the work days.

Health-wise, drinking was always an issue. In the mornings, I would drink about 16 ounces of water, which would drain through in about 1 1/2 hours, giving me a half hour to finish getting dressed and out of bed. At noon, for lunch, one of two women would assist me— Sarah or Sandy. I would drink eight more ounces and try to get another 16 ounces in for supper. Getting undressed at night did not take long. In the morning, because I had a professional job, I had to take time for my makeup. I was still wearing a wig, so that didn't take long. I would take sponge baths in bed usually doing my body in parts: my hair one day, my upper body another day and my legs at another time.

Over the years, I have had many attendants—some that I have hired myself, and others that were sent by an agency. Everyone was so different. It was fun when personalities clicked. Bea was one of my favorites, because she was very focused on getting the job done, but having fun at the same time. Once we got into a conversation about stereotyping in the movies, because of an old movie I was watching on TV.

I asked Bea, "What stereotypes about white people are portrayed in movies?"

Bea laughed, "If a white person hears something going on outside, they run out of the building right away! They get shot, or beaten up—a black person is smarter than that! We stay inside until everything is over!"

Renée was really into politics, so I learned a lot. Mindy, my niece, was an attendant for me while she was in college. She was the only one I would trust with a shower. Other attendants were too serious, and some appeared not to like the job at all. There was only one person I had who once decided to lift my leg with my toe—why? Ouch! The major benefit of using an agency was that if an attendant was sick, or didn't show up, you could always call the agency, and still get to work close to the right time.

Once I went to Madison to speak to a small group of doctors and people on the medical assistance policy committee. There were a lot of younger people who had care needs. For patients who were younger and able to self-direct their own care, we were recommending a nurse review of care plans only once every 6 months instead of every two months. To save money, we recommended having a nurse four times a year less, or upon request as needed for those people that developed a specific need. That would be a savings of $120 per person per year, which was a huge savings, since there were several thousand people being taken care of statewide. There was one doctor on the committee who looked as if he was 93 years old, and said that no one could direct his or her own care like a nurse or doctor. Personally, I knew when I was having skin care problems or other issues. I was sure that when that doctor would need these services himself, he would be able to direct his own care. Anyway, that change in policy was eventually accepted.

Thus, my life changed again. I enjoyed having a woman assist me. A man never really looked at detail or choice, and believed that whatever was easiest worked. Steve helped me two hours at night for a while without pay. Since our divorce was finalized, he felt good about bringing in a small paycheck, now. I could be alone for long periods of time, but I never felt safe if I was alone while I was lying down. I also had more control of what time I wanted to go to bed, because Steve was there. I could go to bed at different times on different nights rather than at a specific time every night if someone else was attending me.

Again, Stevie was transferred to a prison in Pekin, Illinois, where we could visit him a little more often, because it was a four hour drive.

Alicia was now six years old, and into games. Evelyce was three, and didn't understand them, so she would come into my bedroom where we played games on the bed, and mess up our bingo, or Candyland. Alicia would yell at her to get out of the room. Evelyce would run to Grandpa Steve to tell on her. She would make up stories.

"Grandpa, Grandma hit me!"

Grandpa was shocked, since he knew I couldn't lift my arm.

"Grandma hit you?"

Evelyce would enhance her stories.

"Yes Grandpa! Right here!" and point to her arm.

Grandpa played along and yelled at me.

"Grandma, why did you hit Evelyce?"

That would panic Evelyce.

"Oh no Grandpa, I lied."

"What?"

Evelyce continued with her head down.

"I lied."

While Alicia always rode on the back of my chair, Evelyce liked riding on my pedals.

I developed osteoporosis, fragile bones, especially in my wrists causing me to take medication once a week, and had to drink at least eight ounces of water. Then, I had to sit straight up for a half hour, before I could lie down, or eat anything. Arlene, who took the same medication, laid down forgetting she needed to sit up for the half hour, and because of this, helped me to avoid the same problem. She thought that she was going to die! I am still on the medication for the disease, but the medication has brought my bones closer to normal density. I also stopped going swimming, because when people would put me in the pool, one person would go underneath my arms and grab my wrists as another carried my legs. I didn't want to take a chance on breaking anything, especially my wrists. Now, at camp, there is a hydraulic lift by the pool.

Now…where the heck did I put my bathing suit?

~ 25 ~

A cruise, A Move, and Bad News

I always wanted to go on a cruise, but did not really know if the ships were accessible. About the year 2000, Merle and Jeff cruised a lot, and wanted us to go with them on a trip they were planning. The trip came just before I was eligible for attendant care, but it was not covered for a vacation. One of the Easter Seals camp counselors, Sarah (Cheesy), had been giving me a bath once a week, and was going to school at UW Parkside in Kenosha. I asked her if she could fit our trip into her schedule. Steve was glad an attendant was coming with us, because he couldn't handle me alone, especially in an unfamiliar environment.   Merle   liked to travel Royal Caribbean, so we chose to go on the *Grandeur of the Sea*s. We were routed from Chicago through Detroit, and I did not like the Detroit airport. Quite a while passed before someone arrived with a wheelchair to transfer me to the correct terminal, and onto the plane to Miami. Both Sarah and Jeff lifted me into the airplane seat, although the airport staff normally did it. Everything went according to plan in Miami, and even an accessible van met us at the airport.

When we arrived at the ship, I noticed that it looked like a huge hotel, and the accessibility was great! We had barely settled in our cabin, when they called everyone on deck for the lifeboat drill. We put on our life jackets, and went to our designated lifeboat. I hoped that I would remember everything in case of a real emergency. After the drill, we stayed on deck, and watched the shoreline as the ship pulled out of the harbor city block by city block. My eyes focused on the buildings. All of a sudden, I saw the water hitting the beach, and my head turned in the opposite direction—solid water with nothing else in sight! I looked back at the disappearing coastline, and wondered if I had made a mistake!

When Sarah, Steve, and I went back to the cabin, it had a porthole window where we could see the sun was setting just above the water. The window looked like a photograph on the wall. It was picturesque and serene even though it moved up and down a bit. I never got seasick, but Jeff did.

When arrived at our first port, I stayed on the boat, because we were on one of the beaches in Haiti. I knew my wheelchair would not go through the sand. I did not want to transfer into a chair that had big, balloon wheels, nor did I want to board a small tender (boat) which bounced up and down in the waves. So, instead, Merle and I investigated the ship. It had a big shopping area; casino, theater, and a daily newsletter that let you know what was going on in the different areas of the ship. There were several places to eat along with about six bars. There was one dining room located on the nose of the ship so one could see the water. Haiti seemed like a very poor place. The residents had little boats where they used old blue jeans and shirts as sails. As we were all sitting and eating lunch, we saw a huge waterspout in the distance. Weren't waterspouts dangerous? No one else seemed to pay attention. It was very skinny, long, and far away! But, couldn't that be dangerous?

While we were docked, the casino was closed. Of course, Sarah, Jeff, and I went to the casino the first night we sailed, and I taught Sarah how to play blackjack. She was so proud she could play it that by the end of the week, she had earned her first $100 chip.

The next day, we pulled into San Juan harbor in Puerto Rico. I felt like I was a 16th century pirate attacking the majestic stone fort used as a Guardian Point to the Spanish Caribbean. It was much easier to get off the boat here than it was in Haiti, and we traveled down the long harbor until we reached a pier.

I loved Puerto Rico! Sarah and I walked through the harbor area to the older section of the city, which had no curb cuts. We found one broken curb that my electric chair could climb to get into a few of the stores. The houses in the area were next to each other, and very colorful. There was a bright blue house, an orange house, a bright green house, and a yellow house. As we were walking, I couldn't really get onto the sidewalks, but that was okay, because I was going faster than the traffic, and traffic jams were everywhere. The drivers were very nice and patient, and treated me as if I was a car.

Of course, we found a casino. Puerto Ricans played the game differently, but it was still blackjack. When the dealer dealt the cards, all of the players would get their second cards before the dealers dealt their own. I wasn't sure how that affected the odds. Also, when I gave the dealer a tip, I had to put it a little off center on top of my bet.

When it came time to leave Puerto Rico, the sun had set. As we cruised out of the harbor, Steve was in the cabin while Merle and I were on the top deck. Not sure where Jeff and Sarah were. The lights were on around the fort. Merle made a remark.

"Steve should really be up here with you, not me."

But, Steve wasn't feeling well. He loved all the eating on the boat, but all the eating didn't agree with his diabetes so, it was hard to include him in anything except sleeping, reading, eating, watching boxing, and gambling. He always took me anywhere I wanted to go, but never participated in many of the activities.

I really did not feel much of the movement of the ship, and the waves were actually calm throughout our cruise. Since Steve was in the Navy, he thought that he would be bouncing off the walls, but this ship was much bigger, and carried about 3000 people plus the crew. Occasionally, but seldom, would I feel just a little swish under my wheelchair as if two waves had hit at an angle. Steve, just once, basked in the hot tubs that were on the top deck of the ship. When he wasn't eating, he was reading, or sleeping in the cabin.

Sarah went swimming in one of the swimming pools, and I enjoyed going back and forth from the front of the ship to the back of the ship just looking into the water. Every once in a while, we could see a glimpse of Cuba, and we also partially sailed through the Bermuda Triangle. I was glad that we never told Steve until after we were through it, because he would have been terrorized for the whole trip! While I was on the ship's deck one day, a little girl came over to me and said, "My Mom is sitting over there, and she said you were one of her teachers." I even knew someone on the ship!

To send an e-mail to my program assistant, JoAnne, at work, it cost 50 cents a minute. She was surprised to hear from me, and the staff told me she screamed out my name when she saw who sent the e-mail.

BY THE GRACE OF GOD AND YOU
A Chair Does Not a Person Make

St. Thomas was next on our cruise. It was a beautiful little island. It was different, because the cars' steering wheels were on the left, and they drove on the left side of the street. The one clerk I talked to said that most people walked to their jobs. I shopped by myself, and the deals were good! I bought some earrings for my sister, a necklace for my Mom, and a watch and a ring for Steve.

One night, we went to a captain's reception, and on another, to see the 50's singing group, the Platters. Most of the doors were automatic, and I could use everything, except for the elevators, independently. One day, I went on the top deck, and watched ice sculpting - in 87-degree weather! At midnight on another day, I went to the buffet to see all the sculpted food, and ate chocolate.

Our last stop was an island in the Bahamas where people enjoyed the beaches, and then, on to Miami and back home.

In 2002, Merle asked if we would go on another cruise, because there was one huge ship that he wanted us to see. It was still Royal Caribbean, but this time the ship was the *Explorer of the Seas*. It probably held 5000 people counting the crew. Steve was up to going on another cruise, and so was I! Mindy had just turned 20, and she was ready to go! We both hoped the cruise line would allow her to help me in the casino.

Once we decided on all of the "shipmates", Merle and I went to the travel agent. We knew the ship we were going to be on, but costs were higher than before. I knew about what I could spend, but Merle really wanted us to be in a balcony stateroom, so we could feel the warm breeze off the ocean, because the windows on the last ship did not open. I was very surprised when he told us, "I want to pay the difference for all three of you to be on a larger ship and in a balcony room!" Wow! What a friend!

This time, I was better organized about the travel plans. I requested a letter for airport security that I had gel cell batteries, so they knew they would not explode on the plane. Then the airport staff would not have to take my wheelchair apart - and *no one ever* reassembled right! We booked a non-stop flight so we would not have to change airplanes. We also made sure there was a handicapped accessible bus waiting for us at the Fort Lauderdale airport to take us to the cruise ship in Miami. Most everything went smoothly, except that Merle and Jeff had an airplane ticket mix-up, which took a while to fix, but since it was done early, they did not miss the flight.

For the last 20 minutes of our flight, I had "caboose pain." When I first was lifted onto the plane seat, it felt like I had a "wedgie." When I was lifted back into my wheelchair, it felt like something came out of me. I didn't smell anything, so I thought it was okay, and I was happy to be on the ship. We rushed through our paperwork—tickets, birth certificate, credit cards, etc., and finally got into the balcony stateroom. I quickly had Mindy put me on the commode in my chair. I was covered with blood and feces, and had to throw away my slacks. I had hemorrhoids and thought maybe one of them was bleeding, and even though the problem calmed down, it had not stopped by the next morning. Mindy took me to the two Swedish doctors on board the ship, helped them put me on the table. They examined my caboose with a long inserted device.

"We do not think that this is a hemorrhoid problem. The blood is coming from too high up. We're not sure what the problem is. This medication may help you. If it doesn't help you, you cannot get off at the next island. The Grand Cayman Island would be the first chance for you to get to an airport to fly home if needed." I hoped that the pills would work, and I sent an e-mail JoAnne again, asking her to call my doctor. I wanted to let him know what was going on so that my insurance would cover it.

Merle took me on tour of the new ship. There was a basketball court and a rock-climbing wall, which no one should climb on a windy day on a ship. There was a theater where Ricky Nelson's sons performed, an ice skating rink and show, as well as a shopping area where a Mardi Gras parade was held. And, that was just a few things available on the ship!

The next day, I was feeling better, the weather was perfect, and I even took the tender to the beach. I did not stay long, but I did investigate a shopping area on the shore.

It was raining a little by the time we arrived at the island of Jamaica. When we left the dock, a few Jamaicans asked if we wanted dreadlocks put into our hair. I forgot how long they said it would take, and I realized I could just leave my wig with them, but I quickly decided against it. I was pleased to know there was an accessible handicapped vehicle available for hire, but we just decided to walk down the street. I couldn't find a curb to go down unless I backtracked a long way. Four Jamaicans lifted my chair off the curb and onto the curb across the street. I gave them $5 for the help. Steve and I then went into a McDonalds. Their money was also called "dollars," but the cost of a happy meal was over $5000! It took me a while to adjust to such a huge difference in the value of the currency. In the shopping area, a man sang reggae to us. I always enjoyed that type of music, and then, we walked back to the ship.

The next island we went to was the Grand Cayman Islands, and luckily, my bleeding had stopped. There was no dock on this island, and the ocean was very rough. It was not safe for me to be carried onto the tender, because the stairs were going up and down in the opposite movements with the ship. I believe that Mindy had spent some time with dolphins on Jamaica, and decided to spend some quality time in the sun on this island! This ship definitely had more things to do, but the other ship seemed more elegant with many more chandeliers.

The next place with a dock was Cozumel. They had a beautiful new shopping area adjacent to the dock as well as many soldiers and military equipment.

On this trip, this ship was much bigger, like a huge hotel with at least ten stories of multiple inside and Oceanside cabins. Accessibility was great, and I could even get into Merle and Jeff's cabin just down the hall. I particularly enjoyed the cabin. The breeze from the ocean was beautiful in the evening, the cabin had more floor space. The cabin attendants folded our new towels into different animal shapes every day, and using our lost sunglasses on the animal they created.

The food was scrumptious! I particularly remember a chilled, watermelon soup that had a few onions in it which made the flavor burst in your mouth. There was double chocolate, fudge rum cake, too. Mindy bought a cookbook, and made the same cake several times after she returned home.

When we reached the airport, I really enjoyed the "futuristic" train ride going straight to the terminal. The ride was fast, but smooth, and people were standing or holding onto poles rather than sitting.

Unfortunately, my letter about the wheelchair did not work at this airport, and the workers took my wheelchair apart anyway. Many did not speak English, and although Steve spoke Spanish, I was sent back several times for a pass and a tag that I did not need. When I finally got off the plane in Milwaukee, the hand control was hanging when my wheelchair reached me, the clutches were off which meant that the chair brakes were off, and probably rolling around in the belly of the plane! I wanted to cry! Bob and Susie picked us up at the airport, and Bob, without tools, put my wheelchair back together. Thank you Bob!

When I got home, for about 5 months, I forgot about the bleeding that I had. But, at the end of fall, it started again. I was so embarrassed, because it was something I could not control. My doctor suggested I go to a specialist, and I went to see him the day before I had a meeting in Madison, and told him about it. I asked him about it.

"Do you think I can still go to my meeting? I could take care of this when I come back."

"If I were you, I'd go straight to the hospital," he said.

I opted to follow his advice, and colonoscopy was performed. It was found that I had diverticulitis. The doctor wanted to know what pill they gave me aboard ship to stop the bleeding, but I didn't know, and he could only hope the bleeding would stop. I was in the hospital for four or five days. One of the nurses who took care of me was going to be off the following day.

"I'm off tomorrow. I hope I get to see you again."

Did that mean she just wanted to see me again, or that I was so ill that nobody might see me again? Once the bleeding stopped, she admitted something to me.

"You know, I wasn't really sure what was going to happen. You were very weak."

I really didn't know how weak I was until I got better. After I had lost about 3 pints of blood mixed with feces, the bleeding finally stopped. My doctor told me that many people were told not to eat seeds or nuts, but there was no proof that if I did stop eating these things, the problem wouldn't happen again. Occasionally, I had problems with pain in the left upper quadrant of my stomach. If that happened to me, I stopped eating seeds and nuts for a while. Otherwise, my diet has stayed the same. I haven't had any other occurrences of diverticulitis. And, just because someone didn't feel well, didn't mean a person wouldn't go to work and continue living their life. I caught up with my work emails from the hospital.

There were other "movements" occurring. Gavino and Heather weren't getting along, so Heather and the girls moved 300 miles up north to be near Heather's Mom. Now the Grandkids were far away. Eventually, Heather earned a business degree, and a few years ago, remarried. She was doing well. I'm proud of her. It wasn't easy.

In June 2003, Gavino married Natalie. I was hoping he would stop using alcohol and drugs. I took it as a good sign when the judge that married them was the same judge that had sentenced him to jail for a DWI. Gavino teased, "Before the Judge gave me a few months in jail. Now that he performed my marriage, he gave me a life sentence!"

By now, I had a lot of problems at the house dealing with the snow removal, getting the lawn mowed, and having the strength to go up and down my ramp without problems. I really wanted to live in a place that had no stairs or ramps, and had an attached garage.

Louise's sister had moved into a new condo built on the north side of town, and I went to see it. Steve thought it would be a good idea to move there, too, so I started to plan. Within the next few months, I put a down payment on a unit. Luckily, I had caught my condo unit in its construction phase, and the cost of the changes was minimal because no construction changes had to be made. So, I asked for lower light switches and an accessible shower to be built into the master bathroom - all for less than $200 difference! I listed my house for sale in late fall, and hoped that it would sell before my condo would be done, estimating that would be approximately late the next spring of 2004.

At my job, I was working with others on a project to make people more familiar with the problems people with disabilities have doing the simple things and just adjusting to daily life. I still couldn't believe people took 10-minute showers! I thought it was important to inform people, disabled or not, all did the same things, but with a disability, they also had to adjust activities that would allow them to be involved in community events as well as work. Remember, it was not worse having a disability; it was only different. It took time to adjust, because they do things differently.

October was Disability Awareness Month. This article describes what we did that year:

October 2, 2003 *Kenosha News* **It All Has To Come From You** by Liz Berger.

Local event celebrates those with disabilities. Carol Schaufel is a Chicago Cubs fan who plays the harmonica. She also happens to be disabled, but she prefers people focus on the first two attributes. "I think it's important that people don't come to see your chair, that they see you as a person first," said Carol, who has a neuromuscular disorder and uses an electric wheelchair.

Increasing awareness of people with disabilities was one of the goals of an event Wednesday called "Celebrating People with Disabilities—Living and Working in Kenosha." It was sponsored by the Kenosha County Division of Aging Services and other agencies, held at the Kenosha Public Museum during Disability Awareness Month. It featured two speakers who talked about disabilities.

A pictorial display highlighting 11 disabled people, including Carol, who live and work in Kenosha County was at the Museum Wednesday and will be displayed at various locations until the end of the month. Frank Germinaro, principal at St. Mark's School and former director of the Kenosha Pops Band, is featured in the pictorial. He spoke Wednesday about the importance of having a positive attitude. When he was young he suffered from renal disease and got a kidney transplant. Because of his outlook and the support of his family, he is "still going strong." "If you're disabled you need support," he said. "You can't do it on your own." But, he added, "It all has to come from you."

Keynote speaker Tom Hlavacek, Milwaukee office director of the Wisconsin Coalition of Advocacy, said that over the years society has become more accepting of people with disabilities. People used to stereotype disabled people as incapable of doing what nondisabled people could do. He said that attitude changed as disabled people started to assert their rights and society began to acknowledge that they belonged in the mainstream.

BY THE GRACE OF GOD AND YOU
A Chair Does Not a Person Make

"The pivotal event in the history of the disabled people's movement was the enactment of the Americans with Disabilities Act in 1990. The law, however, was more of a milestone event in and to the problem of discrimination." Tom said.

Some people featured in the pictorial spoke privately Wednesday about the experience of living with a disability. Teresa Gilliland, 42, is blind due to a disorder called retinitis pigmentosa. She said she is actually more able today in some ways than 12 years ago when she developed the disorder. "I am a much better listener, more organized," she said. Even her 19-year-old daughter, Tiffany, who helped her Mother around the Museum Wednesday, said that she has developed positive qualities, like patience, as a result of having to help her Mom.

Armando Olivares, 45, has fibromyalgia and cannot work because of it. He said he has had to learn to live with his disability. That means remembering to use both hands when he drinks a glass of water. "It changed my life through the years," he said. "It changes constantly."

Rich Fedor, a student at the University of Wisconsin Parkside who interviewed people for the pictorial, said he learned a lot about disabled people after working with them. "It was really nice getting to know the people for who they are and not just their disability," he said

Moving took a lot of organization. First, I had to tell the construction workers where I wanted the height of the light switches, and choose an appropriate accessible shower for my wheelchair. I met with the condo reps for the color of the rug, style of the kitchen cupboards, and other options. A former client, Armando, interpreted Spanish for our DVR office, and did an excellent job painting the condo with his daughter, Samantha. He became a friend when he joined the local Easter Seals Service Unit in 1999, and since 2002 had been going to Easter Seals camp and WWAAC. Armando had multiple skills that he could no longer use on a competitive basis, because of his fibromyalgia, which caused chronic fatigue and pain. It is very unusual for males to have it, and is more debilitating. He had worked in construction and as a machine assembler. Holding a hammer or paintbrush in his hand was difficult. A five-pound grasp was secure for a short period of time.

As the condo was being painted, the garage door opener was being installed. I monitored the progress of my condo. I was surprised that it was set up the opposite of Patty's condo (Louise's sister), which meant I had to rethink the floor plan for the furniture placement in all of the rooms. I found a beautiful china cabinet at St. Vincent DePaul for only $50 - $110 with delivery. Two Men and a Truck was a highly recommended moving company, and perfect for my needs. One of Steve's friends, Alfredo, and a counselor, Gary, from KAC, along with my son, Gavino, would bring the boxes and other smaller items.

By the time I was supposed to close on the condo, my house had not yet sold. I took a short-term loan out on the value of the house to pay for the condo. Two months later, the house was sold. I was given a date of May 29 to move into my new condo.

Everything was ready to go on May 29. However, Gavino's wife, Natalie, was in the hospital, and her labor had begun, so Gavino couldn't help. The movers loaded up the truck, and Steve and I followed the truck to the condo. I told the movers where to put each piece of furniture as they brought it inside. Everything fit! Armando installed the vertical blinds, while

Alfredo and Gary piled everything they had brought into the middle of the living room floor, which was sorted later.

Gavino's baby was born the next day—my first grandson! Steve and I went to see the baby, the new Daddy, and Natalie. Their little boy was about a week early - which was good for his Mother, and perfect timing for his Dad to avoid some "moving" work.

We were living closer to Gavino's family, now. As the baby grew, I had more of a chance to see all of them. We were very happy when Natalie decided to be baptized with her son. Later, though, I was so mad when I realized that I had erased the video we filmed!

Stevie was released from a halfway house, and moved in with us about a month later. We were trying to find him a place to live, but he wasn't eligible for housing, because of his offenses. He would not be eligible for five years, unless he continued good behavior. There was no other place for him to go, so Stevie stayed here. He seemed to be better. We set the parameters with our guidelines, and he seemed to be following them well, and he took some medication prescribed for him.

That same year, we had another addition to our family born November 5. It was a little "Shidoodle" puppy—a Shih Tzu and Poodle combination. Stevie picked out the only black puppy in the litter. We all had a chance to meet with the puppy a few times, before we bought her. She came to live with us sometime around Christmas. The puppy was just six months younger than Gavino Junior.

We named her Chaparita, which is Spanish for little squirt or little cute girl, and pretty tricky! She had little tiny sharp claws, would get excited, and scratch my chin and cheek area enough to make it bleed causing me to scream. She only did that twice, as she learned more about me, would come to me on her front knees so she wouldn't hurt me with her paws! She learned fast, except training her to go into a dog litter box was hard. She would almost catch on to the idea, but finally, trained Steve to take her outside.

Stevie decided that he wanted to be the one to take Chappy, which was her nickname, to puppy training. That was a bad idea, because puppy was more interested in the treats than learning commands. Stevie learned how to roll over, sit, and shake hands! For a treat, Chappy learned how to stand on her hind legs and turn in a circle. Merle came to visit a lot, and he and Chappy got along well.

Chappy slept with me until she was about a year old. Something unexplainable happened at that time. Whenever I had a lot of pain in my back, I slept sitting up leaning forward on a pillow. One night, I called for Steve to move me, and I heard the door open and close. The dog started barking like crazy, and lifted my head. It was dark, and I thought I saw Steve nose to nose with Chappy less than two feet from me.

"Why are you making the dog bark like that!" I asked him.

The head turned toward me. I could see an unusual smile that somehow I recognized. In the meantime, the dog continued to bark. The figure rose, and backed away from me.

"Who is this? If this is a burglar, is Steve knocked out in the living room? Dare I try to use my voice activation phone to call for help?" I thought.

I tried to yell for Steve again, and the figure had backed all the way to the door. All of a sudden, the door opened, and Steve turned on the light. The sheet like figure immediately disappeared.

"What is that dog barking at?" he asked.

I told Steve what happened, but he didn't believe me. Steve thought that I was dreaming. So, I had to ask Steve the question.

"If I were dreaming, why was Chappy barking?"

He couldn't explain, so he laid me back down, and slept with me for a while when he normally he slept with the lights and television on in the living room. Surprisingly, I was not afraid, and went right back to sleep. Thinking about the incident off and on for a few weeks, I thought that haunting smile was my Dad's silly smile when he was teasing me. Maybe it was Dad who just came to see how things were going.

In summer of 2005, the State of Wisconsin gave Recognition Service Awards to different departments and divisions such as Probation and Parole and DVR. DVR recognized three of their employees on a statewide basis. Kenny drove Stevie and me to Madison, so that I could accept one of the awards. Stevie thought it was very impressive to be able to sit with me in the State Assembly Chambers, and then, next to me on the assembly floor at one of the representative's desks. I received an award that day for my 'contribution and leadership in developing strategies for addressing accommodation issues from both practical and technological viewpoints.' It was said that these strategies would impact employees with disabilities in the Division of Vocational Rehabilitation and the Department of Workforce Development. After the ceremony, Stevie was impressed when he, Kenny, and I had our picture taken with Governor Doyle.

A few months later, Steve and Stevie had left to eat a late lunch, and I was home alone in bed. When Steve and Stevie came home, I heard something outside, but didn't think much about it. A few minutes later, Steve and an FBI agent came into my bedroom.

"When Stevie and I got out of the car, there were two FBI agents outside with guns drawn on us," Steve told me.

They frisked both of them, handcuffed Stevie, and read Stevie his Miranda rights. The FBI told the neighbors who were outside to go away. They brought Stevie inside to his bedroom. One man talked to Stevie alone while the other agent rifled through all of his drawers. A copy of a letter was with them that was allegedly written by Stevie, and addressed to a federal judge. It was Stevie's handwriting, and he was writing threatening letters, again. Steve had done everything that he could to try to keep Stevie out of trouble. For the longest time, every day, he would remind Stevie not to write any letters. It was starting again, and the agents took Stevie directly to the Milwaukee jail. This time, the judge gave him the maximum sentence of eight years.

Steve felt bad as nothing could really be done, but we went to all of Stevie's trials to support him. We still wished that Stevie would go to a mental health prison where he would have been in rehab. He was in Marion, Illinois, for a while, so one of my attendants, and her daughter, Zita, along with Nene, drove Steve and me down to see him. Stevie was transferred to Leavenworth, again, where he would stay until he was released to a pre-release center closer to home with an eventual discharge in 2014.

Steve became discouraged with condo living. When he first heard the word "condo,"

Steve thought it would be great!

"Wow! A lot of movie stars and boxers live in condos!"

But, the people were noisy moving around upstairs, and the condo rules were hard for him to follow after living in our own home for so long.

When we first moved here, we were the only occupants in the entire building. A bad storm allowed rain to enter the electrical box tripping the alarm. The firefighters came to the condo a couple of times. I always thought the alarm notified the fire station, but we had to call. After our second call, the firefighters told us what would happen the next time we called.

"You have to do something about this alarm, or we are going to have to charge you for coming the next time."

The problem was finally fixed only after another couple moved in the building. I couldn't really afford to move again, and I enjoyed the condo living. It was heaven for me not needing ramps, no snow shoveling, lawn maintenance, and a flat exit straight into the garage. Steve's depression was worsening, though.

In 2006, Merle passed away, and a month later, at Christmas, Arlene passed away. Both had been a big part of my life for decades. Merle was the first teacher I met when I taught at Bullen. I felt good that I was able to talk to him the night he died in the hospital.

"Your friendship has always been important to me. I love you," I told him.

He expressed the same to me. Jeff took care of the funeral service and the gravestone, which had a picture of a Royal Caribbean Ship lasered onto the marble along with a picture of his head in the foreground of the ship. Anchors were raised on the corners of the headstone. Etched with his name was "Sail away my friend". I was proud of Merle, because he donated his eyes, bone marrow, and skin. Merle was a very private person, but one thing that he really wanted to do was to donate organs and tissues that would be helpful for others. Although Merle probably wouldn't share this with anyone, Jeff and I thought this letter was mindboggling! It was from the Wisconsin Tissue Bank, Milwaukee. We could not believe how many lives his donation touched. If you decide to donate your tissue, this is how much you can help others.

November 25, 2008

Dear Jeff,

Thank you so much for allowing us the time to share some of the information about Merlin's tissue donation with you. In his death your friend helped many people with the generous gift of tissue donation. We can ensure you that Merlin helped at least 290 people through the gift of donated bone and soft tissue.

The number of people that your friend helped through his tissue donation is beyond anything that we can capture in this letter. We hope it comforts you to know that Merlin has impacted many lives throughout the country.

The information that is included below is bone and tissue donations that have been transplanted. Because we rely on the surgeons and staff to provide us with the information on how and where the bone grafts and tissues were transplanted, we cannot provide you with exact details about the recipients, nor can we guarantee you that this information is all-inclusive.

1. *Some of the many people your friend helped are:*
2. *3 people received the gift of bone or soft tissue for neck fusions*
3. *3 people received the gift of bone or soft tissue for spinal fusions*
4. *A person received the gift of bone or soft tissue for a cancer/trauma surgery to completely replace that piece of their bone and the surrounding tissues*
5. *72 people received the gift of bone, or soft tissue for orthopedic operations, those usually range from repairs of fractures or replacing bone loss from a number of different things: trauma, removal of screws, or bone tumors*
6. *211 people received the gift of bone or soft tissue for dental surgeries most often replacing bone loss for the removal of teeth or facial surgery from a traumatic injury*

It is very hard to put into words the profound impact of Merlin's donation. Although nothing will ever take his place, we hope this information provides you with the knowledge that some good has come from the loss of your friend. If you have any questions please do not hesitate to give us a call...

Arlene was an excellent role model for me from the start, and appropriate, since she worked so hard, and retired from the Navy base always working from her wheelchair. She had been going through a lot of pain for the last couple of years, and was bedridden by this time. She always told me this.

"You know, I was never very busy until you got me involved in everything you were doing!"

And, then, added the following.

"I don't know how you get done all that you do with your limitations! You can't scratch your own nose without help."

We definitely had respect for each other.

~ 26 ~

Mom's passing & Life After

Mom and I still played Scrabble every weekend after Dad passed away. She drove for another two years before her first stroke, and then, stopped driving. However, TIAs became a problem, and eventually, became strokes.

My Mom went into rehab after her first stroke learning how to walk again and take care of herself. While she was in rehab, we saw her three or four times a week, and drove back and forth to St. Luke's hospital. Her personality and accent changed. The hardest thing for her to remember while she was in rehab was to keep her legs uncrossed, so the blood could flow freely. At least nine times during our first few visits, we would remind her about it, and she would have a funny look on her face like her Mother did as if she was saying, "Dah! I did that again!" Mom was able to take care of herself, but also had fallen on occasion, but received therapy for it. Kenny lived with her after rehab for a while to help her, and then, she wanted to live on her own again.

We would giggle at the way she would describe her therapy when she was in the hospital.

"I played baseball today and my teammates would keep throwing the ball over my head! I couldn't catch it," she might tell us.

To keep her mind active, the doctor also wanted her to have many easy crossword puzzle books, and we played Scrabble, too. While she wasn't quite as fast, she was still good at it, and she even applied a seven-letter word or two! Instead of playing three games, however, we would play one. A couple of times, she would catch me falling asleep between turns. Another way to keep her mind active was with Louise, who was always like another daughter to her, and she enjoyed talking with her on the telephone. While in the winter, Steve would bring Mom to visit on weekend days, so that she would not have to worry about shoveling the snow off the ramp at her house.

Mom no longer enjoyed cooking. Although, Meals on Wheels brought food to her for a while, she didn't like the meals, and felt as if it was a waste of food. She did not like meat that well, but they brought it to her anyway. Mom did love Supervalu's Delicatessen, though, and would buy one pork rib at Supervalu's delicatessen providing her with at least three meals.

Mom continued having a lot of chest pains, and was admitted to the hospital multiple times. The doctors could find nothing, so they thought it was GERD (Gastro Esophageal Reflux Disease). During one of her hospitalizations, and when Susie took her home, it was apparent that the pain medication gave her delusions.

"Mom told me that she saw cobwebs in the corners as well as all over the ceiling and flowers growing out from under the rug!"

Susie told me what Mom had said to her.

"Susie, how could you let this house get so dirty?" Mom asked her.

"Mom, there is nothing there!" Susie had told her.

So, to prove that the flowers were there, Mom bent down to touch one, but there were no flowers. When she got in the bedroom, she told Susie that there were a lot of rabbits. Then, Mom pulled down the covers on her bed, saying there were dozens of delicious rolls and donuts. Luckily, I thought, it only lasted a few hours.

Susie was having problems too. She and Bob were visiting a museum in McHenry, Illinois, and when leaving, she slipped on a piece of Plexiglas. Bob couldn't catch her, and Susie broke her kneecap in four places. She had surgery in Illinois—bolts and screws—the works, and spent time in a nursing home receiving 8 hours on a CPM machine (Continual Perpetual Motion stimulator) and 2 hours of physical therapy a day. Most things could be replaced in a human body, but not a kneecap, so they bent her knee degree by degree until the cast was able to be removed permanently and she could bend her knee 90 degrees. Therapy continued for about a year and pain occasionally still exists.

Mom's pain continued, yet still wasn't afraid to be alone. When she was bad, she would call for an ambulance on her own, and unlock the door for the paramedics. We had to call an ambulance once while she was at our house, because Mom just couldn't breathe. After that episode, she told me that she just couldn't handle that pain anymore. To check out her heart, Mom scheduled her surgery for early October. I was always finished with my Christmas shopping by July. So, while waiting for her surgery, she kept busy wrapping all the Christmas presents I bought. Steve told Mom just to relax and not work so hard before the surgery.

"I might not come back from my surgery. Who would finish wrapping these last presents for Carol? I have to finish them!" she had told Steve.

"Oh, Mother-in-law, you will come out of this fine," he replied.

"How do you know? No one knows what the future is. I just don't want Carol to have to worry about this!" Mom retorted.

Mom also told me what others had said about me, and that I was an inspiration to a lot of people, and changed a lot of lives. I was never good at accepting compliments, and never knew what to do with them. This time, I really thought about what she was saying. I knew Mom was proud of both Susie and me. I was also touched by a little note from a new client.

"I know how busy your schedule is, yet every time I come to see you, I always feel that I'm your only client! Thank you for your help."

Clients, students, children, and volunteers always stopped to say "hi" to me. When I was shopping for school clothes for my grandchildren, a student of mine told me he was now a professor at UW Parkside.

Even my doctor had recently asked me a question.

"How do you stop from being depressed?"

"I work with so many people that have so many problems. My problems are nothing compared to theirs. I keep busy. There is no time to be depressed," I answered.

I was blessed to have a lot of support, too. I had good parents, supportive relatives, great friends, understanding coworkers, excellent teachers, and even strangers. I tried to do what I thought was right in any situation, and hoped that I didn't hurt anyone along the way. My favorite thing was to smile at people, if I caught their eye, and most smiled back.

Mom and I talked every night on the telephone, since I moved out when I was 38 years old. She did not think she was going to live after her surgery, but she was ready to go, and was not afraid. I was glad that we had talked a lot, because the morning of the surgery, we had to leave very early for the hospital, and it was foggy. The fog was thicker than I had ever seen it. By the time we arrived in Milwaukee, Steve and I barely made it to her room to say "hi" to her, before she went into surgery. Within five minutes after we arrived, an orderly came to take Mom. Everyone touched her, and gave her a hug. She put her hand out to touch me, before she was wheeled in the elevator, but missed. From the elevator, she threw a kiss, and I caught it.

Mom's four to six hours of surgery took 12 hours. The doctor finally came to us.

"Early in the surgery, she passed away, and we revived her. The main arteries of her heart were fine, but all of the smaller arteries were totally plugged. We did what we could, and put her on life support." The doctor felt that her situation was critical, but hopeful. Steve and I went home. Susie and Bob stayed.

We were back and forth to Milwaukee every day. Most of the time, either JoAnne or Armando would take me to the hospital after work. Susie worked late afternoons and evenings, so she and Kenny would go during the day. Mom never awoke from her coma, but at times it felt like she could understand us when we were talking to her. She did squeeze the hands of some people, and blinked her eyes as if she understood even though her eyes were never open. One side of Mom's body could not move, and Susie thought she may have had another stroke.

About eight days later, her kidneys stopped functioning. The fluid that built up caused stress on her heart. On the 10th day, and after rereading Mom's *Living Will*, the doctor realized maintaining her life this way was not what she wanted, and decided that it was cruel to keep her alive. So, life support was removed.

JoAnne drove me to the hospital that last day. We got to the hospital, and there was no light in her room. I asked at the desk where they had taken her, and the person indicated that she had passed away, and was still in the room. I went into the room alone. I went around the drawn curtain. Mom was covered up to her chin with a sheet. Her eyes were closed, and her mouth was open. I talked to her for a while, and thanked her for a good life. JoAnne came into the room for a while, too, before we went back home.

When we got home, Steve explained that the hospital had called Susie, and let her know that Mom had passed away. Susie had called Steve right away, but I had left for the hospital already. Steve tried to follow us, but could not catch us so he came back home.

Susie and I went to the funeral home for the arrangements. Everything was pretty much done except when Susie brought the dress that Mom wanted to wear. Mom had bought it specifically for her funeral, but the dress did not fit her. Mom had gained 20 to 30 pounds of water weight, and looked very swollen. Mom always had a very good figure. Even at the hospital, her arms and body were hard to recognize. The mortician indicated that he had a white jacket Mom could wear, and he asked Susie if she could bring a blouse from home. The mortician had to put plastic bags between Mom's body and her clothing, because water was seeping from her.

We told little Gavino (Nino), who was three, that my Mom had died.

"Grandma died?" Nino asked.

"No, not Grandma. Great Grandma died," Steve answered him.

Natalie told him that the angels came and had taken her to Heaven.

Little Gavino responded,

"Tupid (stupid) angels. They better not come and get my Grandma!"

Gavino was so little, he sat on my lap, or stood on the pedals of my wheelchair by the casket.

"Thank you for coming!" and he would add, "Come again!"

He was a big help! Susie was still on crutches from her broken kneecap. I gave Evelyce and Alicia each a rose from Mom's flowers.

I dealt with Mom's death better than my Dad's. Maybe it was easier, because Mom had prepared me, or because I did not recognize her with the water weight gain. Steve did not want to wait at the funeral home for me, so Armando took me home after everyone left.

About a year after Mom's death, I fell apart, and so did Susie. Adrenaline is the only thing that helped us through the funeral, because we depended upon each other. We both called her phone after her death just to hear her voice on her answering machine, and it was soothing. We are still dealing with the loss.

A few days after Mom died, and before her funeral, Renée (my attendant that day), was in the kitchen, and I heard her yell.

"What was that?"

She ran into my bedroom. My dog was on my lap, growling, and focusing her eyes over my head in a mirror. Renée looked at the same spot the dog was looking, but I saw nothing in the mirror, or over my head. Renée, who had had a vision of her Father's accident and death when she was eight years old, told me something amazing.

"There is like a hand above your head with four fingers—the fingers have like a falling lighted glitter. It is like giving you a blessing."

Chappy was still growling like a car motor revving up her engine. Renée sat on my bed by the window, and suddenly, she almost fell through it as if she was pushed. Whatever it was left through the window. Chappy stopped growling immediately, and left the room.

"I don't know what that was," Renée said

"It was probably my Mom just saying goodbye," I told her.

"No, it was not your Mother. There were *four* fingers!" she responded.

A couple of days later, I discovered that my friend, who sang at my wedding, had passed away. Ann had cancer many times, and was my friend who was a midget with no thumbs. Although I saw nothing, I'm sure it was Ann saying good-bye. She was important in my life too.

Before she died, Mom had put her money into a revocable trust, so it would not affect my attendant care issues. The downturn in the stock market due to the economy, caused much to be lost. And, then, because her stock should have been put under the trust name, it took a while for it to be resolved. Susie had a big job on her hands as well as Mom's house. Kenny was the only one that could move into Mom's house at the time, and it worked out well for him, because he had a dog and a couple of cats including Merle's cat that he inherited. Kenny could not have his dog in an apartment, and his animals, and Presley, were important to him.

After Mom's stroke, she requested that she wanted Susie and me to divide her assets equally, and then take care of the Grandkids, and other organizations, per her wishes, as we felt appropriate. Gavino was having problems with drinking, and Stevie was in prison. Natalie and Heather both needed vehicles at the time, so I brought them vehicles to take care of the Grandkids. Steve needed a car, and I needed a new van, because a year prior, I had the transmission overhauled. I also transferred my lift from the old van to the new one for the wheelchair.

I gave Eddie my old van as he had always done so much for Steve and me, especially when we had visited Las Vegas. His van was not working, and he was touched by the gesture. Unfortunately, shortly after we did this, Eddie became very sick, and almost died. He said that his recovery was a revelation for him, so he sat down, and wrote notes to all of his friends who meant a lot to him. These notes were to be distributed when he died. He lost both his legs, but why, I don't know. Perhaps due to cancer, they were amputated to his hips the next year, and he was unable to sit up without a safety belt in his wheelchair. He had to give up driving. Armando and I stopped to pick him up one day soon after he could no longer drive, and took him to the casino in Milwaukee. We had a lot of fun, but Eddie got sick. He had an accident in the bathroom, so we came home early. It was good that we had that time together.

 I helped my friend Armando to purchase a vehicle. Ever since 2002, he has always been there to drive me to meetings, as well as actively participating and even taking on the presidency and other positions at WWAAC for many years. Thanks to Armando, I left the house once a month, or so to go gambling, which I did not want Steve to do anymore. He even took me to family weddings, since Steve did not usually like going to gatherings. Even on Christmas, Steve usually went to his friends' houses while my family came to ours.

One of the first times Armando took me gambling, I won, so I went shopping in the Milwaukee casino store. I was trying to hurry when I turned around, and bumped into a display area. Everything slid to my back, and fell to the floor. A clerk and Armando put everything back together. While in the elevator as we headed back to the van, he asked a question.

"When did you buy these 3 potted wooden plants?"

"Huh?" I said.

When I backed into the display, they slid in my backpack, so I made him walk all the way back to the store with me to return them.

"I saw them in your backpack when you left, but wasn't sure if you had paid for them or not," the clerk told us.

"I told you we could have gotten away with them!" he grunted. His disability was causing pain from walking, and he just didn't want to return to the store.

Armando and I formed a close friendship, which was tested again shortly after he got his vehicle. Armando had to go to the dentist, because for several months, he had a lump under his tongue. He had no insurance to take care of it, but a person at the Kenosha Community Center set up a Milwaukee appointment, and he had already been waiting for this appointment for months. I told him that I would go with him. The dentist was very suspicious of the lump, and wanted to remove it for testing immediately. Armando could not raise $350 quickly, so surgery was out of the question. Armando had sixteen siblings, and his Father and two of his brothers had already died of cancer. I could not let him pass up this opportunity, so I put the surgery on my credit card, and he could figure out how to pay me back later. The dentist gave Armando a local anesthetic to numb the area, and he squirmed as the Dentist removed the lump. I knew the anesthetic wasn't strong enough to numb his pain. I couldn't understand how the dentist didn't see it! But, the dentist did a good job, and we found out later the lump was cancerous, but had not spread. Armando went through multiple radiation treatments.

"How many people die because they had no access to medical care?" I wondered when there was no insurance to cover medical care in any form, what might happen.

Fortunately, for the radiation treatments with more to follow, Armando was eligible for other medical care plans.

When it came time to evaluate my eligibility for MAPP which was the medical program that I signed up for in 2001, I met with Jessie, and gave him all my paperwork. I let him know about the trust, and he asked if there was anything else. I remembered the money I had put away when I was teaching. He asked if he could see that paperwork, and I gave it to him. I received a letter from the state that indicated that I owed $80,000, because I was not eligible for MAPP when I applied for services. I knew I had discussed this with a person about the eligibility, but I know I didn't bring in the paperwork, because we were waiting for the Social Security eligibility on my physical condition.

One of the benefit specialists that I worked with indicated that the rules for MAPP had been changed shortly after the first people were made eligible. At first, I thought I could just pay the pretax $80,000 from the portion of paperwork that had not been evaluated, but nothing would be left. Then, a second letter informed me that they had miscalculated, and I owed $250,000 instead of $80,000. I got a lawyer, because I did not know what to do. In the hearing, I found out it was an IRA. It was right on top of the paper. Dah! How dumb could I be? Dad had changed the account for me, and I had never paid attention.

My lawyer worked on the case with the State. The state claimed, "At the time I was made eligible, I would have owed $50,000 to be eligible." This was a good deal for me, so I paid it with the IRA. After cashing it in and paying the penalties, I think I still had $7000 left. About $4000 of that went to the lawyer. I was so happy to have everything finished! I thought the state was fair, but for the first time in my life, I was scared. Not only did I feel stupid, because I messed things up, but I had never been on any type of benefit before. I was proud of that. Now, when I was about to retire, did I actually put myself in jeopardy because I worked? Would I be able to handle my own costs when I retired?

During the couple of months of the investigation, I was wondering if I could really afford to live on my own when I retired. For a month, I tried to pay my own cost, but even if I paid attendants minimum wage of $7.25, I was still short about $500 per month. Now, I was still eligible for MAPP services. What if I had an emergency, or gas prices went up? Early in 2010, I had some information that helped me. I asked for an estimate of my retirement income, and because I had worked for the state over 30 years, not counting teaching, I would get a good pension. It would be enough to pay my bills along with a little extra. I would also get Social Security, which would be enough to cover my attendant care at a decent salary. That was a big relief!

Going forward to 2009, I got really sick. I had a constant cough that I just could not control. There was so much mucus in my lungs that the emergency room staff person told me to put my head backwards, and then stuffed a soft, long, blue multiple anchor shaped device into my throat to my lungs. He quickly pulled it out, which opened the "anchor" tips that carried a lot of gunk out of my body. I struggled to put my head back up as I could not breathe at all. The doctor pushed my head back, again.

"Your head has to be back to open the airways."

It would have prevented my panic if he had explained everything before he proceeded. I spent about a week in the hospital, and actually ended up losing my hearing in my right ear. The doctors never said that the mucus pressure caused the hearing loss, but what else could it have been?

After that, to prevent misinterpretation in staff meetings and clients, I began wearing a hearing aid. I really understood people with hearing impairments better, now, because I couldn't tell from where any sounds were coming. I turned my head to listen, and tried to fill in what I thought a person meant. Not a good idea! Therefore, I started repeating what I thought I heard which solicited corrections in a more positive way. Some of what I thought I heard was funny! I had inner ear nerve damage, and even if someone spoke louder, there were many different meanings from which I could choose. For instance, I couldn't tell the difference between "hat, fat, cat, and pat".

It was interesting that my lung doctor, who was also my Dad's doctor, thought that I may have had polio, because of my weak cough and the gases in my lungs. That was a real diagnosis for the first time in my life. But all the doctors I saw had been adamant.

"You cannot get polio while you are in the uterus!"

My primary doctor didn't think I had polio, however.

My Doctor knew I had a neuromuscular disability, and advised me not to take flu shots, but Pneumonia shots I could have. Flu shots were very hard on people with neuromuscular problems. It was a good thing that I had given flu shots up a long time ago. I was back to square one with diagnosis. Whatever my diagnosis was would not make my disability different.

In September 2009, Gavino was released from the Alcohol and Drug Correctional Center. He moved back in with Steve and me for a while. I hoped that he had learned his lesson, because his fifth DWI resulted with a car accident, and fortunately, only the cars were seriously hurt. I wanted Gavino to become responsible. His Alcohol sessions seemed to help him realize he could control his life if alcohol and drugs were not in his system.

He was fortunate that Natalie decided to move back to Wisconsin with his son just in time for his son to see him before he got out of prison. Little Gavino was five years old, and was so happy to see his Dad again! When Gavino was let into the visitation room by the guards, we were sitting at a table waiting for him. Nino looked up at him as if he was an angel staring at his Dad with a mysterious smile for the first half-hour. His Dad had a chance to hold him, and play with him as well as raid the vending machines.

When he got out of prison, Gavino applied for DVR services and with the help of Rosemeen, he found a factory job on a bus line in a short period. He was able to maintain that job as he worked though his problems of staying sober and clean. The biggest problem was that he started working third shift. Lack of consistent sleep became an issue.

Also in 2009, I went to Madison to accept recognition for 30 years of service to DVR. I received a silver coffee cup and a recognition for my "achievements and accomplishments."

Carol has assisted persons with disabilities to obtain and maintain employment for 30 years! She is an inspiration and a motivating force to everyone she works with. The words used by her colleagues to describe Carol include: courageous, altruistic, exceptional, wise, inspiring, caring, dedicated, poetic, respected, compassionate, astounding, resilient, genuine, go-getter! Thank you, Carol for your lasting commitment to DVR's mission, the people we serve, and your colleagues.

Eddie died in 2009. A few weeks after he passed, I received one of the notes that he had written a few years ago when he almost died.

The note read: *You've always been my dearest friend. I'm very grateful for all the kindness you've shown me. You're a very strong and determined person. Don't change. Ed*

Little Gavino (Nino) was five years old in 2010. Natalie, Gavino, and I took him to his first Cubs baseball game. He sat next to me on a movable chair in the handicapped section—a section one level up behind home plate. The woman brought Nino a ball signed by the ushers in the area.

The woman pointed to the dirty spots on the ball.

"Look, this ball was used on the field. See these dirt marks?"

Unfortunately, the Cubs did not win that day. However, when you're talking about the Cubs, it was never about winning. It was about enduring, enjoying the day, the outdoors, the food, and the excitement. The Cubs lost 9-0. What was exciting about that day was that it was family day, and the kids had an opportunity to run around the bases. As we were watching the game, Nino and I were planning how he was going to run around the bases. I wanted to make sure he knew which were first, second, and third bases. He didn't know, and was surprised, "You mean you don't go…" as he pointed from third to second, and then to first base.

After the game, we all walked to the Wrigley right-field entrance door. The security usually only let one parent go with a child onto the field, but I was approved to go onto the field as well. That was very exciting for me! We walked from the right-field door, over the opposing pitchers' bullpen mound to the dugout by first base. They kids started there, then ran from first, to second, to third, and home. The view from down on the field was amazing. The scoreboard, the vastness, the vines…! It was a great day! Nino even bought a Soriano T-shirt, because it was his favorite player. In the meantime, I tried to put a hex on the opposing pitchers' bullpen, so the opposing teams would lose on a regular basis. Needless to say, it didn't work.

I really gave credit to the Cubs for teaching me patience and the value of persistence. The Cubs haven't won a *World Series* in over a century. It wasn't about winning with the Cubs;

it's important that people kept trying and finish! Enjoying the highs in your life and dealing with the lows. Louise and I still went together to games whenever we got a chance!

At Christmas time, we were at the mall, and I could not get Nino to stop and see Santa Claus. We finally went past Santa, again.

"Are you sure you don't want to stop and see Santa Claus?" I asked him.

He decided that he would do it, since there was no one else in line. As he covered his mouth, Nino whispered to Santa Claus from 6 feet away,

"Am I on the naughty list?"

Natalie shook her head left to right, so Santa would know Nino was good. Nino started smiling ear to ear, as if the world was lifted off his shoulders! He was no longer worried.

When I went to camp that year, Armando took me, so he could see everyone, and say "hello," but he could not stay. Doctors had found what they thought was a different type of cancer in one of his kidneys. His kidney was going to be removed the last day of camp. I spoke to him that day on a cell phone. I felt everything would be okay. Arlene had a similar surgery, and her entire kidney was removed to make sure the cancer could not spread. I knew a lot of people who had only 50% of one kidney which worked, and they were doing just fine. It was a hard thing for Armando to go through, but he always faced things head-on with a smile.

Steve was jealous of my friendship with Armando, but Steve was my main concern. I would always help him, because he had taken care of me for so long. Armando's Mother was getting older, and she was his main concern. Steve was getting older, and had some problems with vision, diabetes, alcoholic history, depression, balance, foot pain, and dementia. If something would happen to Steve, or if he couldn't help me anymore (either by choice or by physical limitations), Armando said that he would help me. We gave each other mutual support, and Kenny told Steve once, "Carol is not married." While it was true, it put things in perspective for Steve, but made him leery.

Gavino had moved back in with Natalie for a while, but it didn't work for various reasons, and he moved back home. He always flirted with my attendants no matter how often I told him not to do it. In one three-week period, he introduced me to three different girls. Fortunately, none were my attendants.

"This is going to be your daughter-in-law!" he told me.

"Yeah, right!" I told him, and added, "I don't want you introducing me to anyone unless you are really serious! When you know what love is, and can make a real commitment, then you can introduce me!"

In 2010, a cute, small, shy girl named Devyn began working for me through Society's Assets. She had completed her CNA (certified nursing assistant) in high school. She started on a weekend, so I was in bed when we met. I had pillows all around me forming a table, which held my laptop on my lap. My legs were always folded up under me.

"I was a little shocked when I met you because I thought you had no legs and that wasn't on the care plan," she told me.

She took the pillows away, one by one. She felt more comfortable when she found my legs. Devyn was very easy to talk to, and we became friends quickly. She didn't have her driver's license yet, so I had a chance to meet her Grandmother, Marge, who would drive her back and forth to her jobs.

Devyn did a good job, even though it took her a while to get everything down. She had some disabilities that put her through a lot when she was younger. Bipolar medication stabilized a lot of the problems, but she still needed to be reminded to complete tasks. She also had attention deficit disorder, but was very strong for her height, and handled me very well. I knew, in time, she would be a very good attendant. She took instruction well, and was not afraid to try different things as she became more comfortable with me. I remembered thinking she was just two years younger than my daughter would have been if I could have carried my baby to term. In some ways, Devyn was very wise, and old for her age. She didn't like drama, and had experienced a lot due to her disabilities. On the other hand, I had to tell her how to prepare meals, and do other things the easy way. We were a team. Ironically, the color of paint I chose for my house 8 years prior was *Devonshire cream.*

It felt good that my attendants had stayed consistent for a while. Lynn, Kristin, and Devyn were sharing the workload. Devyn's Mother came in every couple of weeks for two or three hours to clean. Steve took night duty of lying me down and turning me as well as driving me to and from work.

~ 27 ~

Retiring

In January 2011, I turned 64. This whole year was a surprise to me. I thought that I'd be working until I was at least 70, but many things made that impossible.

Just to name a few, Steve's vision was getting worse, and had a hard time picking me up from work. One eye had no vision for quite a while due to a cataract, and other problems. His other eye also had a cataract, and he could not see the colors of a traffic light. He would drive behind a car, and follow the taillights. By April, Bob used Arlene's accessible van to pick me up, but he was unable to pick me up from work on a regular basis because of his schedule. I could no longer take the city bus alone, because my arm would fall, and I could not get it back into position. I also began having stomach pain, which I thought might be another kidney stone. I didn't want to miss any work, and since the pain only seemed to bother me at night, I slept with my laptop on top of a pillow on my stomach.

A few months later, Gavino had picked up a bureau of drawers curbside. Shortly, thereafter, we noticed some bites on Nino and Steve's backs and arms, and realized that it was bed bugs! That was scary for me, because I would not be able to lift my arms to wipe them off me! We called an exterminator, and while we were waiting, the bedbugs did not bother me except for the last two nights. I found a couple of bites on my face and a couple on my arms. I could not take care of them myself. The exterminator explained that condominiums were not like apartments, but were considered separate housing. Therefore, we didn't have to worry about the bugs spreading to others, but I worried about the bugs spreading to my attendants and family who visited. I didn't want them to invade their homes, so I recommended that after returning home, they remove their clothing, and put them in a hot dryer for 20-30 minutes. We were very lucky that the bugs never spread to anyone else's home.

The most important thing in my decision to retire was Gov. Walker's widespread fast changes for retirement and Social Security, which would take away my ability to live independently. I was extremely happy when 14, fabulous Democratic Senators exiled themselves from Wisconsin to delay a sweeping vote of anti-union legislation. After three weeks, they returned on March 13. A friend of mine and I were there to greet and support them.

When I was first employed at DVR in 1979, I worked with Sen. Wirch who was a Job Service Employee and one of the 14 Senators. I was proud of him and the others, because it was not easy being separated from their families, because of their self-exile from Wisconsin.

Besides the sweeping changes being proposed to eliminate the union, I was told about other changes for retirees. Kathy, a rehab teacher for the blind, called to tell me why she was retiring. We started together, to some extent, when I was first employed by DVR. John was another counselor who had just retired, and was encouraging me to get out while I could.

At the beginning of April, I updated my information on my retirement funds from Madison, and called Social Security. I had to apply, first, for Social Security retirement within a month that I would have received less than $1000, and my retirement would start the following month. I scheduled my appointment at the end of April, choosing June 3 as my retirement date. Once my retirement went through, I could, and then apply for Social Security Disability. Everyone begins Medicare at the age of 65, which I would begin the following January. It took six months to apply for disability, and if I received it during that time, I could receive full retirement up to the age of 66. December was the sixth month from July, and that is when my Social Security began with my state retirement starting July 1. That was enough to live on, and my Social Security would pay for my attendant care, because upon retirement, I lost my medical assistance. Perfect timing! It was as if I was being beat up again to change jobs. God knew what He was doing.

In May, while I was off work, Steve began appointments at the VA for several cataract surgeries. We had to find people to drive us back and forth, because Steve couldn't drive. The doctors decided to do his bad eye first to see if they could give him any vision, before the other eye would be done. Unfortunately, when they took out his cataract, he had to be awake for that surgery. Even with the anesthetic, he could feel a lot of pain, because scar tissue had grown, and attached itself to the cataract area. The doctor had to cut the attached scar tissue off and cut out part of the base where the lens sat in his eye. There was no vision after the first surgery, and Steve thought the same thing would happen to his other eye. In addition, he certainly did not want to mess up the vision that was left in his other eye. I did not think that would be the case, because there was no scar in the second eye, or any other problems with it. Once the doctor changed the second lens, he should be able to see. The second surgery was finally completed in the fall. He could see, and drive again!

In May and June, I worked on a list of attendants who wanted to work for cash. I could do two things:

1. I could be an employer, and take out both state and federal taxes from the gross pay, including Medicare and Social Security, and give them net pay, or
2. I could hire them as domestic workers, or contract workers. I'd report the wages of the worker, give them a 1099 form (over $1800/year was needed), and they would be responsible for their own taxes.

The second option was easier, and more realistic. I asked my attendants if they were interested in staying with me, and discussed taxes and personal finances with them. Fortunately, they all stayed. Some only worked 4 hours a week. Unfortunately, Lynn fell and broke her left knee, so she was out of work for a long time. She eventually returned, and worked for a few hours a week. I had two other attendants, Michaela and Jackie, who were there in case of emergencies, and I began paying my own attendants on July 1.

I was able to hold off surgery on what I thought was my kidney stone problem until the end of June. I couldn't handle the pain anymore, and finally, went to the doctor. The doctor told me it was my gallbladder, and I needed surgery. The surgery seemed to go well, but the whole day I bled heavy from the tube they had inserted into my neck. The whole area around the entry of the tube seemed to be way too big, and at the end of the day, they removed the tube and stitched the hole.

While in the hospital the day of surgery, I watched a very bad storm travel down and over the lake. Even the hospital lost electricity for a while, before the generators finally worked. I always look for the positive, so I was happy the electric power didn't go out while I was having surgery. When I went home the next day, I saw 20 to 30 trees that were downed along the lake, and several others that were destroyed as we drove through the Carthage campus. I received a picture of my gallbladder stones, which looked like about 20 black pearls, just like an oyster! I wondered if I could sell them, and make some money. I had seen JoAnne's bladder stones right after she was in the hospital. They were so pretty and looked like wooden oblong balls, and would have made great earrings!

I did stay involved with a few groups after I retired. I continued with the Department of Aging and Disability, Kenosha Area Disabilities Service Group (which supported Wisconsin Easter Seals camps and monitored a free loan closet at the Kenosha Job Center), and Fun & Fit - a once a year recreational and informational, hands-on activities for people with disabilities. They could try rock climbing, kayaking, line dancing, and others. You could even buy raffle tickets to win a night at the accessible cabin in the Bong State Recreational Area. Other accessible cabins were available throughout the state, which people with disabilities could rent for about $30 per night. Check with the State Parks Department if you are interested.

It took me a while to recover from the gallbladder surgery. I called LaVerne from the Department of Aging and Disability to let her know that I would not be at any meetings until fall. LaVerne knew that Angie (my DVR case coordinator) was planning a retirement party for me in July. I think Angie wanted the party to be a surprise, but she called to ask me how I was, and then, told me about the party. I was not busy on the evening when the party was scheduled, but needed to reschedule my attendant so I could be there. Approximately 40 people were present—some from work, some from Easter Seals, some family, Louise, and her niece, Joy, as well as some counselors I admired from KAC. Two of my clients had heard about the party, and stopped by to say goodbye. One client, John, who had been a volunteer for me a long time ago, stopped in with Gary, and John had made me an award for my "excellent work." Another came with someone from the Department on Aging and Disability who just had to tell me that he had an interview for taking driver's license pictures for the Department of Motor Vehicles.

Angie had arranged a very touching program, and many people spoke about my accomplishment. A few who spoke were my former supervisor, Willie; Maggie, a placement person; and Sandy, the person who fed me at lunchtime. Nino just couldn't wait.

"And my Grandma is the best Grandma in the world!" He gave me a hug!

"Awe!" everyone gushed.

David, my nephew, and his wife had a baby in February, brought the baby with them. John Collins, who was a former County Executive, and who presented the volunteer awards for Easter Seals Banquets, spoke, too. He always liked to roast me! The baby was really looking at John intensely when he was talking, and all of a sudden, the baby babbled, "Blah, blah, blah, blah." The people at our table were giggling, but I did not want to embarrass John, and so I said nothing. (I guess he'll find out about it now!)

I received a lot of e-mails and messages from people who couldn't be there. Rosemeen,

Kathy, JoAnn, and others said they did not learn about the party in time to make plans. I received a plaque from Gov. Walker who congratulated me on my dedicated 31 years of service. My friend, Les, sent an awesome e-mail. Lisa, a former student, client, and quadriplegic due to a drunk driver, sent me an e-mail that made me cry.

"...whenever I have a problem, I think, 'What would Carol do?' I know what Carol would say, 'Just soldier on!'"

I took the picture of my gallstones to the retirement party, and placed them behind the cake to make sure that everyone would be able to see them. Everyone, including me, needed some sympathy once in a while.

I had also thought about doing some things for Kenosha Achievement Center, or helping Maggie with some of her paperwork - just to keep busy after I retired. But, in truth, it felt good not to be busy for a while. I took it easy, and racked up 3 million points in Scrabble on Pogo, but that ended when the program was not compatible with Java any longer.

By the end of 2011, Devyn and Gavino became friends, and eventually they started going together. Gavino had always seemed young for his age, because he had started drinking and using drugs, long before he came to live with me. Gavino was doing much better taking on responsibility, and it was good having Nino around every other weekend. I helped Nino with his homework after he got out of school. He would read a book that was supposed to be timed, but we'd talk so much about the content, the time was way off. The books he would read created very interesting conversations—especially if the books were about animals or Disney stars!

Gavino was holding down his new job well, but he was still on third shift, and sleep was difficult for him. He handled it better than I could have—job, girlfriend, kids, exes, and helping his parents. Devyn lived at home with her Mother, and there were personal concerns. With her Mother's approval, Devyn moved in with us. Gavino was happy.

"Devyn also was concerned about who would take care of you, Carol, if she had no transportation to get back and forth to this job."

Shortly after Devyn moved, she became ill, needed an antibiotic, which caused an allergic reaction by interacting with her other medications, further, causing a debilitating condition. Devyn couldn't focus, process instructions, nor could she walk. I called her Mother asking if something like this had ever happened before. Her Mother came over, but did not recognize any of the symptoms, so she took her to the hospital immediately. Three days later, she was able to function, left the hospital, and has been happy that she never had a problem like that again.

Gavino had handled Devyn's drug interaction well, and then he came to me.

"I want to marry Devyn. I know what commitment means and the different problems we could have. I want to be with her."

He was much more responsible, understood the more serious side of life, and himself. They became engaged, but neither was ready to set a wedding date. They moved out about six months later, but continued working with me. Gavino brought her back and forth to work. How proud and lucky I was to have a son that now understood commitment.

"Is this God's gift of the daughter I couldn't have?" I remember thinking.

BY THE GRACE OF GOD AND YOU
A Chair Does Not a Person Make

About seven months after I retired, my wheelchair stopped working. It was nine years old, and had a good, long life! I was lucky enough to get a loaner wheelchair to use while we were waiting for medical/insurance approvals and the fittings that needed to be made. The full process took seven months. This was the longest time I ever had to wait for a wheelchair, but I think it was more of a part of a divine plan.

The biggest problems were that my loaner, motorized wheelchair had no solid side—just armrests, and no place to hang a backpack to carry needed articles. I usually tucked my purse between the side of my wheelchair, and my body for back and hip support. Now, I had to carry my purse under my foot on my pedal. I started having pain, as well, so I was not getting out of bed as much. The neighbor across the street who worked at the Kenosha News for many years, and knew my story, let me know that she was writing a book called *Dandelions in the Dining Room*. She told me the process to get a book published, and that she thought I should write one. Curiously enough, Kenny had also started writing an autobiography, and it was very good! I was inspired! Marge, Devyn's Grandmother, had asked me many questions about my life when she was driving Devyn back and forth to work here. She also thought I should write one.

"You should write a book!" she told me.

Since I was bored and sitting on my bed a lot, I began the book on my computer. David had completed a computer degree, and showed me a few more things to make it easier. He showed me how to set up chapters, and update the information every time I started a new chapter. I decided to give it a try. I wrote the introduction and the first five chapters at one time. I wondered if it was interesting enough for anyone to want to read. I gave it to my neighbor. Susan definitely thought my information was important to share. I started working on it on a regular basis, and took breaks as different things came along. Because I was uncomfortable in an unfamiliar chair with no commode, I did not go to camp that summer, giving me even more time to finish my book.

When I had all my technology on my home computer, I looked pretty funny! I had a telephone wire and microphone on my left ear, and a headset on my right ear for my DragonDictate. I always thought a person looked really smart with one of these devices on their head, but when a person had on both pieces of technology, I looked pretty silly.

After my wheelchair had been fitted by Brian, he read the two-page introduction of my book, and encouraged me to complete the book. He apologized that it took so long for the wheelchair to arrive, since we needed some special features on the wheelchair, such as a pedal that fit under my bed. Then, just as he was about to deliver the completed chair, he had an accident, and a few weeks recovery, before he could deliver it to me. I guess I still had more time to finish writing.

Trish, another retired coworker, was having some serious health problems. We talked for 45 minutes, and she helped me choose the book title. We had been in high school together, and she died just a few weeks after we talked. Thank you, Trish!

Some friends and clients had accessibility issues that they never had before. Companies were not making standard-size wheelchairs, and the wheelchairs were too big to fit on the standard van lifts. Another thing I noticed was that motels were starting to remodel their rooms, and the new beds were too high for people with disabilities. Sitting in my wheelchair, the bed height came up to my elbow! How could I roll into a bed that high? I looked under the ADA rules, and bed height was one of the few things with no standard measurements! I found a lot of complaints online, and noted this was a new issue for many people with disabilities. Previously, bed heights were always 21 to 23 inches from the floor. I never had problems staying at other places in the state for my job. What will they be changing next? I've even heard able-bodied people complain that they had to slide off the beds until their feet hit the ground.

I finally received my new wheelchair, and it was heaven! My back and legs were finally getting better. The book was about half done, and I figured I would have it completed by January 2013, which didn't happen.

I decided that I was going to call Lloyd to see how comfortable he would be if I shared our story in the book. The last time I had spoken to him was back in January. His birthday was September 15, and called at the end of August. I couldn't believe how long the telephone rang with no answer. I thought maybe he was fishing in Idaho or visiting family in Florida. I tried calling again closer to his birthday, and, yet again, after his birthday. I knew that something was wrong when I tried again in early October. This time, the phone was disconnected! I went straight to the Milwaukee Journal, and looked to see if his name was in the obituaries. He died August 13, 2012. I knew that he had a lot of brothers and sisters, and called the first name in the obituary. I needed to know what happened to him. His sister-in-law told me that he had been tested for some recent problems with seizures. Lloyd was at their house the day before he died, and they suspected that he had died from a severe seizure during the night.

I lost a lot that day - more than I can express in words. Although he never married, he was always there when I needed him. Lloyd was a special person, and after his death, I stopped writing this book for a few months. I thought about his seizures. What would my life be like if we had gotten together? He would have died first, but would I have been prepared? For the first time, I knew God's plan was followed. Knowing how He made me do everything else in life, he could have easily convinced me to be with Lloyd if He wanted.

I noticed that I wasn't as tough as I used to be. I no longer could stop from crying watching a movie or attending a funeral by biting my tongue. Heck, I could even cry from watching a TV commercial about abused animals!

During the previous year, I had some problems with my vision again. My eye doctor said that I was getting cataracts.

"You won't have to worry for about 20 years," he had said to me.

However, despite what he had told me, I returned because it was as if I had a piece of wax paper forming already over my right eye.

"You have the fast-growing kind of cataract," he explained to me, and I promised to keep him informed on any new changes in my vision.

I was worried about having to have cataract surgery while I was awake. (I'm such a chicken)! My Dad had cataract surgery on both eyes. For one surgery, he was awake, for the other, he was put to sleep. I asked my doctor to explain the difference.

"Why?" I asked him.

"If there are any concerns with the heart, or other medical reasons, the patient can't be put to sleep under an aesthetic. They keep the patient awake, and just give enough anesthetic to numb the pain," he had replied, and I wondered how long it would be before I would need surgery.

Susie, my sister, who was working as a receptionist at Aurora part-time, had been laid off, and all of the part-time jobs in that category were eliminated by the employer. While she was looking for a job, her grandson needed a babysitter, so she took that job while looking for a permanent job. Running after a small child gave her extra exercise to change dress sizes from size 16 to a size 10! Was I ever jealous!

In October, Michelle Obama came to speak in Racine on behalf of Barack Obama's November re-election campaign. Rosemeen and her daughter, Rehnaz, were going to get tickets, and wondered if I wanted two of the tickets, so that I could go. Rehnaz was a Friday volunteer in my office to get a variety of experiences. She was now President of the National Honor Society, and invited to the next inauguration, because of her involvement in the National Young Leaders Organization. I thought that would be fun, and Armando agreed to drive. It was kind of a cool, drizzly day, but a lot of enthusiasm inside! We got there early, and spent a long time waiting due to security procedures. Being some of the last people allowed into the building, we were seated in the first three rows. I enjoyed watching the Secret Service, before Mrs. Obama appeared on stage. Each one checked their assigned sections very fast in case anything was different. Michelle's speech was so motivating; we supported her speech, so change would happen.

When Mrs. Obama finished speaking, she came towards me. The crowd flowed from my right, and someone pushed the button on my chair, which jammed my wheelchair into the one in front of me. I was afraid someone was going to get hurt. To my surprise, the person that accidentally turned on my chair was one of my former clients. I backed up, and asked her to turn off my chair. Michelle had passed, shook hands with Rosemeen, and gave Rehnaz a hug telling her she could be anything she wanted to be and not to give up her dreams! Armando was further down standing in the second row. He felt the rush of people coming up behind him. He was glad the crowd was close, because it stopped him from falling. He reached out his hand, and Michelle shook it. Overall, it was a very good experience, and a great day. I was uncomfortable with the Secret Service, but since there was a lot of music, it was not a concern.

A few months ago, our dog, Chappy, gave us a scare. She had turned eight years old in November, and this April, she needed surgery to stop the pain that was caused by being born with bad back knees, and a deformity of her right knee. The surgery was going to cost about $3000. I couldn't afford it, and I didn't want to put her to sleep. My lifelong friend, Louise, mentioned Chappy's problem to one of her sisters. They obviously discussed Chappy extensively, because Louise called me back.

"Janet said that she wanted to pay for Chappy's surgery. She has helped other people whose dogs needed surgery. That is what she likes to do. She doesn't want you to pay her back, just let her know the cost and who to write a check to."

What a blessing! Chappy crawled under the china cabinet, and cried whenever it rained. I spoke with Chappy's doctor, and he called in a special orthopedic surgeon for her, because of the deformity. Chappy's doctor had just had rotor cuff surgery, and did not feel he could perform that delicate of an operation at the time. Everyone in Chappy's clinic remembered her, because she was such a horrible patient when she was spayed! She yowled all night as if she was getting killed, and even louder, when anyone came near her the next day! This time she did much better. She was sent home after one night instead of two. We were supposed to keep her tied down for about six weeks, so that she could not run or twist her leg wrong by mistake until May 11. She healed amazingly well. Chappy was ready to run when we finally let her loose! On Memorial Day weekend, we went to a family picnic. She scared us half to death as she chased the soccer ball whenever the ball went out of bounds. I didn't think she understood the concept of the game, since she ran the ball away from people instead of giving it back to them. She was only 12 pounds, but she would chase any size ball just to get into any game available. Chappy had a lot of fun, ran all day, and slept all the way back home, and through the night!

In the past, we had birthday parties for Chappy with about four or five dogs in the neighborhood that came for Lynn's Chicken Delicious cake, while their owners ate pineapple upside down cake. Chappy would hoard all of her presents under my bed, as well as hide under there herself when Lynn's big German Shepard came around. Chappy also loved McDonalds, and always got a dog biscuit there. I was with her once when we went to Burger King. Chappy started crying and crying! I asked Steve what was wrong.

"No dog biscuits here and Chappy knows!" she had a stressful day!

It was raining this month, so I was forced to finish my book. Rehnaz was excellent with computers, and called to ask me if I wanted help with the picture section. Perfect! God only knows I could not finish this by myself, and I believe He wanted this part of my life done.

When the sun finally did shine, I took a walk around my block. I very seldom saw any neighbors, but there was one woman sitting on a chair in the middle of a driveway. She spoke to me, and I stopped for a while. Her name was Sandi, and discovered that we were both retired, but that retirement from teaching was hard for her. I told her I was enjoying mine, and just finishing my book.

"My daughter-in-law is a professional proofreader," she told me.

"Wow! Ouch! God's bat got me again!" I thought.

Sandi gave me her daughter-in-law's phone number. I became more motivated.

Time had passed, when I realized that Alicia was grown.

"What? Alicia graduated from high school?" I couldn't believe it!

All the memories of sleepovers, the zoo, the State fair, games, and ghost stories ran through my head. At Six Flags, I remembered that Nino won a stuffed yellow robot five times his height for making it to the top of that wobbly ladder. Evelyce was always there to help, and feed me without complaint. She also was an excellent motorized wheelchair driver without making me feel like I was riding a bucking horse. You should also know that Nino, at nine, was beginning boxing lessons—the third generation! However, I'm not convinced he will continue.

~ What's Next? ~

Everyone has a story; life happens to everyone. Hear the stories. Grow from them. Isn't that beautiful? Everyone who touches our lives, remain with us as overflowing tears, warming love, giggly smiles, knight-like memories from strangers who saved us, and breaths of learning. By feeling, we live. I tried to live by these two sayings:

1. Today is a gift. It is all we have, and it is precious.
2. Don't cry because something is over, but smile because it happened. Celebrate each life experience while you can - good or bad - in order to progress to the next step of growth.

To me, death is a fulfillment of life. Live life! Enjoy it. Share it. Give of yourself until it hurts, and then give again. Love, and allow yourself to experience being loved. Use the gifts God gave you. Your potential is limitless. Be positive! Your attitude has power. Live your dream. Trust that you are what you were meant to be! It doesn't help to sit on the sidelines. Affect someone else's life today, even if you just catch a person's eye on the street and smile. The person will smile back. Be yourself. Be real. Be you! Just "be!"

Find the positive in people. Don't be afraid of failure. Try—who cares what people think, it's your life. Unfortunately, anyone can acquire a disability at any time. Save your energy with whatever technology you can, so you can live life. Remember, work is important, but it is not everything. Not all good things will happen to you. Hurt is inevitable, but don't hurt anyone intentionally. You only know you are living when you feel. Go live life. Give yourself permission, i.e., if you have to eat with your feet—by all means, eat with your feet! Just don't wear a dress doing it!

Choose your battles wisely—some aren't worth fighting. Very little that we do is completely right or completely wrong. Live life your way—for all that "stuff" with which you have to contend. Make your mistakes farther apart, and you'll know that you are making progress. Forgive yourself for your mistakes—they are going to happen. Misconceptions and myths will always be out there. Don't buy into them. Your disability isn't 115% of your life. Get it down to 10%, then work and plan with that in mind. Having a disability is just different, but not worse.

God doesn't promise anyone a rose garden, but he certainly gives you a garden of memories—from dandelions to orchids. I had been blessed with good and caring parents. My sister and her family brought me joy and support. Steve was a blessing in disguise. Under his tough exterior, he was always there when I needed him despite his pains, dementia, and age. We gave each other a good life plus kids and Grandkids. Gavino has grown into a man facing the responsibilities of life with a positive attitude. Know what you can have control over your life, and what you can't. Gavino is helping his Dad (us) more. We couldn't get along without him. He even introduced me for the first time as his Mom! The Grandkids, of course, are a joy!

I pushed my laptop and yearbooks to the side with my mouthstick. My book was done. Would it be helpful or interesting to anyone? Would people understand that everyone is more alike one another than different? I hope so.

I called Steve to lie me down, and get me comfortable. He turned off the light.

"What's next?" I wondered.

I did not know, and could not guess what God had in store for me, but I'd still like to do three things:

1. Meet Betty White for lunch (better do that soon! She'll be 92!)
2. Travel through my last 11 states (I may skip Alaska—sounds too cold!)
3. Experience a full eclipse of the sun (I've wanted to do that forever!)

My eyes were getting heavy. I heard the rain tapping on my window as I drifted …into… sleep…………..

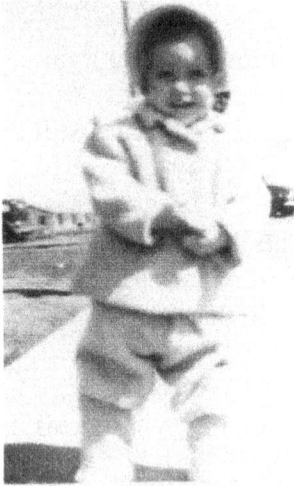

C
A
R
O
L

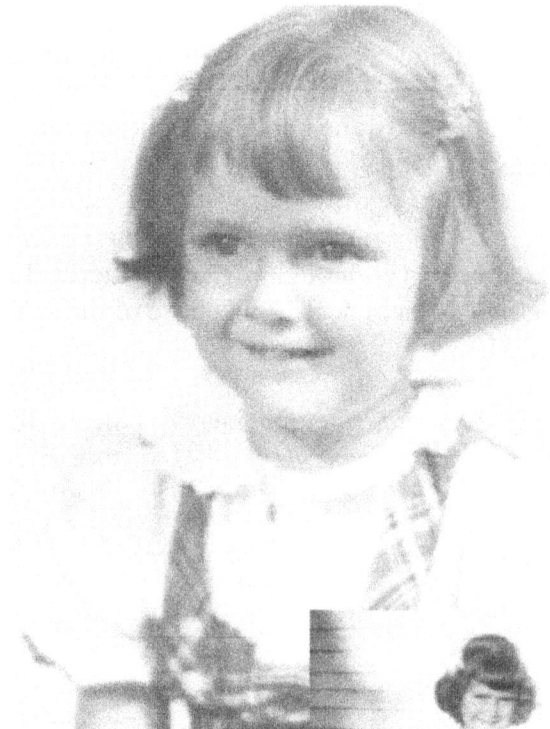

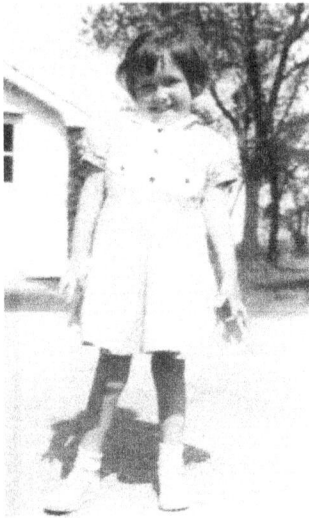

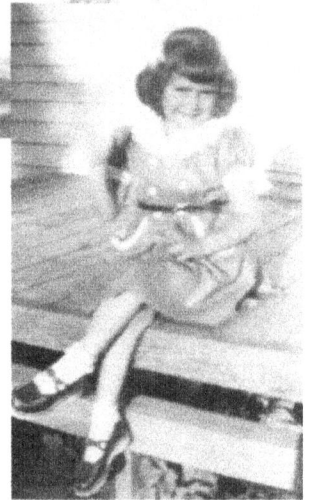

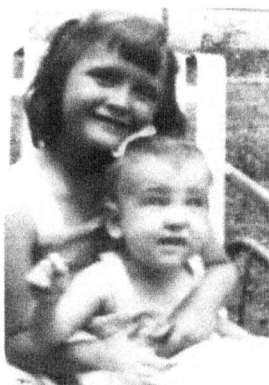

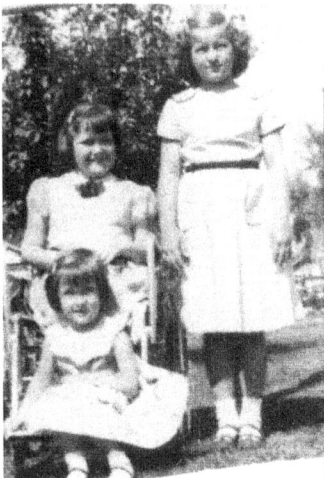

Carol & Susie with

Patty

and

Buddy

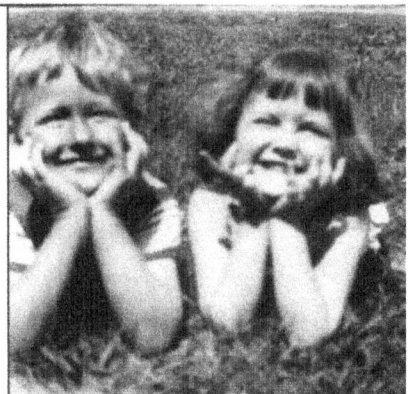

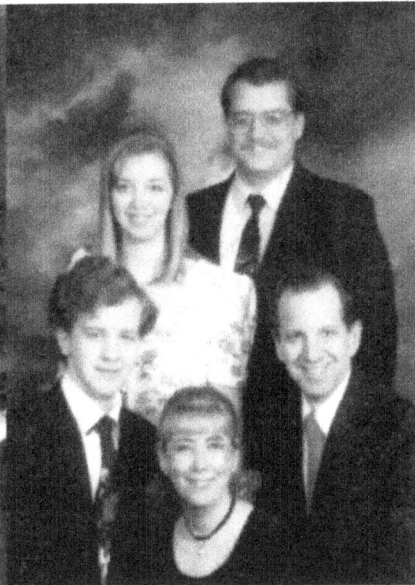

Above: Sister Susie's Family

Ken

Mindy

David   *Bob*

Susie

Left: *Miss Betty, School Secretary*

1st grade classmates, left to right,

Carol, Barbara, Louise & Marilyn

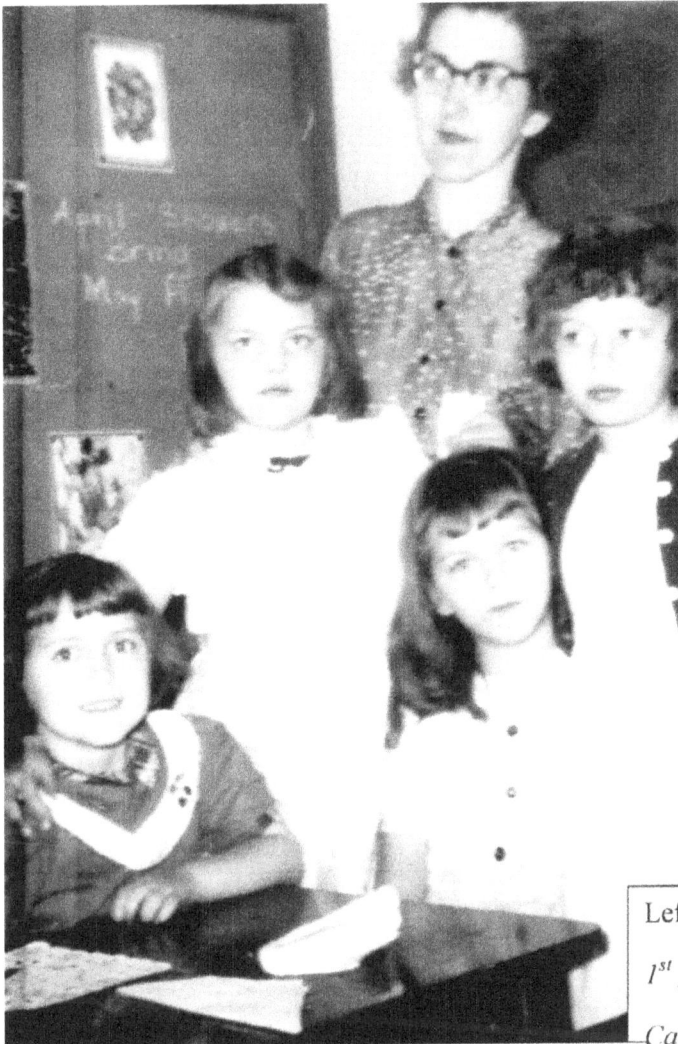

Below: *Mrs. Strange's 2nd & 3rd grade classes.*

Left to Right: *Randy, Susan, Marilyn, Carol, Larry,*

?, Jim, Ronnie, Dickie, Frankie and Jimmie

Below:
*Friends Eddie
& Wife Carol*

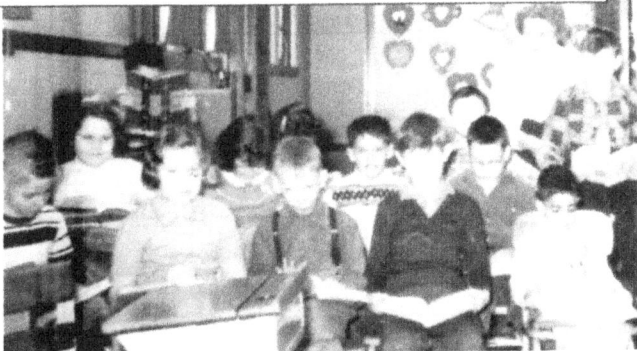

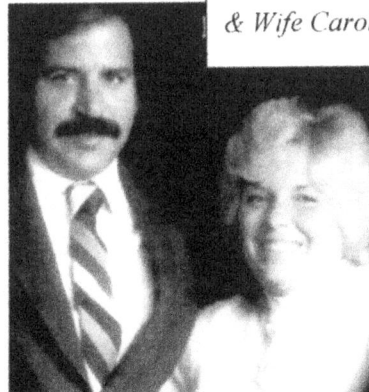

BY THE GRACE OF GOD AND YOU
A Chair Does Not a Person Make

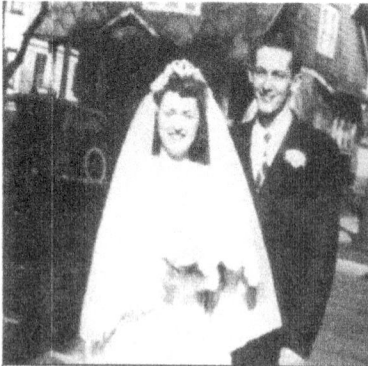

Mom and Dad's Wedding-top

And last picture we took together

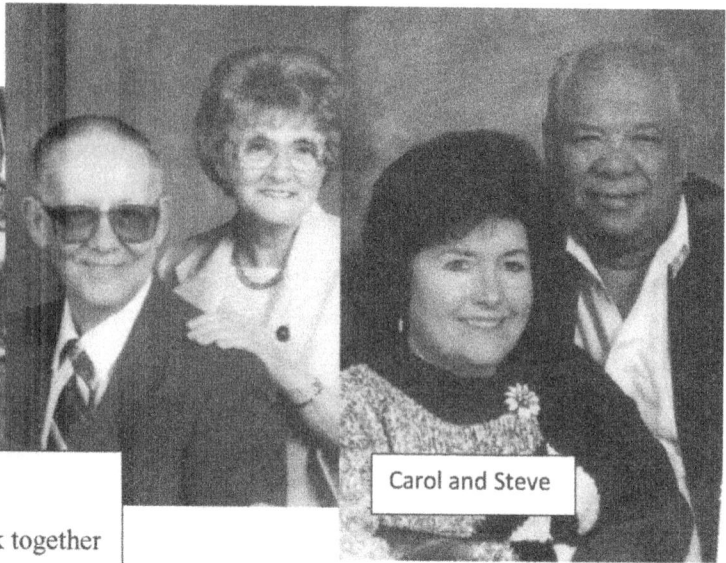

Carol and Steve

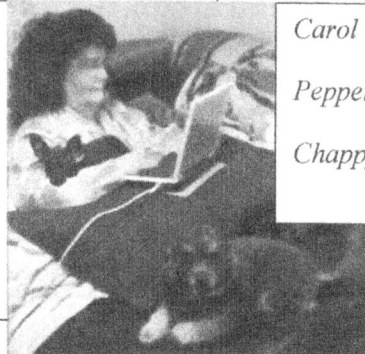

Carol working on book in bed with

Pepper, Nino's Dog in my arms and

Chappy front right.

Grandkids:

Alicia, Evelyce and Gavino, Jr.

Son and fiancé/attendant:

Gavino and Devyn

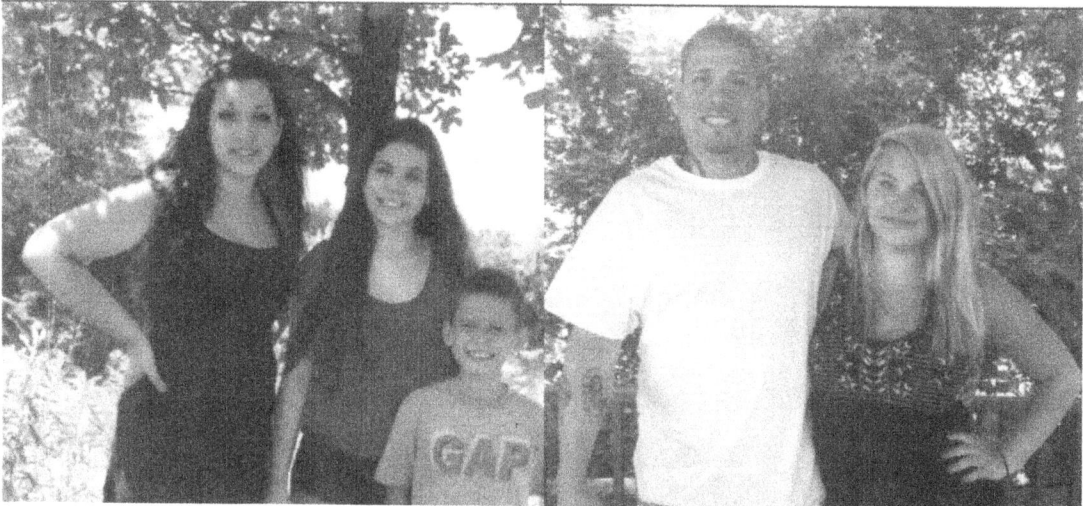

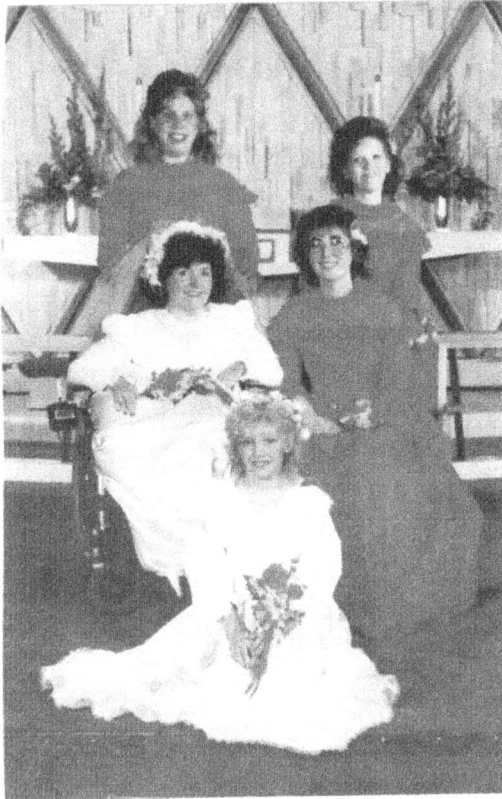

Wedding. 1989

Patty-friend

Louise-1st grade friend

Carol-bride

Susie-sister

Mindy-niece

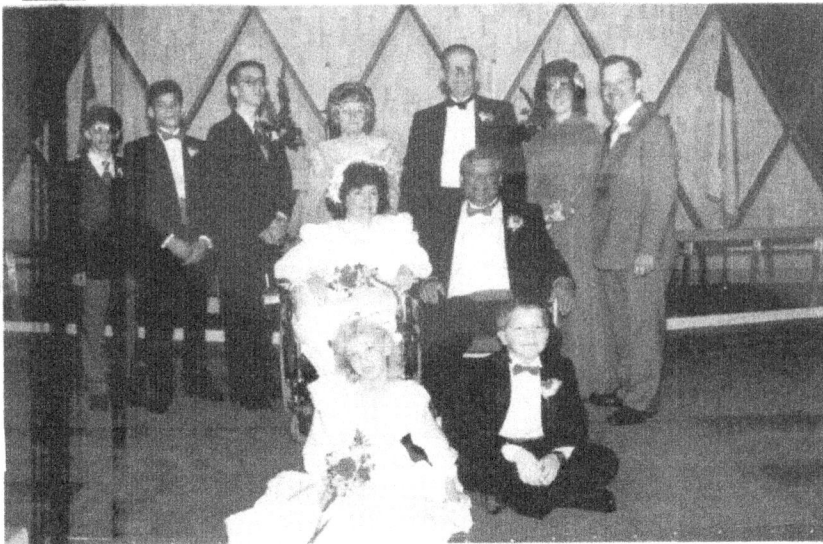

Back row—left to right

Stevie, Gavino`~ sons

*Ken-*nephew, *Mom & Dad*

Susie and Bob (Susie's

Husband)

Middle Row—

Carol & Steve

Bride & groom

Front row:

Mindy, niece

David, nephew

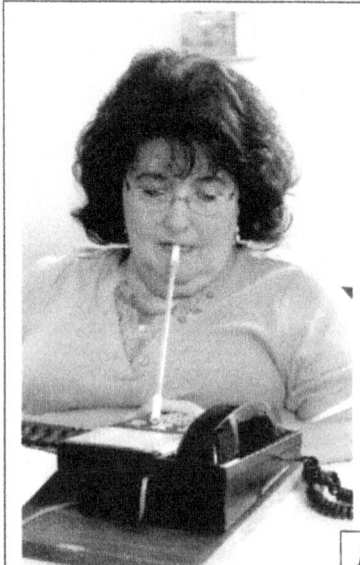

Merle on Gravestone

SAIL AWAY MY FRIEND

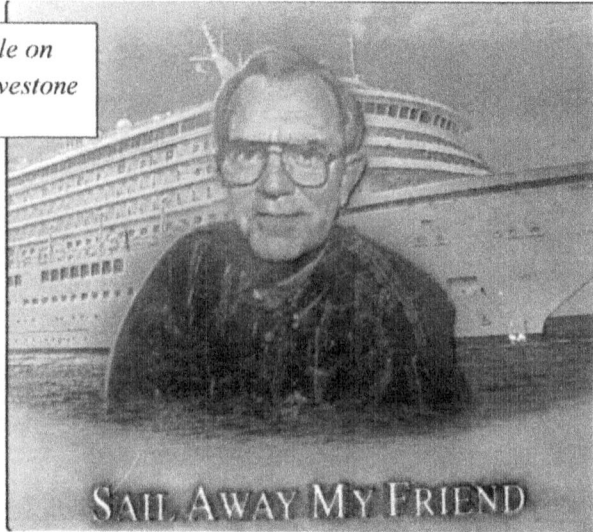

Carol is using mouth-stick at work. Computer keyboard is on Carol's right.

Mary-friend from school.

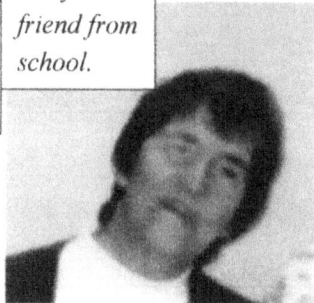

Armando

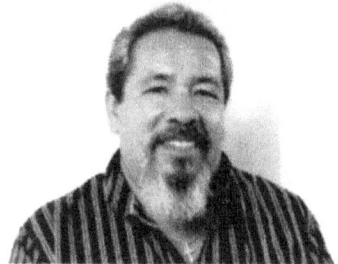

Lloyd   Carol   Kristi

At Muscular Dystrophy Camp

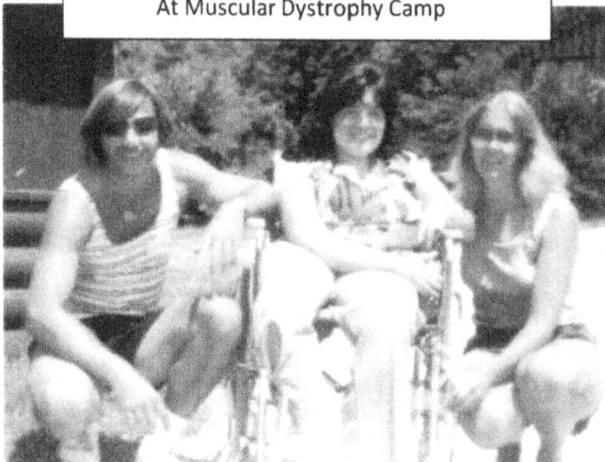

Carol in 2009 at age 62

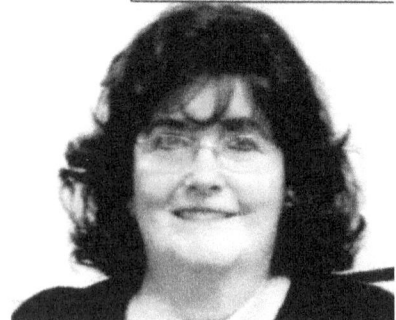